ATKINS

EAT RIGHT, NOT LESS

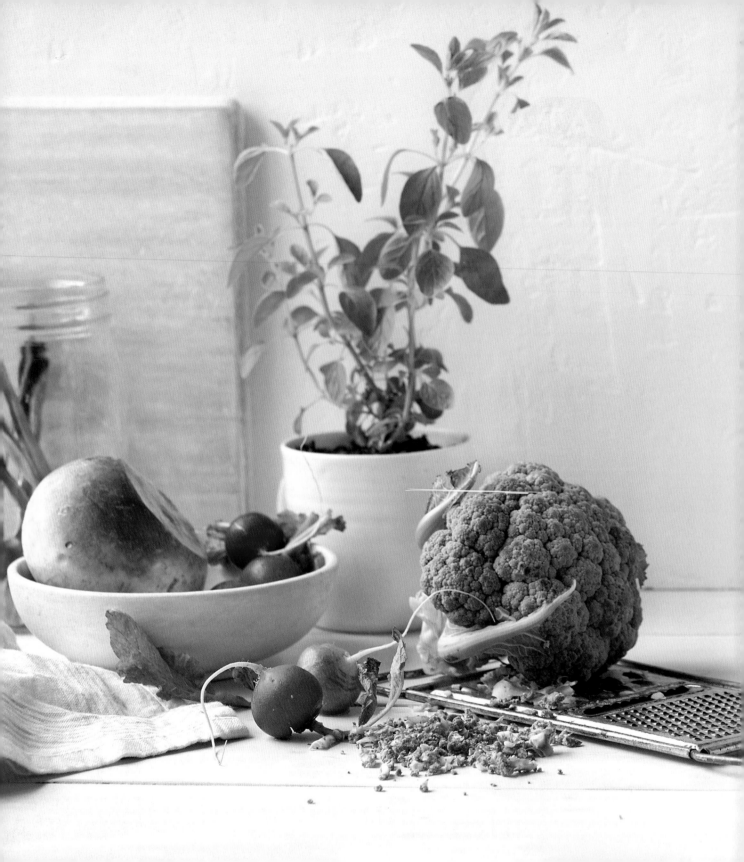

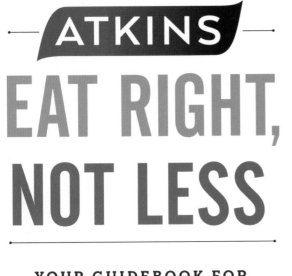

ATKINS

EAT RIGHT, NOT LESS

YOUR GUIDEBOOK FOR LIVING A LOW-CARB AND LOW-SUGAR LIFESTYLE

COLETTE HEIMOWITZ

TOUCHSTONE

New York London Toronto Sydney New Delhi

TOUCHSTONE

An Imprint of Simon & Schuster, Inc.
1230 Avenue of the Americas
New York, NY 10020

First Touchstone hardcover edition December 2017

TOUCHSTONE and colophon are registered trademarks of Simon & Schuster, Inc.

For information about special discounts for bulk purchases, please contact Simon & Schuster Special Sales at 1-866-506-1949 or business@simonandschuster.com.

The Simon & Schuster Speakers Bureau can bring authors to your live event. For more information or to book an event, contact the Simon & Schuster Speakers Bureau at 866-248-3049 or visit our website at www.simonspeakers.com.

This publication contains the opinions and ideas of its author. It is intended to provide helpful informative material on the subjects addressed in the publication. It is sold with the understanding that the author and publisher are not engaged in rendering medical, health, or any other kind of drawing inferences from it.

The author and publisher specifically disclaim all responsibility for any liability, loss or risk, personal or otherwise, which is incurred as a consequence, directly or indirectly, of the use and application of any of the contents of this book.

Interior design by Laura Palese

Photography by Ellen Silverman

Prop stylist: Alistair Turnbull/Food stylist: Nora Singley

Manufactured in the United States of America

10 9 8 7 6 5 4 3 2 1

Library of Congress Cataloging-in-Publication Data

Names: Heimowitz, Colette.
Title: Atkins: eat right, not less : your guidebook for living a low-carb and low-sugar lifestyle / Colette Heimowitz.
Description: New York : Touchstone, 2017. | Series: Atkins ; 6
Identifiers: LCCN 2017025540| ISBN 9781501175442 (hardback)
Subjects: LCSH: Reducing diets. | Nutrition. | Low-carbohydrate diet—Recipes. | Sugar-free diet—Recipes. | Health. | BISAC: HEALTH & FITNESS / Weight Loss. | HEALTH & FITNESS / Nutrition. | COOKING / Health & Healing / Weight Control.
Classification: LCC RM222.2 .H3457 2017 | DDC 641.5/6383—dc23 LC record available at https://lccn.loc.gov/2017025540

ISBN 978-1-5011-7544-2
ISBN 978-1-5011-7545-9 (ebook)

I WOULD LIKE TO DEDICATE THIS BOOK

**to the brilliant and creative team
at Atkins Nutritionals,**

who believes that Atkins is not just a diet but a way of eating that has the power to improve not just your health but all aspects of your life. The Atkins team has worked tirelessly and passionately to incorporate the latest scientific research into Atkins' proven way of eating, develop innovative products to support this lifestyle, and sustains our robust community of people dedicated to living a low-carb lifestyle.

IN ADDITION,

**I would like to dedicate this book to the
late Dr. Robert C. Atkins,**

who established the nutritional principle of eating right, not less, which remains the core of the Atkins way.

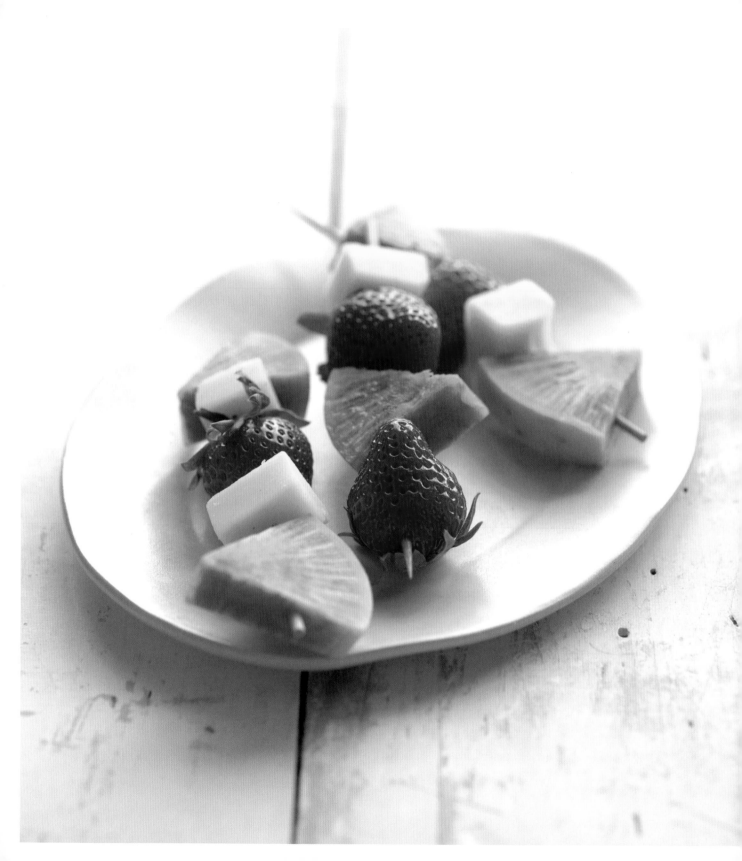

CONTENTS

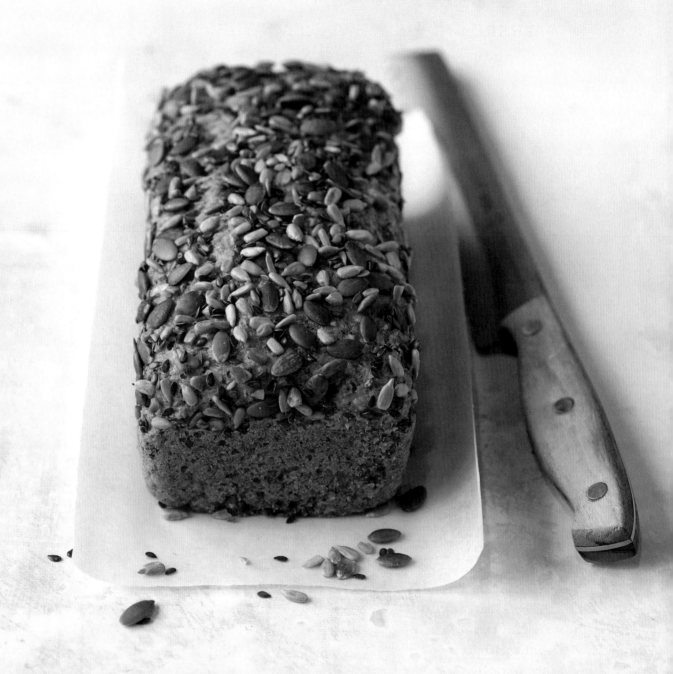

INTRODUCTION

THERE HAS NEVER BEEN A GREATER INTEREST

in food and its role in health—and

ATKINS IS A LEADER IN THIS MOVEMENT.

———•———

THIS JOURNEY STARTED MORE than forty years ago, when a cardiologist named Dr. Robert Atkins disrupted conventional wisdom by developing an approach to better health and losing weight based on eating right, not less. He discovered that when you take simple steps to cut back on carbs and sugar, you transform your metabolism from one that *stores* fat into one that *burns* fat.

Meanwhile, "conventional wisdom" had us cutting calories and fat to lose weight, which turned into a vicious cycle that left us feeling deprived and then overeating. For years, we've been told that fat is the main culprit in the obesity epidemic. We ate low-fat cookies and drank skim milk. And we kept getting fatter. But fat is not the enemy. There is another culprit, one that hides in plain sight, concealed in many of the "healthful" foods we eat and drink. And guess what: it's sugar and excess carbohydrates.

Sugars and foods that become sugars in the body are arguably responsible for one of the biggest health epidemics we face today. According to the World Health Organization, 1.9 billion adults are overweight; in the United States, one-third of adults are obese, 29 million

people have diabetes, and 86 million are prediabetic. In fact, someone is diagnosed with diabetes *every 30 seconds*. The US Department of Agriculture (USDA) confirms that the typical American now eats a staggering 131 pounds of added sugar (including table sugar, high-fructose corn syrup, and other caloric sweeteners added to food products) a year. And that's in addition to naturally occurring sugar in fruits, vegetables, grains, dairy products, and other foods. It is also a whole lot more than your grandparents and probably your parents consumed when they were your age.

But sugar is just the tip of the empty carbohydrate iceberg. If you cut out sugar but continue to eat lots of refined grains, such as white flour, white rice, and most breakfast cereals, you aren't going to have the dramatic weight-loss and health gains that people experience on Atkins. That's because those kissing cousins of sugar quickly convert to glucose, aka sugar, in your bloodstream. They are known as hidden sugars, and from your body's perspective, they are processed just the same as sugar. With Atkins, you'll completely rebalance your intake of protein, fat, and carbohydrates.

You'll be eating dramatically fewer carbs but more protein and fat.

Because you'll be eating fewer carbs and primarily carbs that are full of fiber, your blood sugar levels will remain relatively constant. That, in turn, will minimize hunger and cravings, making it easy to eat this way. Since you can eat foods cooked in olive oil, vegetables topped with a pat of butter, and salads garnished with avocado and olives, you'll find the fare filling and satisfying.

It's Time To Rethink "Diet"

Today, thanks to the movement started by Dr. Atkins, nearly three out of four adults are actively managing their carb intake. But although 64 percent of Americans would like to lose weight, the majority of them don't want to feel forced to adhere to a program. *Diet* has become a four-letter word that is neither healthy nor sustainable. Yet almost 150 million people have adopted this low-carb approach to eating in some form—they want balance, moderation, and variety, and they want to make the right food choices that will have a positive impact on their health and life. The world is ready to embrace what those of us at Atkins have known to be true all along: eating right—not less—helps you lose weight *and* improve your overall health and wellness. I've seen the transition from diet to lifestyle firsthand.

When I was studying to become a nutritionist, if I had been asked whether the following statements were true or false, I would definitely have said they were true:

- The only way to lose weight is to cut calories.
- To lose weight, you must eat small portions and forgo snacks.
- Hunger is the price you pay for paring pounds.
- Eating high-fat foods makes you fat.
- Atkins doesn't provide enough vegetables.
- It's virtually impossible to maintain weight loss permanently.

In the years since then, I've learned that in every case, these statements are *false*. Atkins has opened my eyes to a different but highly effective way of eating.

Eat Right, Not Less

Consider this book your guide to living a low-carb, low-sugar lifestyle. I'll give you an overview of how Atkins works and all the positive health benefits that you have the potential to achieve. Then I'll help you create realistic goals, which will help you decide exactly how you want to do Atkins. Whether you want to start small or prefer a more structured plan, Atkins is *not* hard. Start by making small choices, such as eating more fresh, colorful vegetables, flavorful protein sources, and healthy fats; reducing your sugar intake; and swapping out refined carbohydrates (which contain those insidious hidden sugars—and I'll show you how to find them) for high-fiber carbohydrate sources.

For many of us, diets have been a temporary solution. This is *not* a diet book. This book is about changing your mind-set about eating and food, and I'm going to share simple solutions that will allow you to embrace and sustain a low-carb, low-sugar lifestyle. With Atkins, you eat right, not less. This book is packed with useful information showing you how to do just that, plus 100 delicious low-carb and low-sugar recipes perfect for every occasion, including breakfasts you can grab and go, whole meals in minutes, holiday favorites, and makeovers of popular recipes for when you're craving comfort food, salty snacks, chocolate-y desserts, pasta, pizza, and more. Preparing and eating food should be a joyful ritual of mouthwatering flavors, and you'll be proud to share these recipes with family and friends.

About Me

I spent ten years in private practice working in physicians' offices, directing patients' nutrition programs. For the last twenty years, I have been working in one capacity or another for Atkins. I spent four of them at the Atkins Center for Complementary Medicine, where I worked for Dr. Atkins as a nutritionist with thousands of patients to help them slim down and deal with health problems. In my next sixteen years at Atkins Nutritionals, I've observed and advised thousands of members of the Atkins community in their weight control efforts. When it comes to eating habits and weight reduction, I've seen and heard it all. Now I'm excited to have the opportunity to guide you in your evolution toward making the right food choices, as you transform yourself and pave a way to better health. You can also communicate with me through the community at Atkins.com.

This book is about **changing your mind-set** about eating and food, and I'm going to share **simple solutions** that will allow you to embrace and sustain a **low-carb, low-sugar** lifestyle.

What I have learned is that not all of us need a "program" to succeed, but everyone needs a clearer perspective on his or her carbohydrate consumption. Though some of us need tight guardrails, others just want a guidebook for success: success in meeting and maintaining your goals concerning your health and the health of your loved ones, success in taking charge of your life, and, yes, success in attaining the body you've always wanted. There is a sense of accomplishment that you experience by taking control of your health—and therefore your future—that spills over into every aspect of your life.

Doing Atkins your way allows you enormous variety in the kinds of foods you can eat when you are aware of the impact that excess carbs have on your health. When you are able to control the quality and quantity of carbs you consume to suit your individual metabolism and needs, you can sustain this way of eating for life. Whether you want the instructions for a well-constructed Atkins or just the information you need to reduce your carb intake on your terms while savoring a variety of foods, I hope I can help you learn how to make doing Atkins second nature.

Are you ready? It's time to get started!

PART ONE

EAT RIGHT, NOT LESS

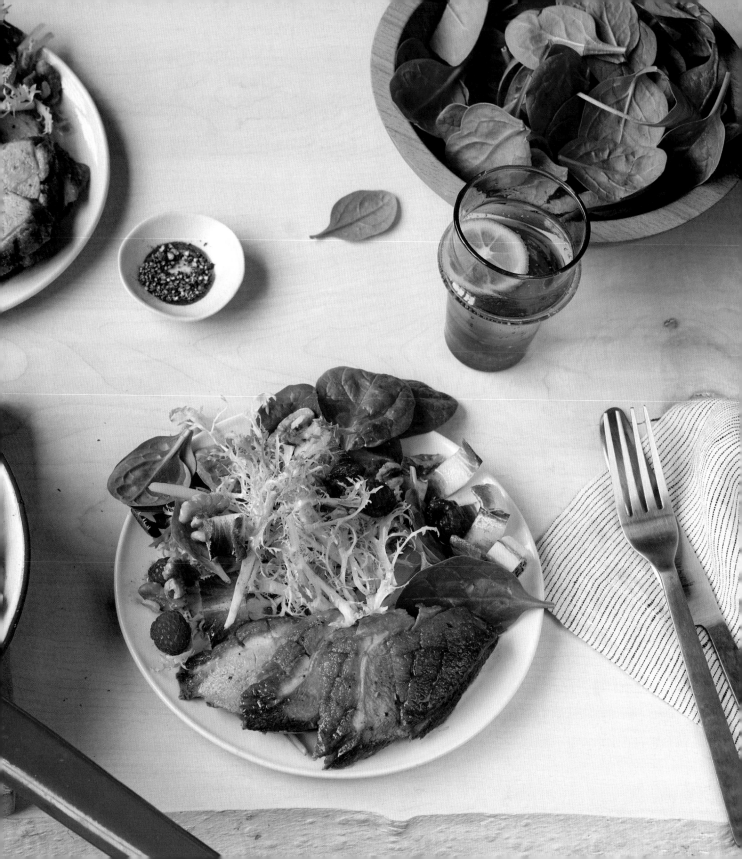

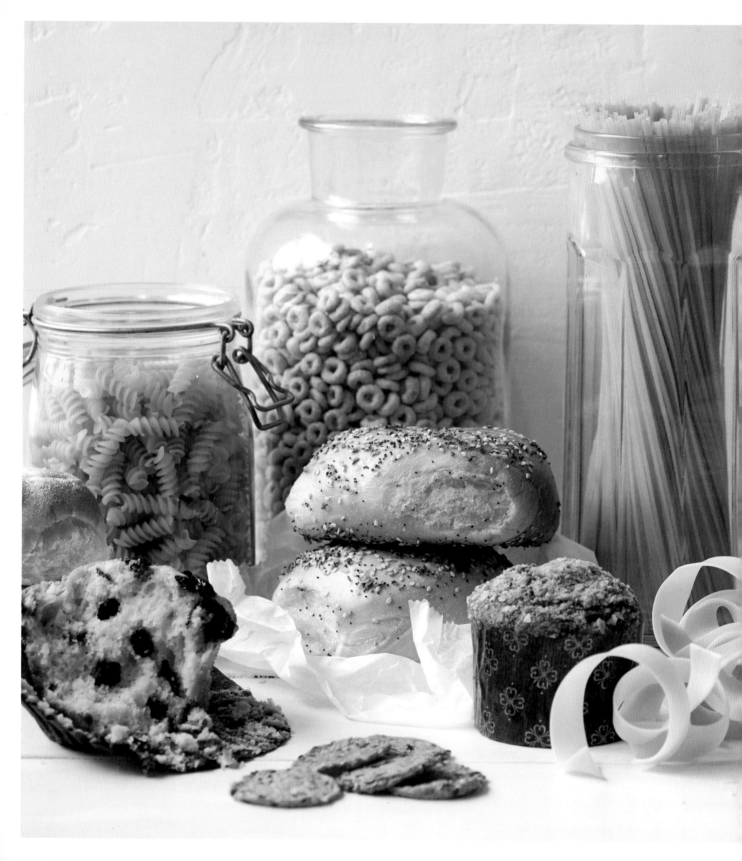

1

THE
HIDDEN
SUGAR
EFFECT

IT'S A HARD FACT TO SWALLOW:

68.8 percent of Americans are overweight or obese,[1]

and the coming generation has a shorter life expectancy than their parents'.[2] It comes down to what we've been putting into our mouths. The way we have been eating—where 50 to 60 percent of our calories come from carbohydrates[3]—has contributed to this health epidemic.

BACKED BY SCIENCE

Atkins is **backed by more than eighty** published, **peer-reviewed studies** conducted over the past few decades. You can see a full list of these studies in **Appendix F,** page 305.

FORTUNATELY, **THERE IS A SOLUTION.** Atkins' proven nutritional approach offers a better, smarter way to help you become healthier and fit. In this book, I'm going to show you how to live a low-carb, low-sugar lifestyle that involves making simple choices that will optimize your health, plus I've included 100 delicious low-carb, low-sugar recipes to help you along your way.

GET TO KNOW YOUR SUGARS

- **ADDED SUGARS:** These include sucrose, also known as table sugar, which is typically extracted from sugarcane or beet sugar and added to foods to make them sweeter (you'll find a list of some of the most common added sugars on page 9).

- **NATURALLY OCCURRING SUGARS:** These are naturally found in fruits, vegetables, grains, legumes, dairy products, and other foods.

- **HIDDEN SUGARS:** Carbohydrates that convert to sugar in your bloodstream.

ARE DIETARY GUIDELINES WORKING?

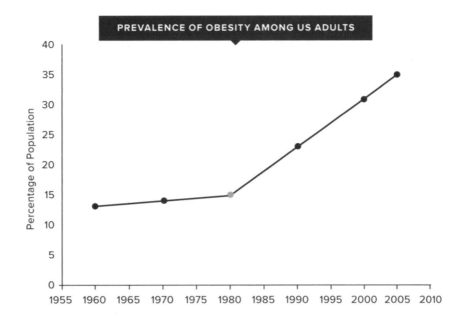

PREVALENCE OF OBESITY AMONG US ADULTS

Percentage of Population (y-axis: 0, 5, 10, 15, 20, 25, 30, 35, 40)

x-axis: 1955, 1960, 1965, 1970, 1975, 1980, 1985, 1990, 1995, 2000, 2005, 2010

Americans now eat less sugar and fewer refined carbs than they did in 2001, but it's still too much. Since 1970, they have also dramatically increased their consumption of fruits, vegetables, grains (including whole grains), and nuts, while decreasing their consumption of meat, eggs, whole milk, and butter, all according to the Dietary Guidelines for Americans (DGA) advice.

Yet since the Dietary Guidelines were first released, adult obesity rates have doubled, and they're set to increase by another 50 percent by 2030. Childhood obesity and diabetes diagnoses have tripled. One-third of adults are obese.

Source: Public Meeting for Oral Testimony on the Scientific Report of the 2015 Dietary Guidelines Committee. On March 24, 2015, the HHS and USDA hosted a public meeting in Bethesda, MD, to hear oral comments on the Advisory Report. **Adele Hite, of the Healthy Nation Coalition.**

An objective reading of the **health status of Americans** since the inception of the Office of Disease Prevention Health Promotion's Dietary Guidelines would indicate that **they are failing.**

First of all, let's examine how the current carb-centric way of eating brought on this obesity-driven health crisis.

Carbohydrates, protein, and fat are called macronutrients. They provide energy, and your body needs them to function, but the customary way of eating, and even typical calorie-cutting "diets" (the diet status quo for the last thirty years), are high in carbohydrates that convert to sugar, leading to blood sugar "highs" and excess sugar that is stored as fat. After your body scrambles to remove the excess sugar, it can lead to blood sugar "lows," during which you feel tired and hungry and crave more carbs and sugar. Carbohydrates are the only macronutrients that have this profound effect on your blood sugar. Here's why: The human metabolism can circulate only 5 grams of glucose at one time, which is equal to about 1 to 2 teaspoons of sugar. If your blood is required to circulate much more than that, the resulting blood sugar high forces your body to "dump" the excess sugar, leading to fat storage and weight gain. We call this the Hidden Sugar Effect.

Think of it this way: a typical breakfast of a bagel and a cappuccino can convert to ten times the amount of sugar in your bloodstream than your body can easily process. You don't see the sugar in carbs, but your body feels its effects and has to work hard to get rid of it. After years and years of consuming excess sugars and excess carbohydrates that convert to sugar, it becomes harder and harder for your body to handle the constant increase in blood sugar, which can eventually lead to prediabetes and type 2 diabetes. In fact, according to an article published in the *Journal of the American Medical Association*, if you combine the population diagnosed with prediabetes and diabetes, there are currently 52 percent of us with this deadly disease.[4]

Remember that bagel and cappuccino you had for breakfast? Once you process the sugar in your blood and your body dumps the excess, you may be stuck with low blood sugar and cravings for more carbs. By keeping an eye on the

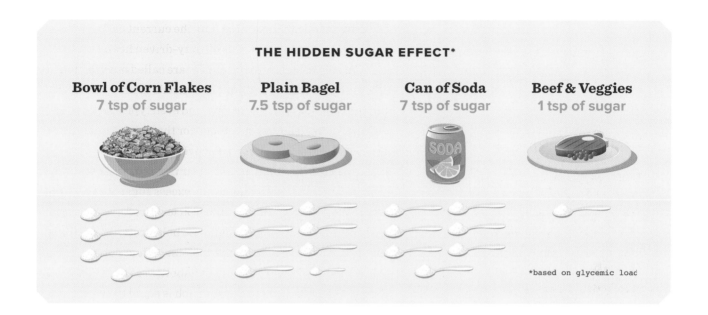

THE HIDDEN SUGAR EFFECT*

| Bowl of Corn Flakes | Plain Bagel | Can of Soda | Beef & Veggies |
| 7 tsp of sugar | 7.5 tsp of sugar | 7 tsp of sugar | 1 tsp of sugar |

*based on glycemic load

quality and *quantity* of the carbohydrates that you eat, you can prevent this blood sugar roller-coaster ride. I'll show you exactly how to do this, but first, let's discuss sugar.

Though you probably know that foods such as white rice and white bread convert to sugar in your bloodstream, nine out of ten Americans are unaware of all the other foods that convert to sugar. So-called healthful foods such as fruit juice; low-fat, fruit-sweetened yogurt; whole wheat bagels; and flavored oatmeal cause spikes in blood sugar similar to those produced by eating a candy bar! And the carbohydrates found in quinoa, ancient grains, and brown rice, when eaten in quantities larger than a ½-cup serving, may also cause blood sugar spikes.

I'll show you on page 25 how you can incorporate these healthier whole grains into your diet wisely so that you lessen the impact on your blood sugar, but what is important to understand right now is that sugar is sugar. Translation: an organic pressed juice or smoothie has the same impact on your blood sugar as a can of soda. Welcome to the world of hidden sugars.

DID YOU KNOW ?

BACKED BY SCIENCE

Of course, you know that **tempting treats** such as donuts, cookies, and candy contain sugar, but more **sugar** than you know is hiding in plain sight everywhere, even in foods that are often deemed "healthy." In fact, four out of five Americans have no idea that added sugars, carbohydrates, and natural sugars all cause your **blood sugar** to rise and, in excess, lead to weight gain, prediabetes, and **type 2 diabetes.**

THE HIDDEN SUGAR QUIZ

*To get a better understanding of hidden sugars,
let's start by testing your knowledge of which foods have a
bigger effect on your blood sugar. You might be surprised!*

WHICH HAS THE BIGGER EFFECT ON YOUR **BLOOD SUGAR?**	ANSWERS (NO PEEKING!)
A strawberry frosted cupcake **OR** a small baked potato	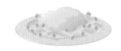 They **both** have the same blood sugar–raising effect as 6.3 teaspoons of sugar.
A chocolate bar **OR** a serving of macaroni and cheese	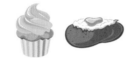 The **macaroni and cheese** has the same blood sugar–raising effect as 11 teaspoons of sugar, compared to 9 teaspoons for the chocolate bar.
A sports drink **OR** a small bowl of corn flakes	The **corn flakes** have the same blood sugar–raising effect as 6.6 teaspoons of sugar, compared to 4 teaspoons for the sports drink.
A chocolate bar **OR** ¼ cup raisins	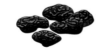 The **raisins** have the same blood sugar–raising effect as 9.3 teaspoons of sugar, compared to 9 teaspoons for the chocolate bar.
A bagel **OR** a muffin	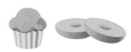 They **both** have the same blood sugar–raising effect as 7.5 teaspoons of sugar.

SUGAR IS NOT SO SWEET

Eating sugar and excessive carbohydrates that convert to blood sugar in your body leads to obesity, but studies also link excess sugar consumption to an increased risk of cancer, diabetes, gastrointestinal problems, eye diseases, osteoporosis, coronary heart disease, and other inflammatory diseases. Too much sugar may also affect your brain and could be associated with poor memory formation, learning disabilities, depression, and even dementia.

Before you throw your hands up in despair thinking about all the hidden sugars lurking out there, it's important to understand that not all foods are full of them. You can feast on Pear and Manchego Mesclun Salad with Caramelized Onions (page 195) or Lemon Pepper Shrimp with Snow Peas (page 233), and you'll be consuming only 2 to 2.5 teaspoons of hidden sugars, while feeling far more satisfied than you ever would after scarfing down 1 cup of macaroni and cheese. Meals and snacks that contain adequate amounts of protein, healthy fats, and high-fiber carbohydrates have very few hidden sugars and help prevent blood sugar spikes and fat storage (i.e., weight gain) while keeping your energy levels steady.

Now that you have made it through the tricky part of learning what hidden sugars are, how they impact your blood sugar, and how to identify them, you should begin to have a better idea of how much of your diet they currently make up and their potential effect on your overall health.

How to Find Added Sugars

There are more than fifty names for sugar! Next time you're at the grocery store or perusing your pantry, you might be amazed at how many foods feature these names on their ingredients lists. Here are some of the most common:

Agave nectar	*High-fructose corn syrup*
Barley malt	*Honey*
Beet sugar	
Brown sugar	*Malt syrup*
Cane juice	*Maltodextrin*
Caramel	*Maltose*
Coconut sugar	*Molasses*
Confectioner's sugar	*Muscovado*
Corn syrup	*Rice syrup*
Dextrose	*Saccharose*
Fructose	*Sucrose*
Glucose	*Turbinado sugar*

A BETTER WAY
TO EAT

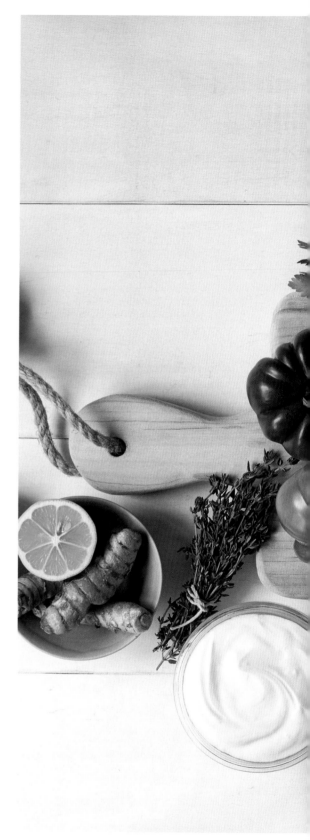

I WILL SHOW YOU how Atkins works and how carbohydrates, protein, and fat function in your body. I will also show you how you can make simple changes to cut back on your carb and sugar intake, giving you the potential to reap major health benefits. You'll learn how this way of eating can help you reduce blood sugar spikes while putting less wear and tear on your metabolism, helping you avoid weight gain as you age. In addition, you'll reduce your chances of getting diabetes while experiencing steady energy levels.

This is not a diet book where you are forced to comply with a one-size-fits-all diet plan. You have seen how traditional diets continue to impact our rising obesity rate and associated health problems, and you have possibly experienced those effects firsthand. My goal is to show you how Atkins' low-carb, low-sugar nutritional approach is truly a better way to eat, with proven recommendations that are tailored to you and your needs.

My goal is to show you how Atkins' **low-carb, low-sugar** nutritional approach is truly a **better way to eat.**

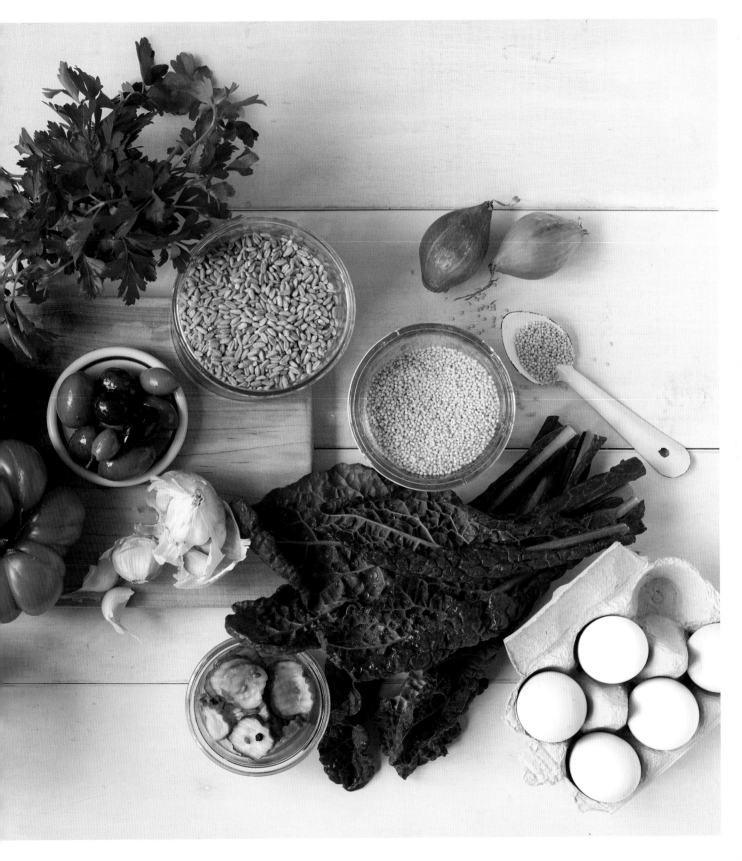

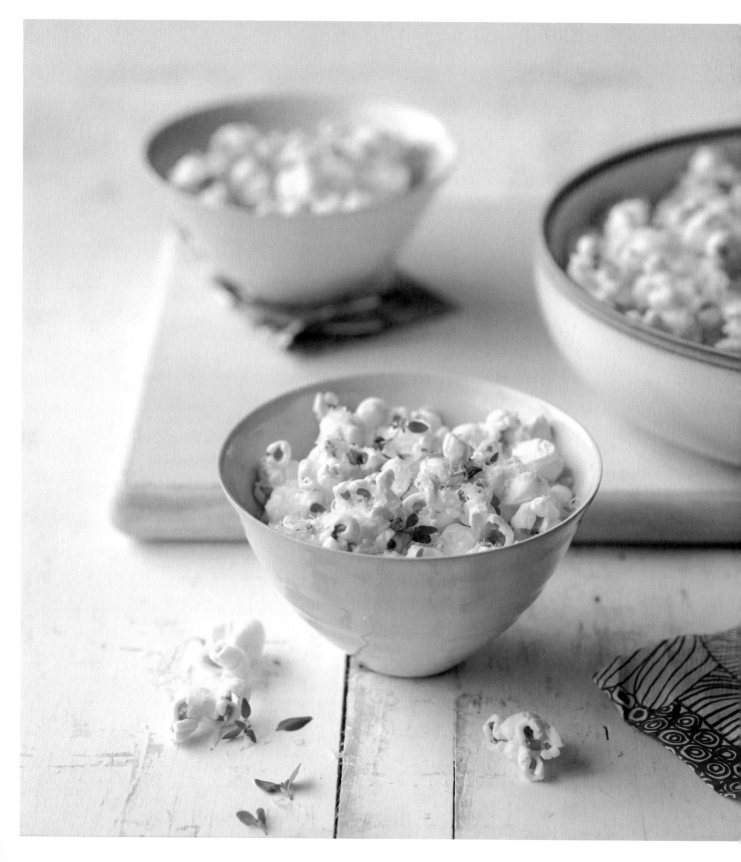

2

HOW
ATKINS
WORKS

When you reduce your
CARBOHYDRATE AND SUGAR INTAKE,

as you do with Atkins, while consuming an optimal combination
of protein, healthy fats, and fiber-rich, low-sugar carbohydrates—eating right,
not less—you flip the switch on your metabolism so you burn both dietary
and body fat for fuel. In other words, you burn fat instead of storing it.

R EDUCING CARB AND SUGAR INTAKE has been proven to improve health and to help lose weight or maintain weight while feeling constantly energized and experiencing less hunger and fewer cravings. There's a reason why this way of eating has become a lifestyle for almost 150 million people.

This is because your metabolism burns two different types of fuel for energy: carbohydrates or fat.

As you have learned, when you consume mostly carbo-hydrates (plus the hidden sugars in them) and cut calories, your body burns those carbs and sugar for fuel, leading to blood sugar spikes, fat storage, fatigue, hunger, and more. Let's dig a little deeper into how Atkins works and why eating right, not less, makes so much sense.

FEEL THE BURN

Metabolism refers to the process of how your body turns food into **energy.**

ATKINS' MANY HEALTH BENEFITS

In addition to weight loss, a low-carb, low-sugar lifestyle has been shown to impact health in the following ways:

- Decreased risk of developing prediabetes and type 2 diabetes
- Decreased risk of developing cardiovascular disease
- Improvements in brain health
- Steady energy levels
- Improvements in epilepsy and related diseases
- Decrease in inflammation markers

HOW DOES ATKINS WORK?

LOW-CALORIE/HIGH-CARB DIET	VS	ATKINS

 UP AND DOWN SUGAR LEVELS

 STEADY SUGAR LEVELS

 INCREASED
- FAT STORAGE
- HUNGER/CRAVINGS

 LESS
- FAT STORAGE
- HUNGER/CRAVINGS

 BURN SUGAR & STORE FAT

 BURN FAT & LOSE WEIGHT

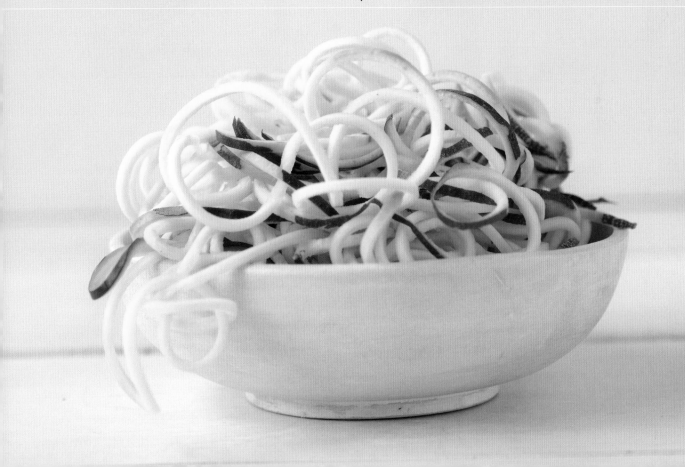

GET TO KNOW YOUR
MACRONUTRIENTS

T HE ADAGE "YOU ARE WHAT YOU EAT" is true, and with Atkins, it all comes down to macronutrients: carbohydrates, protein, and fat. Macronutrients provide your body with energy (calories), and they are necessary for your body to function properly. The amount of carbs, protein, and fat in any food is measured in grams. Here's more about macronutrients.

Carbohydrates

These are broken down by your body into glucose (sugar) and used as energy. Any excess carbs are stored as fat. Carbohydrates are found in all plant foods, including grains, cereals, nuts, potatoes, bread, and pasta. All vegetables and fruit are considered carbohydrates, but their carb counts vary a lot. Berries, for example, are relatively low in carbs, while bananas are not. In general, leafy greens, along with many other vegetables, are low in carbs, while potatoes, sweet potatoes, and grains are higher. Dairy products also contain some carbs, in the form of milk sugars. On Atkins you count grams of Net Carbs, rather than grams of total carbs, because fiber is a form of carbohydrate and has minimal impact on blood sugar levels.

Protein

Your body needs protein because it contains the amino acids that are the building blocks your body uses to repair and regenerate body tissues and cells. It helps maintain a healthy immune system and manufactures hormones. Plus, digesting and metabolizing protein burns twice the calories than digesting and metabolizing carbohydrates does. Protein is found in seafood, poultry, eggs, meat, and dairy. Soy products, nuts, and beans also contain protein as well as carbohydrates.

Fat

Your body uses fat to help improve brain development and cell function, protect your organs, and help you absorb the fat-soluble vitamins A, D, E, and K, plus micronutrients in vegetables. Consuming fat stimulates the burning of body fat, and, like protein, fat keeps you feeling full longer. Since it carries flavor, it also makes food more palatable and satisfying.

HOW TO "EYEBALL" YOUR PROTEIN PORTIONS

Calculating how much protein you eat is simple. There's no need to count calories or grams or weigh your food. You need only about 4 to 6 ounces of cooked protein at each meal. Just use these visual comparisons, and soon you'll find that it's quite easy to "eyeball" how much protein you need.

1 ounce
meat, poultry, tofu, etc.

=

Small matchbox/ remote car key

3 ounces
meat, poultry, tofu, etc.

=

Slim paperback book

8 ounces
meat, poultry, tofu, etc.

=

Deck of cards/cell phone

3 ounces
fish

=

Checkbook

1 ounce
hard cheese

=

An individually wrapped American cheese slice or four dice.
(Note: Limit cheese to 4 ounces daily)

What is a Net Carb?

Net Carbs are calculated by subtracting grams of dietary fiber from total carbohydrate grams on a food label. You can download the Atkins Carb Counter for free at www.atkins.com. This guide provides the Net Carb counts of practically every food.

Nutrition Facts

Serving Size 1 Bar (38g)
Servings per Container 5

Amount Per Serving	
Calories 150	Calories from Fat 90

	% Daily Value
Total Fat 9g	14%
Saturated Fat 2.5g	13%
Cholesterol 0mg	0%
Sodium 170mg	7%
Total Carbohydrate 17g	6%
Dietary Fiber 10g	40%
Sugars 4g	
= 7 Net Carbs	

THE SKINNY ON FAT

All dietary fat is not created equal. Here's what you need to know.

- Monounsaturated fats (MUFAs): are found in olive oil, canola oil, and walnuts and most other nuts, as well as avocados. MUFAs are usually liquid at room temperature. *Cook with heart-healthy olive oil, add creamy avocados, and eat walnuts and most other nuts as garnishes or snacks.*

- Polyunsaturated fats (PUFAs): liquid both at room temperature and in the refrigerator. They're found mostly in oils from vegetables, seeds, and some nuts. *Sunflower, safflower, flaxseed, soybean, corn, cottonseed, grape seed, and sesame oils are high in PUFAs. So are the oils in fatty fish such as sardines, herring, and salmon.*

- Essential fatty acids (EFAs): two families of dietary fats that your body can't produce on its own. Both omega-3 and omega-6 EFAs are PUFAs essential to your health and well being. Omega-3s are found in the fat of shellfish and cold-water fish. Omega-6s are found primarily in seeds and grains, as well as in chicken and pork. Unless you're eating a very-low-fat diet, you are most likely getting more than the recommended amount of omega-6s. *Eat foods (or supplements) rich in omega-3 fatty acids, such as shellfish, cold-water ocean fish, and fish oil (salmon, tuna, sardines,* herring, and anchovies, as well as nonfish sources such as flaxseed, almonds, walnuts, and canola oil). Limit your consumption of corn, soybean, cottonseed, and peanut oils, which are all high in omega-6s.*

- Saturated fatty acids (SFAs): tend to remain solid at room temperature. Butter, lard, suet, and palm and coconut oils are relatively rich in saturated fat. *Fine to consume as part of Atkins' way of eating because we know that the body burns primarily fat on Atkins, and we know from published research that the level of saturated fat in the blood does not increase when you are following Atkins.*

- Trans fats: the only dietary fats you should truly avoid. A high intake of trans fats is associated with an increased heart attack risk, and most recently they have been shown to increase the body's level of inflammation. Typically found in foods you should already be avoiding, including battered fried foods, baked goods, cookies, crackers, candies, snack foods, icings, and vegetable shortenings. Check the list of ingredients, where trans fats are listed as "shortening," "hydrogenated vegetable oil," or "partially hydrogenated vegetable oil." *If you see any of these words in the ingredients list, consider an alternative.*

THE BASICS OF ATKINS

ONCE YOU GET THE BASICS OF ATKINS under your belt, you will realize that it is really quite a simple plan to follow. Before you get started, here are a few other things that will help you have a better understanding of Atkins.

Atkins is *not* a "no-carb" plan. From the very beginning, you will be eating high-quality carbohydrates (many in the form of vegetables) that are rich in nutrients and phytochemicals and high in fiber, which means they are naturally satiating. In fact, with Atkins, you actually eat more servings of vegetables than most Americans do.

You don't need to count calories on Atkins. The quality and quantity of the protein, fats, and carbohydrates that you eat while on Atkins are most important. The only thing you count on Atkins is your daily grams of Net Carbs, which helps ensure that you are eating the high-quality, nutrient-rich foods that keep you full and satisfied, so your calories naturally fall into a healthy range.

Atkins is *not* a high-protein plan. Though you'll be eating adequate amounts of protein, Atkins' typical intake of about 65 to 175 grams (12 to 22 ounces) of protein a day, depending on your height, is not considered high protein. I like to think of Atkins as a nutritional approach that features "optimal" amounts of protein. The ideal amount of protein should make you full after your meal, not uncomfortably stuffed and not hungry until your next scheduled meal.

Atkins has built-in portion control. You will be eating foods that are rich in protein and good fat and high in fiber, helping you achieve your goals while controlling your hunger. This is because these foods are naturally self-limiting. Almost everyone has probably scarfed down half a package of cookies or a bag of chips in one sitting, but have you ever overdone it on hard-boiled eggs or steamed broccoli?

MORE MUSCLE IS BETTER

Muscle is more **metabolically active** than fat. This means that every pound of muscle you have uses more calories for **energy** than every pound of fat, even when you're **at rest.**

WHY VEGETABLES
MATTER

*When you do Atkins, you'll be eating 12 to 15 grams of
Net Carbs of what we call Foundation Vegetables (page 291)
a day. Thus, you will probably eat more veggies than
you ever have before, and for some very good reasons:*

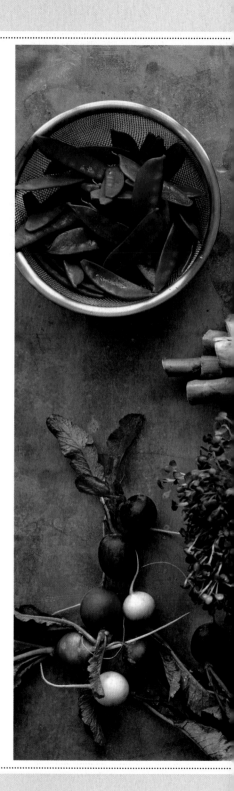

VEGETABLES HELP KEEP YOU FULL FOR LONGER. The fiber and
water in vegetables fill you up far more efficiently than do processed
carbs that are low in fiber. Combining vegetables with protein and
healthy fats will keep you satisfied until it's time for your next meal.

VEGETABLES KEEP YOUR ENERGY LEVELS BALANCED. The fiber
in vegetables also helps regulate your blood sugar. If you're eating
all your allotted vegetables each day, you shouldn't experience the
late-afternoon energy slump (and cravings for sugar) that you may
encounter when eating processed carbohydrates.

VEGETABLES PACK A POWERFUL NUTRITIONAL PUNCH. Vegetables
tend to be low in calories and high in fiber, which means you may
tend to consume fewer calories, while still feeling as satisfied as—if
not more satisfied than—when you rely on packaged foods and
foods devoid of nutrients.

EATING VEGETABLES MAY ADD YEARS TO YOUR LIFE. Numerous
studies[1] show that a diet rich in a variety of colorful vegetables may
help decrease the hardening of arteries, help lower cholesterol
levels, and help prevent inflammation, a component of many
degenerative diseases, including obesity, diabetes, heart disease,
and Alzheimer's disease. Researchers believe that the antioxidants
(vitamins C and E, plus selenium and the carotenoids) may be partly
responsible for this effect.

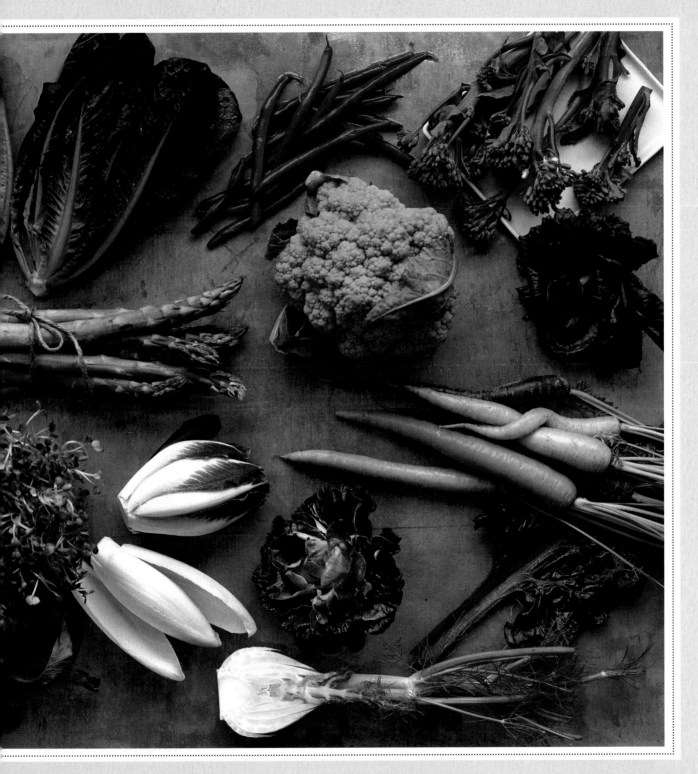

LIVING A LOW-CARB LIFESTYLE
ON YOUR TERMS

HE AVERAGE PERSON CONSUMES 251 to 300 grams of carbohydrates a day, but very few of us actually realize that. Those carbohydrates, especially when consumed in the form of sugar and refined carbohydrates, have a negative impact on both your health and your waistline.

Just one in three Americans knows that you should consume 100 grams of carbohydrates or less in a day. This is where Atkins comes in. Reducing carb intake is a healthy way to live, and I'll show you how you can customize your daily carbohydrate intake based on your needs and a choice of three options: Atkins 20, 40, or 100.

Atkins 20®

Atkins 20 is the classic Atkins plan that has been so successful for millions of people over the past four decades. If you have more than 40 pounds to lose, have a waist circumference of over 35 inches (women) or 40 inches (men), or are prediabetic or diabetic, this is the plan for you. You'll see results quickly. Even after just a few days, your clothes may fit better. As you approach your weight-loss goals, you'll add plenty of fruits, veggies, and eventually whole grains.

HERE'S HOW ATKINS 20® WORKS:

- **START WITH** 20 grams of Net Carbs of carbohydrates a day, with 12 to 15 grams of Net Carbs of carbohydrates coming from Foundation Vegetables (see page 291).
- **EAT** three 4- to 6-ounce servings of protein each day.
- **EAT** 2 to 4 servings of added fat each day.
- **BUDGET** the remaining 5 to 8 grams of Net Carbs from the entire acceptable carbohydrates food list (see pages 289–299).

Atkins 40®

If you have less than 40 pounds to lose, you want a wider variety of food choices, or you are breast-feeding, Atkins 40 is for you. On this plan, you can enjoy a full range of carbohydrate food options combined with a variety of proteins and fats—while still losing weight at a steady pace and feeling satisfied, never hungry. Your carbohydrate choices includes vegetables, fruits, controlled portions of whole grains, and even potatoes, right from the beginning.

HERE'S HOW ATKINS 40® WORKS:

- **START WITH** 40 grams of Net Carbs of carbohydrates a day, with 12 to 15 grams of Net Carbs of carbohydrates coming from Foundation Vegetables (see page 291).

- **EAT** three 4- to 6-ounce servings of protein each day.

- **EAT** 2 to 4 servings of added fat each day.

- **BUDGET** the remaining 25 grams of Net Carbs from the entire acceptable carbohydrates food list (see all appendixes).

Atkins 100®

If you would like to start experiencing some of the positive benefits of reducing your carb intake by gradually making small, smart changes to your eating habits on a daily basis, start here. If you like the changes you are making and feel ready to make more, you can always take it to the next level and try Atkins 40 or even Atkins 20 if you have a significant amount of weight to lose.

HERE'S HOW ATKINS 100® WORKS:

- **START WITH** 100 grams of Net Carbs of carbohydrates a day, with a minimum of 12 to 15 grams of Net Carbs of carbohydrates coming from Foundation Vegetables (see page 291).

- **EAT** three 4- to 6-ounce servings of protein each day.

- **EAT** 2 to 4 servings of added fat each day.

- **BUDGET** the remaining 85 grams of Net Carbs from the entire acceptable carbohydrates food list.

IT'S TIME TO EAT RIGHT, NOT LESS

No matter what Atkins plan you choose to follow, stick with these tips for eating right, not less:

- **FAT IS YOUR FRIEND, BUT DON'T GO OVERBOARD.** Stick with three 1-tablespoon servings of healthy fats a day.

- **PROTEIN KEEPS YOU SATISFIED.** Go for 4 to 6 ounces of protein at each meal, maybe a little more if you are tall.

- **GET YOUR VEGGIES IN AT EVERY MEAL.** The fiber from the minimum of 12 to 15 grams of Net Carbs of vegetables that you're eating every day will help fill you up.

- **DON'T SKIP MEALS.** If you do, you'll feel ravenous by the end of the day and be more likely to overdo it at your next meal. Focus on eating three meals and two snacks a day.

- **DON'T CONSUME ALL YOUR CARBS FOR THE DAY IN ONE MEAL.** Spread out the recommended amount of carbs over your meals and snacks.

See Chapter 4 for detailed information on each of these plans.

HOW MANY CARBS
ARE YOU *REALLY* EATING, ANYWAY?

D O YOU HAVE ANY IDEA how many carbohydrates you eat on a daily basis? Not many of us do, but you might be amazed when you discover that it is way more than you think. You can start by figuring out how many grams of Net Carbs you are eating now. You can do this by recording everything you eat in a food journal (or one of the many online tools or apps available) for a few days. Remember, Net Carbs are calculated by subtracting grams of fiber from grams of total carbohydrates on a food label. This is a valuable exercise to do anyway; once you start reading food labels, you may be surprised at exactly what and how much you are eating, especially foods containing hidden sugars, such as low-fat sweetened yogurt or instant oatmeal.

Now that you have a rough idea of how many Net Carbs you are consuming daily, start making some small, healthy changes. You can use this as an excellent excuse to clean out your pantry of processed foods (cookies, candy, chips, and all those other things you know you shouldn't be eating anyway); you can learn more about what foods to toss and what foods to keep beginning on page 32. Focus on lean sources of protein such as poultry, meat, fish, and eggs; make sure you

KEEP A FOOD JOURNAL

Not only will it help you keep track of your meals and snacks, how many and what kind of carbs you are eating, as well as your portion sizes, you can also use it to record when you are eating and even why. Sometimes we find ourselves eating out of boredom or due to stress, and recording such moments in your food journal can help you begin to understand and recognize your hunger cues. For more tips on how to get started, see page 110.

add healthy fats (olive oil, almonds and other nuts and seeds, and avocados) and eat plenty of fresh fruits and vegetables. You can find sample meal plans in Chapter 4 and Acceptable Foods lists in the appendixes to help get you started. Begin with these smart carb swaps and you should start experiencing some of Atkins' positive benefits.

SMART CARB SWAPS

Small changes lead to big results when you start with these smart nutrient-rich carb swaps.

SWAP	▶	FOR
White rice		**Brown rice** or **fiber-rich grains** such as quinoa, which have more nutrients and are higher in protein
White bread or potatoes		**Nutrient-rich whole grain bread,** or double your serving of fiber-rich veggies
Tortillas or bread slices		**Leaves of lettuce** or romaine (they're naturally low in carbs and will turn your taco or sandwich into a wrap)
Hamburger bun		**Portobello mushroom** (rich in potassium and the perfect low-carb vehicle for a juicy burger)
Fruit juice		**Fresh fruit,** which is higher in fiber and more filling
Low-fat fruit-flavored yogurt		**Full-fat Greek yogurt,** which is higher in protein and lower in sugar. Top with a few blueberries to get your fruit fix.
Crackers		**Almonds** or **pistachios,** which are more satisfying than high-carb crackers and give you an extra boost of protein and heart-healthy fats
Low-fat or fat-free salad dressings (which tend to have sugar added)		**Oil- and vinegar-based** dressings
Breakfast cereal		**Whole grain oatmeal** or, even better, a couple of **scrambled eggs**
Candy		**Fresh fruit** or an ounce of **dark chocolate,** both lower in carbs, and the chocolate is rich in heart-healthy flavonoids

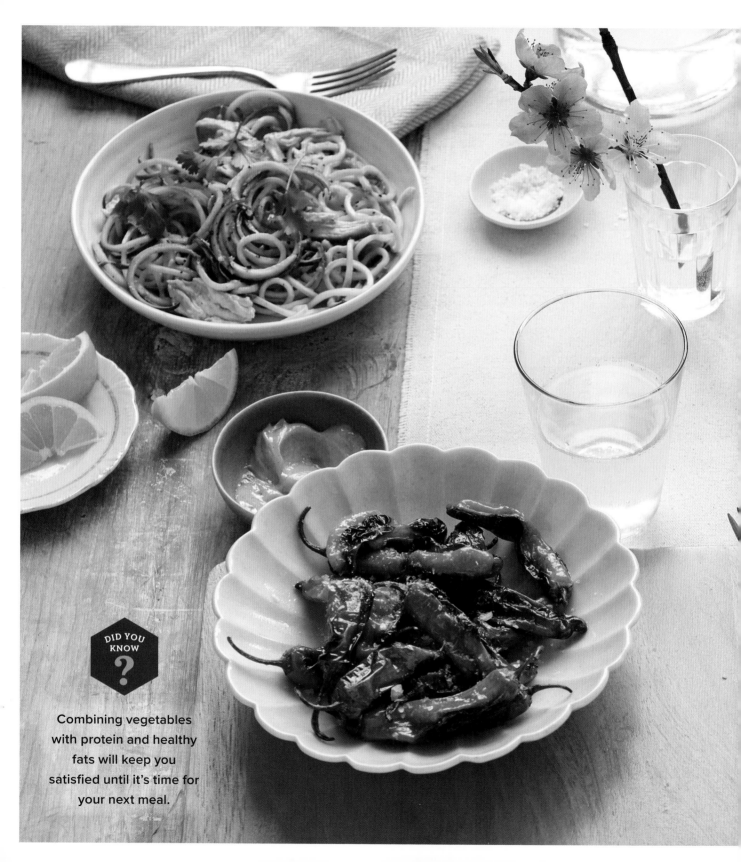

DID YOU KNOW

?

Combining vegetables with protein and healthy fats will keep you satisfied until it's time for your next meal.

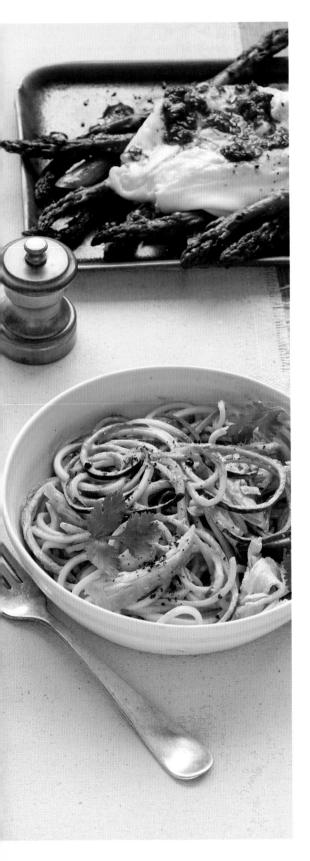

ATKINS
YOUR WAY

E VEN IF YOU ARE NOT ready to take the leap into a full-blown low-carb lifestyle, with Atkins you can start at your own pace. Now that you know how Atkins works, in the following chapters I will show you how you can get started and pick the Atkins way of eating that works for you (with additional details on each option). I'll also tell you about more smart carb swaps; nutrient-rich snacks to keep your energy levels on an even keel all day long; food lists; meal plans; low-carb tips for eating out at restaurants, on the road, and even on vacation; and mouthwatering low-carb, low-sugar recipes.

HOW TO ID HIDDEN SUGARS

Net Carbs are a very good way of determining the effect a certain food will have on your blood sugar. Stick with foods that contain 15 grams of Net Carbs or fewer.

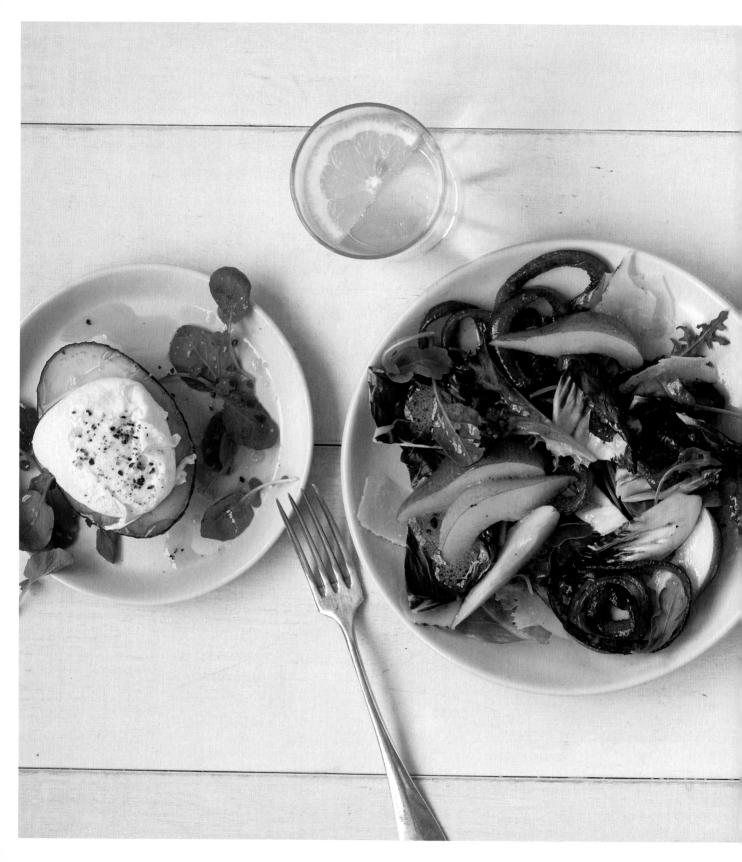

3

LET'S
GET
STARTED

IF YOU ARE READING THIS BOOK,

most likely it is because you are interested in a better
way of eating—one that has the power to improve your health, boost
your energy, and help you feel and look better.

I'm going to show you how
you can **get started** on making
small steps toward **embracing
a low-carb lifestyle** and all the
amazing food you *can* eat.

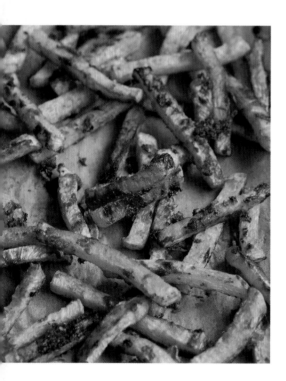

IN THE PREVIOUS CHAPTERS, I have shown the negative
impact certain foods may have on your health, as well
as how Atkins works in a positive way to optimize your
health. Now it's time to talk about the fun stuff—I'm going
to show you how you can get started on making small steps
toward embracing a low-carb, low-sugar lifestyle and all the
amazing food you *can* eat.

Before you skip to the recipes in the second half of this
book, first things first: having the right food available is
your secret to success. It's time to clean out and organize
your fridge, freezer, and pantry and toss all foods containing
hidden sugars, added sugars, and processed carbohydrates.
Once you have a clean "low-carb" slate, it's time to go grocery
shopping. I will give you some important shopping tips so
that you can stock your kitchen with fresh, delicious, and
naturally low-carb foods—carbohydrates rich in fiber, plus
protein and healthy fats—that you will love to eat. And
you will definitely want to keep reading to discover some
essential tools and gadgets to help you along the way.

When you finish this chapter, you will have everything
you need to get started on the Atkins plan of your choice
based on your goals (you will learn more about Atkins 20,
Atkins 40, and Atkins 100 in Chapter 4) and all the tools and
food you need at your fingertips so you can start cooking
some of the mouthwatering recipes in this book.

HOW TO SET S.M.A.R.T. GOALS

If you are ready to embrace a better way of eating by reducing your carb and sugar intake and making small, healthy changes you can live with, it helps to set some goals so you can stay focused. You need to make sure your goals are S.M.A.R.T.: Specific, Measureable, Attainable, Realistic, and Timely. This proven strategy will improve your chances of success. Here's how to get started:

SPECIFIC: You have a greater chance of achieving a specific goal than a general goal. A goal that is too general would be "I'd like to eat fewer carbs." A specific goal is "I'd like to reduce my carbs to 100 grams of Net Carbs a day, five days a week."

MEASURABLE: Next you need to establish your criteria for success. If your goal is to reduce your carb intake to 100 grams of Net Carbs a day, this is something you can easily measure by tracking your daily grams of Net Carbs in a food journal or the Atkins app (see page 42) to gauge your starting point and your progress.

ATTAINABLE: You want to make sure you can actually achieve the goal you set, or you may become discouraged and quit. For example, cutting back to 100 grams of Net Carbs a day may be more attainable for you than deciding to cut back to 20 grams of Net Carbs a day right away.

REALISTIC: Get real! You want to challenge yourself, but you also don't want to set yourself up to fail. Perhaps cutting back to 100 grams of Net Carbs seven days a week is an unrealistic expectation, maybe due to your travel or work schedule. Start with 100 grams of Net Carbs a day five days a week and commit to achieving that!

TIMELY: Your goal should have a deadline so that you have a timeline by when you hope to accomplish it. At that point, you can evaluate your progress and set new goals.

Now that you understand the process of S.M.A.R.T. goal setting, your options are endless. Here's one more tip that will help you stay focused on successfully achieving your goals: review them daily! You can program reminders in your smartphone or even jot them down and post them on your computer or refrigerator. Display them wherever you think you will see a powerful and inspiring reminder.

CREATING YOUR OWN
LOW-CARB KITCHEN

———————— • ————————

WHEN YOU TOSS THOSE TEMPTING treats that have been contributing to blood sugar spikes, constant cravings, low energy, mood swings, and more, you will begin to feel so much better. Start by giving your kitchen a low-carb, low-sugar overhaul. I will divide your kitchen into the categories of fridge, freezer, and pantry so you have step-by-step instructions for each. Giving your kitchen this kind of attention will set you up to begin eating right, not less.

Fridge

TOSS THESE NOW

- Your first (and easiest) step is to toss anything that is expired (hello, salad dressing that's three years old).

- Next, toss anything that doesn't look or smell good, including vegetables that are past their prime. Don't worry, I will show you some tricks for not letting food go to waste in the future.

- Now it's time to read some labels. You would be amazed at the sugar lurking in foods such as barbecue sauce, salad dressing, low-fat yogurt, spaghetti sauce (you should probably toss that two-week-old, half-full

jar anyway), jams, and jellies. Now, I am not suggesting you throw out perfectly good food, but you could at least delegate a section of your fridge as a "high-sugar/high-carb" zone if you have other household members who will eat it. Once those foods are gone, if you are on Atkins 20 or Atkins 40, I would suggest replacing them with low-carb options. Sauces (such as barbecue, pasta, and steak sauces) should not contain more than 3 grams of Net Carbs per serving.

- Now that the shelves and drawers are cleared out, this is your chance to wipe down your fridge and clean up all those mysterious spills so you are truly starting with a shiny, clean slate.

WHAT TO KEEP

- Fortunately, many things in your fridge may be naturally low in carbs already, including most vegetables, some fruits, meats, eggs, dairy products, and oils.

- You can also keep condiments such as salsa, hot sauce, mustard, low-sugar or sugar-free salad dressings, mayonnaise, horseradish, pesto, lemon or lime juice, and soy sauce or tamari.

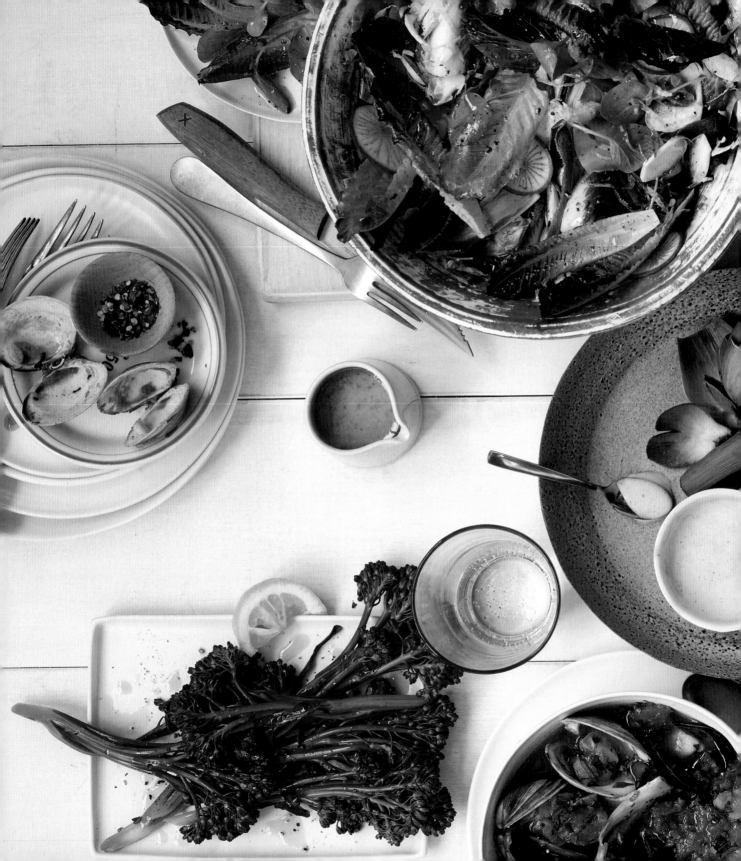

Freezer

- Start by tossing anything that's expired, freezer-burned, or impossible to identify (including that mysterious thing wrapped in foil that has been lurking in the darkest depths of your freezer for years).

- It's time to read the labels again. Depending on their sugar and Net Carb content, you might need to say so long to processed frozen food, such as waffles, breakfast pastries, pizza, pasta, chicken nuggets, ice cream, and more.

WHAT TO KEEP

- Keep frozen broccoli, cauliflower, bell pepper, and spinach. Watch out for frozen vegetables that are high in carbs, such as potatoes and corn.

SMART LOW-CARB CHOICES FOR YOU *AND* YOUR FAMILY

If you are doing Atkins 100 or you have other members in your family who would like to make more healthful choices, look for foods that contain less than 5 grams of sugar and less than 15 grams of Net Carbs per serving. If there is any added sugar, make sure it is one of the last three ingredients on the ingredients list.

- Frozen berries are naturally low in carbs. Check the labels on other frozen fruit.

- Protein such as frozen meats, shrimp, seafood, and more are all perfect to keep.

Pantry

TOSS THESE NOW

- Canned soups are typically high in carbs, but you can keep tomato soup or chicken and vegetable soups, broccoli or vegetable cream soups, as well as squash soups, which are typically lower in carbs. Canned fruit is usually packed with added sugar and syrups, but you can keep canned fruit packed in its own juices; just drain off the juice before eating.

- It's time to toss breakfast cereal and instant oatmeal, unless you use a high-fiber bran or flax cereal with 15 grams of Net Carbs or less. Toss all those sneaky snacks: crackers, chips, cookies, and more. Replace them with cheese chips or flax chips that contain less than 3 grams of Net Carbs or less per serving if you are on Atkins 20, 5 grams of Net Carbs or less if you are on Atkins 40, or snap pea chips that have 15 grams of Net Carbs or less if you are on Atkins 100. Next time you go to the store, seek out high-fiber seed crackers, which are typically low in Net Carbs.

- This is also a good excuse to go through your spice rack and toss anything that smells stale or that is years old.

- Since most of the food in your pantry is nonperishable, you can donate anything that is not opened to a local food bank. And if you have family members who will revolt in protest if you donate or toss those tempting treats, store them on a shelf that is easily accessible to them but not you.

WHAT TO KEEP

- You probably already have some great low-carb options in your pantry, including:

Canned seafood (tuna, salmon, crab)

Sardines

Anchovies

Canned tomatoes

Salsas

Pasta sauce or tomato sauce without added sugar or 5 grams of sugar or less per serving

Canned green chilies

Tomato paste

Canned pumpkin

Chicken stock or broth

Beef stock or broth

Vegetable stock or broth

Nuts

Roasted red peppers (rinse if there is sugar in the ingredients)

Sun-dried tomatoes in oil (a little adds lots of flavor)

Artichoke hearts

Jars of pesto or other vegetable-based sauces

Other canned low-carb vegetables and beans (read the labels)

Dill pickles

Italian pickled vegetables

Nut butters

Olives

Your "Get Started" Atkins Grocery List

Once you have cleaned out your fridge, freezer, and pantry, you should have a better idea of what low-carb foods you will need to buy to stock your kitchen. You can start with this general grocery list. In upcoming chapters, you will be able to add to and customize this list in much more detail based on how you decide to do Atkins

(in Chapter 4, I'll give you more meal plans and Acceptable Foods lists to help you) and which recipes you want to start cooking—there are so many to choose from, I guarantee you will be inspired!

Let's Talk About Carbs (Again)

Let's remember that Atkins is not about eliminating carbs. What you have learned so far is that certain carbs have a negative effect on your blood sugar and your health, but there are also foods that are crucial to your well-being that truly make this a lifestyle. Think of these foods as the foundation of your new way of eating. Initially there may be some carbs you will need to steer clear of and others you will eat in moderation, ensuring that those you do eat are high-fiber carbohydrates balanced by sufficient protein and healthy fats. In reality, this is the way everyone should be eating. Now let's start working on that low-carb grocery list.

PRODUCE

You can eat a huge assortment of veggies on Atkins, and this list is just the tip of the iceberg; it includes colorful vegetables and plenty of other salad essentials. You should consume a minimum of 12 to 15 grams of Net Carbs of vegetables a day, which is about 6 cups of raw vegetables and 2 cups of cooked veggies, but you can mix and match to suit your needs. The Net Carb counts of these vegetables range from 0 to a little over 5 grams of Net Carbs per serving, and I have organized this list in order from the smallest amount of Net Carbs to the largest.

HOW TO READ A FOOD LABEL[1]

Nutrition Facts

Serving Size 1 Bar (38g)
Servings per Container 5

Amount Per Serving

Calories 150   Calories from Fat 90

	% Daily Value
Total Fat 9g	14%
Saturated Fat 2.5g	13%
Cholesterol 0mg	0%
Sodium 170mg	7%
Total Carbohydrate 17g	6%
Dietary Fiber 10g	40%
Sugars 4g	
Protein 8g	
Vitamin A	0%
Vitamin C	0%
Calcium	6%
Iron	6%

* Percent Daily Values are based on a 2,000 calorie diet.

INGREDIENTS: ALMONDS, CHICORY ROOT FIBER, SOLUBLE CORN FIBER, SOY PROTEIN ISOLATE, SOYBEANS, PEANUTS, DRIED BLUEBERRIES, POLYDEXTROSE, SUNFLOWER OIL, PALM KERNEL OIL, WHEY PROTEIN CONCENTRATE, APPLE JUICE CONCENTRATE, CONTAINS LESS THAN 2% OF: NATURAL FLAVOR, RAISINS, DRIED APPLES, WHEY POWDER, RICE STARCH, SALT, SOY LECITHIN, OAT FIBER, CITRIC ACID, VANILLA POWDER, SUCRALOSE. 120202
CONTAINS ALMONDS, SOY, PEANUTS, MILK.
MADE IN A FACILITY THAT ALSO USES EGGS, OTHER TREE NUTS, WHEAT.

SERVING SIZE Watch out! The amount shown on the label, as well as calories per serving, refers to a single serving, and many packages contain more than one serving.

TOTAL FAT You can consume higher levels of saturated, polyunsaturated, and monounsaturated fat on Atkins because you are burning fat, instead of carbohydrates, for fuel. You should, however, avoid trans fats, because they have been shown to increase levels of "bad" LDL cholesterol while decreasing levels of "good" HDL cholesterol. If the ingredients list includes hydrogenated or partially hydrogenated oil, the product contains trans fats.

TOTAL CARBS Remember to subtract grams of fiber from total grams of carbs to get Net Carbs. You will see grams of sugar, but keep in mind that food labels do not distinguish between added sugar and naturally occurring sugar. You will have to dig deeper into the ingredients list to discover that.

DAILY VALUE The Daily Value (DV) is the recommended amount of each nutrient for average adults and is based on a 2,000-calorie diet. If the DV of a nutrient is 5 percent or less, the food is considered to be low in that nutrient; if it is 20 percent or higher, it is considered high.

INGREDIENTS This includes everything in the food product in order of highest content. This is where you'll find added sugars and trans fats, as well as naturally occurring sugars and whole or refined grains.

Sprouts

Chicory greens

Endive

Olives, green or black

Watercress

Arugula

Radishes

Spinach

Bok choy

Lettuce, all types

Turnip greens

Hearts of palm

Radicchio

Mushrooms

Artichoke

Celery

Pickle, dill

Broccoli rabe

Broccoli

Sauerkraut

Avocado

Daikon radish

Red/white onion

Zucchini

Cucumber

Cauliflower

Beet greens

Fennel

Okra

Rhubarb

Swiss chard

Asparagus

Broccolini

Bell peppers

Eggplant

Kale

Scallions

Turnips

Tomato

Jicama

Yellow squash

Cabbage

Green beans

Leeks

Shallots

Brussels sprouts

Spaghetti squash

Kohlrabi

Pumpkin

Garlic

Snow peas

MEAT

You can have any kind of meat on Atkins. Here are some options:

Beef

Ham

Lamb

Pork

Veal

Venison

Cornish hen

Chicken

Duck

Goose

Pheasant

Quail

Turkey

Ostrich

Avoid chicken nuggets, breaded cutlets, and anything that has been deep-fried, stuffed, breaded, battered, or coated in flour.

SEAFOOD

You can also have any kind of fish or shellfish on Atkins.

FISH	SHELLFISH
Flounder	Clams
Herring	Crabmeat
Salmon	Mussels*
Sardines	Oysters*
Sole	Shrimp
Tuna	Squid
Trout	Lobster
Cod	
Halibut	

Oysters and mussels are slightly higher in Net Carb counts. Avoid anything deep-fried, stuffed, breaded, battered, or coated with flour.

DAIRY PRODUCTS

You can stock your fridge with these essentials. Eggs are a versatile and tasty part of Atkins, and you'll find some "eggs-cellent" recipes in this book.

Large eggs

Heavy cream

Light cream

Half-and-half

Sour cream, full-fat

Mayonnaise

Unsweetened almond milk

Plain coconut milk

Unsweetened soy milk

You can use liquid cream or half-and-half in your coffee. Watch out for packaged creamers; many are full of sugar or high-fructose corn syrup.

CHEESE

Here are some cheeses to start with:

Parmesan

Romano

Goat

Blue cheese

Cheddar or Colby

Gouda

Mozzarella, whole milk

Swiss

Cream cheese, full-fat or plain

Feta

Havarti

Jarlsberg

String

Laughing Cow

FATS AND OILS

There are no carbs in these, just fat. A typical serving size is 1 tablespoon.

Butter

Mayonnaise (watch out for added sugar)

Coconut oil

Olive oil

VEGETABLE OILS (look for cold pressed or expeller pressed):

Canola

Walnut

Soybean

Grape seed

Sesame

Sunflower

Safflower

Use olive oil for sautéing only. Walnut or sesame oil should not be used for cooking but can be drizzled on cooked veggies or salad.

BEVERAGES

Always check the Nutrition Facts for high sugar content. You can pump up the flavor of water with a few squeezes of lemon or lime.

Clear broth/bouillon (or you can make your own nutrient-rich bone broth from our recipe on page 161)

Club soda

Decaffeinated or regular coffee and tea, sugar-free iced tea

Diet soda

No-calorie flavored seltzer

Herb tea without added sugar

Unflavored soy/almond milk

WATER, INCLUDING:

Filtered

Mineral

Spring

Tap

HERBS AND SPICES

All fresh herbs work great with Atkins, and there are minimal amounts of carbs in dried herbs. If you need to restock your spice rack, this list is a great place to start, but your options are endless. Just watch out for spice mixes that contain added sugar.

Basil

Cayenne pepper

Cilantro

Dill

Oregano

Tarragon

Parsley

Chives, fresh or dehydrated

Ginger, fresh

Rosemary, dried

Sage, ground

Black pepper

Salt

Garlic

SALAD DRESSINGS

Look for dressings with 3 grams of Net Carbs per serving or less. Even better? Make your own salad dressing—you can take your pick from the recipes in Chapter 9.

Red wine vinegar

Caesar

Ranch

Lemon and lime juice

Blue cheese

Balsamic vinegar

Italian/Creamy Italian

French

NONCALORIC SWEETENERS

You should count each packet as 1 gram of Net Carbs. Try not to consume more than three per day.

Sucralose (Splenda)

Stevia (Truvia)

Saccharin

Xylitol

SMART SHOPPING
STRATEGIES

THESE HELPFUL TIPS WILL HELP turn your grocery shopping excursion into a streamlined and effective experience.

Start with a plan. Review your schedule for the week; this will help you determine what meals and snacks you need to shop for. For example, if you know you have an evening full of pickups and drop-offs for kids' after-school activities, pick a recipe that uses a slow cooker so that you have an appetizing low-carb meal waiting when everyone gets home. If you have a busy day of meetings and you know you'll be eating lunch at your desk, make sure you cook an extra serving or two for dinner the night before, so you can take leftovers to work. If the weather looks nice, pick a meal that you can prepare on the grill.

Make a list. This helps you stay focused and avoid impulse buys. Shopping list apps make it a breeze to update your list whenever you need to. Some apps allow you to link your list with family members so everyone can update the list in "real time."

Pick a shopping day. I always like to do my grocery shopping for the week on Sunday. Pick a day when you won't be rushed trying to get everything you need and when you will have plenty of time to prep your food for the week.

Never shop when you're hungry. Make sure you're hydrated, and have a low-carb snack before you go, so you're not tempted by impulse buys simply because you are starving. (You'll find a list of quick and easy low-carb snacks in Chapter 5.)

Shop the perimeter of the store. This is where the foods that make up the "foundation" of Atkins are located: fruits, vegetables, dairy products, meat, and fish. I start in the produce section and fill my cart with a rainbow of colorful vegetables. From there I hit the deli counter for roasted meats and cheeses, then the meat and seafood counter, and finally the dairy section.

Steer clear of the center aisles. The center aisles usually feature the food you are trying to avoid—the processed stuff that is high in carbs and packed with hidden sugars. I usually need to hit the center aisles only for canned tuna and salmon, canned vegetables, broth and bouillon, spices, oils, and condiments.

PREPPING FOR THE WEEK

O NCE YOU GET HOME FROM the grocery store, you're not quite done! Spending a little time up front to prep your food for the week is another secret to success with Atkins. It makes it much easier to make healthful choices.

Slice and dice. Wash and cut up the veggies you bought, and store them in clear containers so you can grab a handful of veggies for a quick snack or throw together a salad in minutes. This is also the key to not letting those beautiful veggies go to waste.

Prep your leafy greens. Give them a spin in a salad spinner and store in a clear container or zip-top plastic bag with a paper towel to soak up any extra moisture.

Cut up your cauliflower and broccoli. Remove the outer leaves from a head of cauliflower or broccoli and cut into florets. Store the florets in a loosely sealed plastic bag so it's easy to grab a handful any time you want to roast or stir-fry them. If you want to make cauliflower or even broccoli "rice," pulverize the head of cauliflower or broccoli with a food processor and store in individual, sealed plastic bags or containers. You may also be able to find frozen or fresh cauliflower rice in your grocery store's frozen or produce section.

Shred or spiralize. If you bought zucchini or summer squash, you can spiralize or shred it in advance, drain the liquid, and store in an airtight container so you have fresh low-carb "noodles" that you can use in place of pasta or as a side dish. You can even add them to soups or an omelet. If you don't feel like making your own, you might be able to find packaged spiralized vegetables in your grocery store's produce section.

Check your eggs. This is a great opportunity to make one of the best (and portable) low-carb snacks ever, in my opinion: hard-cooked eggs. Hard cook and store a dozen in their original carton in the fridge, and you'll have everything you need for a quick egg salad, deviled eggs, or a grab-and-go protein-packed snack.

Prep your poultry. If you have the time, bake, sauté, or grill a batch or two of chicken thighs or breasts in advance, which can be a lifesaver for you during the week. Once your chicken is cooked, let it cool slightly and divide into 4- to 6-ounce portions and store in the fridge. Now it is ready for salads, wraps, soups, or the low-carb recipe of your choice. After three to four days, freeze any leftover chicken until you're ready to eat it. You can use the same cook-in-advance method for ground beef or turkey.

LOW-CARB KITCHEN GADGETS

*These handy tools will make prepping, cooking, and storing
your low-carb ingredients and meals a breeze.*

SPIRALIZER: This gadget cuts vegetables into long noodles or strips, resembling spaghetti. "Zoodles" (noodles made from zucchini) are your answer to pasta.

SLOW COOKER: If you want a delicious, hot, low-carb meal waiting for you after a busy day, you need a slow cooker. Prep the ingredients and throw them into your slow cooker in the morning, set the timer, and your meal is ready when you are. It's perfect for soups, stews, casseroles, curries, and roasts.

IMMERSION BLENDER: This handheld tool lets you blend ingredients or puree food right in the container you are preparing it in. You can puree soups or use it to make whipped cream, mayonnaise, vinaigrettes, or smoothies.

SALAD SPINNER: This is used to wash and remove excess water from your salad greens, because who needs a soggy salad?

MINI FOOD PROCESSOR: This gadget takes up hardly any room on a shelf or your counter and can dice, chop, and puree your ingredients in minutes.

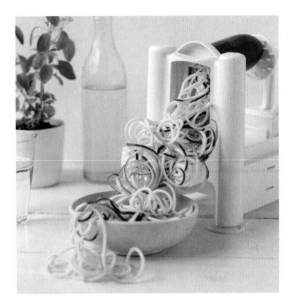

STORAGE CONTAINERS: You will need these to store and transport leftovers. You can also use them to store cut-up veggies in the fridge, perfect for low-carb snacking.

COOKBOOK HOLDER: You might want a nice stand to display this book in your kitchen so you can easily refer to the tasty low-carb recipe of your choice while you are cooking.

ESSENTIALS FOR A LOW-CARB, LOW-SUGAR LIFESTYLE

Discovering a better way of eating and moving more
may inspire you to incorporate some other healthful habits into
your life. These tools will help you do all of that.

ATKINS APP: Atkins provides this free tool, which has a host of helpful features, including:

- **Food search.** You can find nutritional info for grocery items, restaurant meals, and Atkins-friendly recipes and products.

- **Meal tracker.** You can track your daily grams of Net Carbs, and it also includes popular brands and restaurant dishes and a breakdown of fats, protein, and Foundation Vegetables.

- **Progress tracker.** This helps you stay on track with your goals.

- **Atkins overview and Acceptable Foods lists.** If you ever need a refresher on what Atkins is all about or need to review a food list on the fly, you'll find the information right in the Atkins app. Plus, you have access to Atkins' database of more than 1,000 low-carb recipes.

ATKINS CARB COUNTER: This guide gives you the Net Carb counts of practically every food. You can download it for free at Atkins.com.

FOOD JOURNAL: There are many food journal apps you can choose from; some even let you upload photos of your meals and snacks so you have a visual diary of what you eat each day.

ACTIVITY TRACKER: A variety of activity trackers allow you to track your daily steps, workouts, and even sleep. You can even sync your device with the Atkins app.

WATER BOTTLE: It's easy to mistake thirst for hunger, which is why it's important to stay hydrated. Plus, water helps flush toxins from your body and is important to your overall good health. You should drink at least eight (8-ounce) glasses of water daily to prevent dehydration. This is much easier if you have a water bottle by your side and refill it often.

EXERCISE
HAS ITS BENEFITS

A TKINS WILL HELP YOU IMPROVE your health and boost your energy, even without having to exercise. But there are many benefits to getting out there and moving more—that is, if you're interested in maintaining your weight, sleeping better, managing stress, improving your mood, boosting your energy, building muscle (especially because a pound of muscle burns more calories at rest than a pound of fat), and decreasing your risk of heart disease, diabetes, and metabolic syndrome. The American Heart Association recommends the following:[2]

FOR OVERALL CARDIOVASCULAR HEALTH:

- At least **30 minutes of moderate-intensity** aerobic activity at **least five days per week for a total of 150 minutes**

OR

- At least **25 minutes of vigorous** aerobic activity at least **three days per week for a total of 75 minutes;** or a combination of moderate- and vigorous-intensity aerobic activity

AND

- **Moderate- to high-intensity muscle-strengthening activity** at least **two days per week** for additional health benefits.

FOR LOWERING BLOOD PRESSURE AND CHOLESTEROL:

- An average of **40 minutes of moderate- to vigorous-intensity** aerobic activity **three or four times per week**

Exercise is anything that gets your body moving and your heart pumping, including walking, jogging, biking, exercise classes, stair climbing, and playing sports. Strength and stretching exercises are also good for building and strengthening muscles and increasing overall stamina.

The reason I call this a **"guidebook** for living a low-carb and low-sugar lifestyle" is that I'm here to **gently guide you** in the direction you want to go.

BECOME MINDFUL ABOUT HOW YOU EAT

Did you know that it takes about 20 minutes for your brain to register that you are full?

If you scarf down your meal too quickly or while you are distracted, whether it is because you are eating lunch in front of your computer again or you are busy updating your social media status, you may end up overeating. Some studies[3] are beginning to suggest that eating more slowly and thoughtfully may actually help you make healthier food choices. This is called mindful eating, when you bring your full attention to the ritual of eating and enjoying the flavors and the experience.

Listening to your body's physical cues will lead to recognizing your body's hunger signals, which should help you begin to understand when you are actually eating because you are hungry instead of for emotional reasons or out of boredom.

Fortunately, you have an advantage with Atkins, because the powerful combination of adequate amounts of protein, high-fiber carbohydrates, and healthy fats naturally helps you feel more satisfied and able to recognize and control your hunger signals. Slowing down and being mindful of how and what you eat with Atkins has its benefits, such as:

- Controlling your appetite
- Preserving muscle tissue
- Regulating your blood sugar
- Improving your cholesterol
- Decreasing your risk of heart disease
- Preventing diabetes
- Keeping your energy levels steady all day long

MOVING FORWARD

IF YOU HAVEN'T ALREADY, TAKE a little time to review the tips on how to set S.M.A.R.T. goals. This will help give you focus and direction. Feel free to share your goals with friends and family; maybe you can inspire them to join you on your journey toward a better way of eating, because research[4] has shown that you are more likely to be successful at making healthy changes to your lifestyle when you have support and motivation of friends and family. Once you have set your goals and you've started overhauling your fridge, freezer, and pantry, following my grocery shopping tips, and figuring out everything you need to do to prep and organize your food for the week, you will be on your way toward living a low-carb lifestyle on your terms.

The reason I call this a "guidebook for living a low-carb, low-sugar lifestyle" is that I'm here to gently guide you in the direction you want to go in, so you have all the facts you need to decide exactly how you would like to incorporate Atkins into your life. If you're ready for a little more structure, Atkins 20 or Atkins 40 may be the approach you choose. Or you can start with Atkins 100, which is a way to ease slowly into reducing your carbs with small, healthy changes. As you can see, there are plenty of options to choose from, so let's learn more about them.

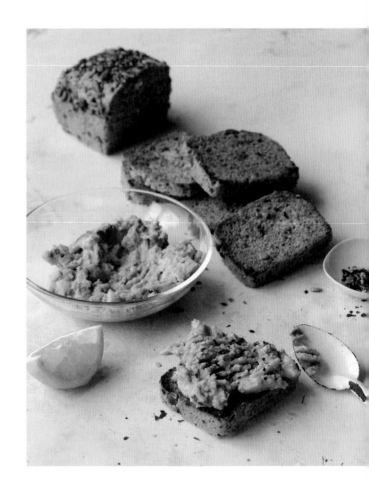

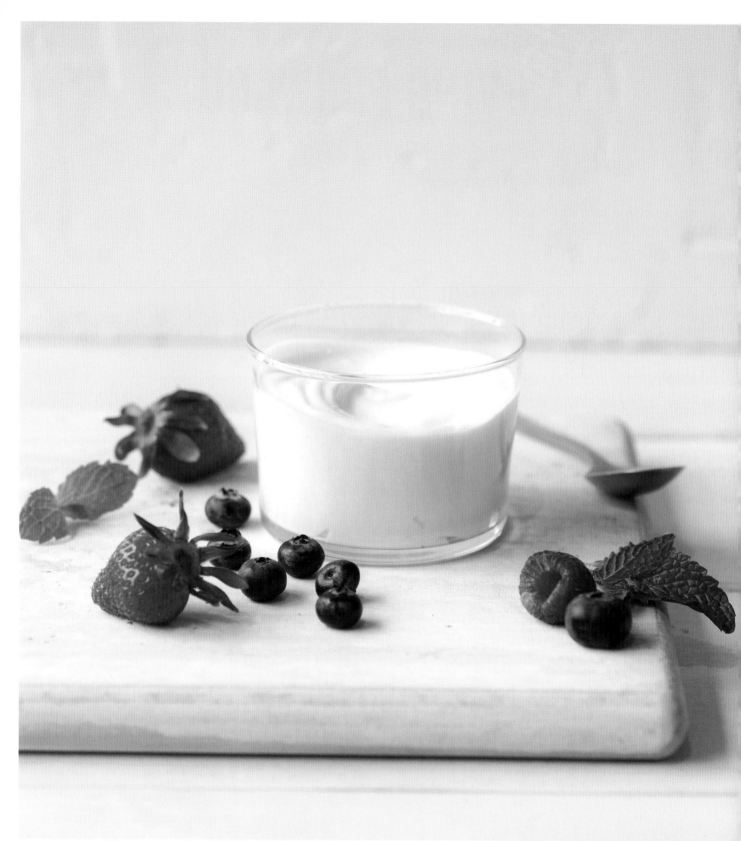

4

ATKINS
YOUR WAY:
ATKINS 20, ATKINS 40, or ATKINS 100

In this chapter, you'll learn all about Atkins 20,
Atkins 40, and Atkins 100.

It's important to learn about these options because
Atkins is a way of eating that can be customized to your needs, and
you can easily move between Atkins 20, Atkins 40, and
Atkins 100, depending on your goals, which may change over time.

OVER THE YEARS, I'VE LIVED every aspect of the Atkins lifestyle, from classic Atkins 20 to Atkins 100 and everything in between. This way of living has benefited me in many ways. First, I do not have any signs of heart disease or diabetes (I lost both parents and two siblings to complications of those diseases), I am at a healthy weight, I never became overweight as everyone else in my family did as they aged, and I have great energy.

Once you decide how you want to do Atkins, you will be able to fine-tune your grocery list and meal plans based on the Acceptable Foods lists for each option. No matter which way you go, there are plenty of delicious food choices so that you will never feel deprived, plus ways you can customize Atkins to your needs.

DAILY TARGETS BY PLAN

STARTING POINT	ATKINS 20®	ATKINS 40®	ATKINS 100®
NET CARBS (grams) = total carbs minus fiber	20	40	100
PROTEIN	3 servings of 4–6 oz per serving	3 servings of 4–6 oz per serving	3 servings of 4–6 oz per serving
HEALTHY FATS	3 servings of added healthy fats per day: butter, salad dressings, olive oil, etc.	3 servings of added healthy fats per day: butter, salad dressings, olive oil, etc.	3 servings of added healthy fats per day: butter, salad dressings, olive oil, etc.
CARBOHYDRATES	LIMITED: 12–15g Net Carbs from low-carb vegetables, AKA foundation vegetables (see p. 291 for list). Remaining carbs from whole milk dairy (hard cheeses, sour cream, cream) or low-carb products	ALL FOOD GROUPS: 12–15g Net Carbs from low-carb vegetables, AKA foundation vegetables (see p. 291 for list). Remaining carbs from fruit, nuts, legumes, dairy, and/or whole grains	ALL FOOD GROUPS: 12–15g Net Carbs from low-carb vegetables, AKA foundation vegetables (see p. 291 for list). Remaining carbs from fruit, nuts, legumes, dairy, and/or whole grains

	ATKINS 20®	ATKINS 40®	ATKINS 100®
ADDING CARBS BACK INTO YOUR DIET	Add in 5g Net Carb increments starting with lower carb foods and gradually progressing to higher-carb foods • Nuts and seeds (not chestnuts) • Berries, cherries, and melon (not watermelon) • Whole milk yogurt and fresh cheeses, such as cottage cheese and ricotta • Legumes, including chickpeas, and lentils • Tomato and vegetable juice "cocktail" (not fruit juices or dried fruits) • Higher-carb vegetables, such as winter squash, carrots, and peas	Add 10g Net Carbs when you're within 10 pounds of your goal weight by increasing your serving size or adding more variety If you're still losing, you can continue to add 10g Net Carbs each week until you find the level of carb intake where your goal weight is maintained	Continue to consume 100g Net Carbs daily to maintain weight. If you gain weight, lower carbs.

MAINTAINING YOUR RESULTS

	ATKINS 20®	ATKINS 40®	ATKINS 100®
VEGETABLES	12–15g Net Carbs from low-carb vegetables, AKA foundation vegetables (see list on p. 291)	12–15g Net Carbs from low-carb vegetables, AKA foundation vegetables (see list on p. 291) Remaining carbs from fruit, nuts, legumes, dairy, and/or whole grains	12–15g Net Carbs from low-carb vegetables, AKA foundation vegetables (see list on p. 291) Remaining carbs from fruit, nuts, legumes, dairy, and/or whole grains
PROTEIN	3 servings of 4–6 oz per serving	3 servings of 4–6 oz per serving	3 servings of 4–6 oz per serving
HEALTHY FATS	3 servings of added healthy fats per day: butter, salad dressings, olive oil, etc.	3 servings of added healthy fats per day: butter, salad dressings, olive oil, etc.	3 servings of added healthy fats per day: butter, salad dressings, olive oil, etc.
ADDING FOODS BACK INTO YOUR DIET	PROGRESSIVE: There are five important points to understand as you begin to reintroduce foods: • Count your carbs • Introduce new foods one at a time • Experiment with new foods so you don't get bored • Don't forget foundation vegetables • Write it down Continue to add carbs in 5g Net Carb increments until your weight stabilizes. Maintain carb intake to reach your goal.	ALL FOOD GROUPS: Continue to avoid/limit sugar, refined carbs, and any "trigger" foods that cause you to consume too many carbs Continue to add carbs in 10g Net Carb increments until your weight stabilizes. Maintain carb intake to maintain your weight.	ALL FOOD GROUPS: Continue to avoid/limit sugar, refined carbs, and any "trigger" foods that cause you to consume too many carbs.

HOW TO GET STARTED ON
ATKINS 20

ATKINS 20 IS BASED ON Atkins' classic nutritional approach, which has been popular and effective for forty years. Atkins 20 consists of four levels. You will start by consuming 20 grams of Net Carbs a day and gradually increase the amount as you reintroduce various foods. If you decide that Atkins 20 is the way to go, most likely you are ready to commit to giving the way you have been eating a total makeover. You are willing to embrace a clear-cut, step-by-step structured plan that leaves little room for guesswork and helps you kick carb and sugar cravings to the curb while eliminating blood sugar spikes and energy and mood swings and improving your overall health and wellness.

To start, you reduce your carb intake to 20 grams of Net Carbs a day, which, over the years, has been proven to be highly effective. In fact, for some people, going "cold turkey" with carbs that quickly convert to sugar and added sugar may be the only thing that works. I've seen this firsthand with many of the folks I've worked with and talked to over the years (reducing carbs has certainly helped me control my cravings and my killer sweet tooth), but science also shows this

Atkins 20 is a clear-cut, step-by-step structured plan that leaves **little room for guesswork** and helps you kick carb and sugar **cravings** to the curb.

to be true. Some studies suggest that reducing your consumption of these foods, and replacing them with protein, healthy fats, and fiber-rich carbohydrates low in sugar means you end up craving them less, if at all.[1] In fact, this way of eating has been shown to reduce your cravings in all food categories, including fatty, salty, high-carb, and fast food, not just sugar and sweets.

Ready to get started? It's quite simple, actually. Just stick with the list of Acceptable Foods for each level, and you can expect some big changes as you learn how to eat right, not less!

ATKINS 20®	LEVEL 1 >>>>	LEVEL 2 >>>>	LEVEL 3 >>>>	LEVEL 4 >>>>
	20–25g Daily Net Carbs	25–50g Daily Net Carbs	50–80g Daily Net Carbs	80–100g Daily Net Carbs

ACCEPTABLE FOODS:

	LEVEL 1	LEVEL 2	LEVEL 3	LEVEL 4
Foundation vegetables, proteins, healthy fats, and most cheeses	●	●	●	●
Nuts and seeds	●	●	●	●
Berries, cherries, or melon	●	●	●	●
Whole milk greek yogurt, ricotta, or cottage cheese	●	●	●	●
Legumes	●	●	●	●
Tomato juice	●	●	●	●
Additional fruits	●	●	●	●
Starchy vegetables	●	●	●	●
Whole grains	●	●	●	●

Your Personal Carb Balance

You will eventually discover the maximum daily grams of Net Carbs you can eat while continuing to improve your overall wellness, keep your appetite and cravings under control, and stay energized. This is called your Personal Carb Balance, and it is affected by your age, gender, activity level, hormonal status, and other factors.

See Appendix A for the Acceptable Foods list for Atkins 20, Level 1, page 289.

Atkins 20—Level 1

In Level 1, your goal is to shift your body from burning primarily carbs for fuel to burning primarily fat for fuel, and you will do so by reducing your daily grams of Net Carbs to 20.

You'll follow this level for a minimum of two weeks, but if you are motivated by fast results and appreciate the structure and food choices, you can follow it for much longer.

TIPS FOR LEVEL 1

- **Eat three meals and two snacks a day.** There is no reason you ever need to feel hungry on Atkins, especially when you eat a delicious and filling meal or snack every three to four hours (check out the snack recipes in Chapter 7). Pair your carb snacks with either fat or protein. The key is to never let yourself get to the point when you're starving; that's when it's much harder to resist your craving for salty or sweet foods.

- **Eat 20 grams of Net Carbs a day.** This includes 12 to 15 grams of Net Carbs that come from Foundation Vegetables. From the very beginning, you'll be filling your plate with more colorful nutrient- and fiber-rich vegetables than the average American eats, and you can pick other carb foods from the list of Level 1 Acceptable Foods (see Appendix A).

- **Make sure you get enough protein.** Protein is a natural metabolism booster. Shoot for three 4- to 6-ounce servings a day.

- **Don't fret about fat—too much.** Fat pumps up the flavor of your food. A serving size is 1 tablespoon, and you should eat two to four servings of added fat daily.

- **Drink at least eight 8-ounce glasses of water daily.** Water is great for your skin, digestion, and overall health.

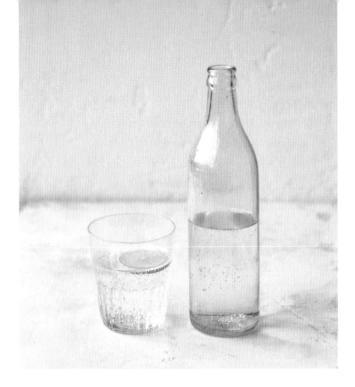

- **Watch out for hidden sugars.** Read food labels carefully, looking for grams of added sugar, particularly in foods such as marinara sauce, ketchup, marinades, and salad dressings. In restaurants, request oil and vinegar or a creamy dressing for salad, and request sauces on the side.

- **Use sugar substitutes—in moderation.** That means no more than three packets a day.

- **Stick with the list.** Follow the Level 1 Acceptable Foods list, and you're good to go! If you decide to stay at this level for longer than two weeks, you can also add nuts and seeds.

After two weeks, if you're ready to explore more food choices while continuing to eat right, not less, and progressing steadily toward accomplishing your goals, you can move to the next level.

YOU BOOZE, YOU LOSE?

Although I don't recommend drinking alcohol in Level 1 of Atkins 20, as long as you count the Net Carbs as part of your daily total, an occasional glass of wine is just fine once you transition to Level 2, as well as if you're doing Atkins 40 or Atkins 100. Although alcohol is not stored as fat, your body burns it as fuel first, which postpones any fat burning. Once your body processes the booze, you're back to burning fat for fuel. You can drink scotch, rye, vodka, and gin, but watch what you mix them with. Seltzer, diet tonic water, and diet soda mixers don't contain sugar, but juice, tonic water, and nondiet soda do. And a drink or two may lower your resistance to that pile of nachos or a slice of pizza. To counteract the cravings, pair your drink of choice with one of our low-carb savory bites or appetizers in Chapter 10.

Atkins 20, Level 2

In Level 2, you're continuing on the journey toward discovering your Personal Carb Balance. You'll start at 25 daily grams of Net Carbs and increase your overall carb intake in 5-gram increments. You might level off anywhere between 30 and 100 grams of Net Carbs a day.

TIPS FOR LEVEL 2

- **Keep eating those veggies.** Fill your plate with a minimum of 12 to 15 grams of Net Carbs a day of Foundation Vegetables. Sure, vegetables contain carbs, but they are the kind of carbs you should be eating.

- **Start adding carbs back one by one.** If a certain food triggers the cravings you're trying so hard to kick, hold off on that food and try another. For example, if you've decided to try almonds, or maybe chickpeas or strawberries, and suddenly your hunger is uncontrollable and you feel your blood sugar swings start to return, wait to reintroduce them. How the body reacts to certain carbs is different for everyone.

- **Watch your hunger.** Hopefully you're starting to learn how to recognize your hunger cues. When your stomach starts grumbling, have a low-carb snack or eat your next meal earlier than you otherwise might have.

- **Go slow with fruit.** Once you start eating fruit, such as berries, cherries, and melon, you may find that it spikes your blood sugar and/or causes cravings. A quick fix is to pair the fruit with fat or protein. For example, you can have berries with heavy cream, cottage cheese, or Greek yogurt or melon with prosciutto or provolone cheese.

When you're ready to start reintroducing even more foods, you can move to Level 3.

Atkins 20, Level 3

At this point, you are getting closer to meeting your goals and determining your Personal Carb Balance. This level sets the stage so that eating right, not less, can become a way of life for you.

You'll gradually increase your daily Net Carb intake in 10-gram (or 5-gram, if you prefer) increments, continuing to introduce new foods and gauging how they affect your progress toward your goal.

TIPS FOR LEVEL 3

- **Add foods one by one.** Keep an eye on your progress as you reintroduce foods; your age, sex, activity level, and metabolism may determine how they affect you.

- **Watch for your trigger foods.** As you continue to add foods back that you haven't eaten in a while, some foods (i.e., a banana, corn, or brown rice) may trigger cravings and uncontrollable hunger. If this is the case, cut them out for a couple of days and then try again.

- **Be patient with plateaus.** The journey toward accomplishing your goals is not always a linear one, and it's totally normal to experience stalls in your progress. If you feel you are on a plateau, reduce your daily Net Carb intake by 10 grams.

If you have accomplished your goals, are in control of your cravings and hunger, and are ready to learn how to maintain the results you have achieved, it's time to move on to Level 4!

SCIENCE SUPPORTS ATKINS

See **Appendix F** for the peer-reviewed independent published **studies that support** Atkins 20, 40, and 100 (page 305).

See Appendix B for the complete Acceptable Foods list for Atkins 20, Level 2 (page 295).

See Appendix C for the complete Acceptable Foods list for Atkins 20, Levels 3 and 4 (page 298).

YOUR CARB CRIB SHEET

At this point, you are adding more and more foods that are higher in carbs to your Atkins menu—more fruit, plus starchy vegetables and whole grains. Here are some tried-and-true tips I have found to be very helpful.

FRUIT

This sweet treat adds a burst of juicy flavor to your meals, but it may make your sweet tooth go out of control if you're not careful.

- **START WITH** lower-carb fruits, such as berries, cherries, and melon, and progress slowly by swapping one serving of berries or melons for a serving of higher-carb fruit. In other words, don't go bananas over bananas.
- **STICK WITH** two servings of fruit a day, including berries.
- **TREAT FRUITS** higher in carbs as a garnish; for example, add orange slices to your salad or sliced grapes to cottage cheese.
- **PORTION OUT** your fruit. Cut an apple or pear into slices and share them with a family member or save what you don't eat for later.

STARCHY VEGETABLES

Up until now, you've been enjoying a wide variety of Foundation Vegetables. Now you can start adding starchy vegetables, which are also rich in fiber and antioxidants but higher in carbs. Treat them as an accompaniment to your Foundation Vegetables.

- CRUNCH ON raw carrots (I love to snack on them with hummus), add grated carrots to tuna or chicken salad, or include them in a cabbage slaw.
- PINING FOR POTATOES? Steam and mash potatoes and cauliflower (a Foundation Vegetable) together.
- GET CREATIVE with side dishes by sautéing ¼ cup of peas with sliced scallions and thinly sliced spinach leaves or stir-frying asparagus, mushrooms, and peas together.
- ROAST ONE CUT-UP POTATO or sweet potato with an assortment of cut-up Foundation Vegetables, such as mushrooms, zucchini, and cauliflower.

WHOLE GRAINS

Last but not least come whole grains. Not everyone can tolerate grains and products made from them, and you've also learned about the hidden sugars that convert to sugar in your blood, so it's best to proceed slowly as you learn how your body reacts to them.

- DON'T CONFUSE whole grains with refined grains, such as white flour and white rice. You'll still want to limit baked goods, including bread, pita, tortillas, crackers, and cereals made with refined grains, but you can find low-carb versions of these products in Appendix E.
- START SMALL. Eat small portions of whole grains, or use them as a garnish. Once again, on Atkins 20, whole grains shouldn't be the star player in your meals but part of the supporting cast.
- SPRINKLE some cooked wild rice or quinoa on top of a tossed salad as you would sliced almonds.
- TOSS some cooked brown rice or whole wheat couscous with sliced mushrooms, red bell peppers, zucchini, and cooked chicken, beef, or pork. This is a nice alternative to a traditional stir fry.

*See Appendix C
for the complete
Acceptable Foods list
for Atkins 20, Level 4
(page 298).*

Atkins 20, Level 4

When you reach this level, you have succeeded in making significant changes to your eating habits. You should be feeling good, both physically and emotionally. Embracing this better way of eating—a nutritional approach that truly works—will allow you to achieve results that are sustainable for life. You've learned how your body reacts to certain carbs—which foods you can continue to enjoy, which you should eat in moderation, and which you might choose to eat only occasionally. You've also discovered (or rediscovered) how to listen to your body and recognize cravings before they hit, as well as how to satisfy your hunger before it gets out of control. You're in this for the long haul, and now you know exactly how to do it.

TIPS FOR LEVEL 4

Don't forget the basics:

- **Continue to consume** 12 to 15 grams of Net Carbs a day of Foundation Vegetables.

- **Remember to drink** plenty of water (eight 8-ounce glasses a day).

- **Stick with** two servings of fruit a day.

- **Consume** two to four servings of added fat a day.

- **Eat 4 to 6 ounces** of protein at each meal.

- **Start or keep moving.** Regular physical activity provides a host of health benefits. Why wouldn't you want to take advantage of the boost in energy you may be experiencing?

- **Adjust your carb intake as needed.** You might need to tweak your daily carb intake if you increase or decrease your activity level.

- **Watch your portions.** You can ensure you don't overdo it on nuts or cheese by preportioning servings of these foods in advance.

You Can Always Go Back—to Level 1

Once you have successfully progressed though all four levels of Atkins 20, you can enjoy the results you have achieved and the healthy habits that have become a part of your life. But sometimes life gets in the way. Maybe you've had a stressful week at work, or, even better, you're on vacation. During times like these, it's easy to believe that you'll be just fine having a cookie or doughnut or a fruity tropical drink. Then you get overly confident and think, "Well, if I can handle one cookie, another one or two will be just fine." Sometimes that may be the case and you're able to bounce right back into your low-carb lifestyle without any undue effects. On the other hand, those foods have the potential to bring back all the cravings you've been trying to conquer. Watch out for carb creep! If you see your hard-earned results start to go south, there is a simple solution: return to Level 1 for a week or two to jump-start your progress and stabilize your blood sugar levels.

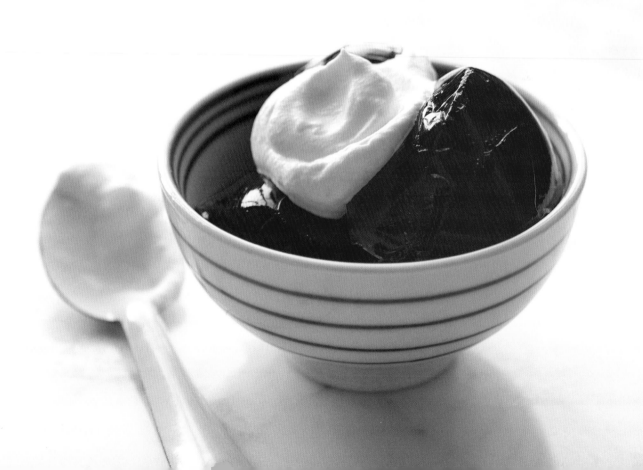

ATKINS 20 is easy to do, especially if you start out by following this meal plan (and the Acceptable Foods list), which features two weeks' worth of low-carb meals and snacks you can prepare in minutes, as well as tasty recipes from this book. Feel free to substitute the recipes in this meal plan for others in this book.

ATKINS 20 MEAL PLAN — WEEK 1

	MONDAY	TUESDAY	WEDNESDAY
BREAKFAST	Egg-filled Avocado with Prosciutto	Creamy Avocado Smoothie	Cauliflower Rice Scrambles
SNACK	Tuna-stuffed Deviled Eggs	Asparagus with Burrata Cheese and Kale Pesto	2 stalks celery, 2 tbsps Ranch Dressing
LUNCH	Ropa Vieja Soup	Baby Kale and Blue Cheese Salad with Warm Hazelnut Dressing	Old Bay Shrimp Salad
SNACK	Low-Carb Flax Meal Bread, 1 oz cheddar cheese	Tuna-stuffed Deviled Eggs	Avocado Toast
DINNER	Chimichurri Steak Bites, Watercress Bacon Salad with Ranch Dressing	6 oz salmon, Steamed Artichoke with Homemade Lemon Mayonnaise	Fried Sage Chicken and Zucchini
TOTAL NET CARBS	21g	20g	20.5g
TOTAL FV	15g	14.9g	11.9g

THURSDAY	FRIDAY	SATURDAY	SUNDAY
Power Mug Muffin with Cinnamon Butter	Salmon Eggs Benedict	Avocado Toast	Birdies in a Basket
Basic Bone Broth, 2 stalks celery	Asparagus with Burrata Cheese and Kale Pesto	Prosciutto-wrapped Shrimp with Kale Mayonnaise	½ Hass avocado, 2 tbsps mayonnaise, Cilantro Parmesan Crackers
Mixed Power Greens with Prosciutto-wrapped Chicken Tenders	Smoky Habanero Chili, ½ Hass avocado	Mixed Asian Greens with Shredded Sesame Chicken	Crispy Duck Spinach Salad with Warm and Tangy Turmeric Dressing
Bourbon Pecan Pâté, Cilantro Parmesan Crackers	Hot Crab Dip, 2 stalks celery	Tuna-stuffed Deviled Eggs	2 Salted Caramel Cheesecake Bites
Italian Stuffed Cabbage, For dessert: Double Chocolate Brownies	Lemon Pepper Shrimp with Snow Peas	6 oz bone-in pork chop, Cheesy Scallion Cheddar Cauliflower Mash	Roasted Fennel and Cod with Moroccan Olives
20.9g	19.3g	20g	20.4g
12.1g	12.9g	12.5g	12.5g

ATKINS 20 MEAL PLAN
WEEK 2

	MONDAY	TUESDAY	WEDNESDAY
BREAKFAST	Cauliflower Rice Scrambles	Avocado Toast	Egg-filled Avocado with Prosciutto
SNACK	Manchego Mini Muffins	Asparagus with Burrata Cheese and Kale Pesto	Tuna-stuffed Deviled Eggs
LUNCH	Roasted Fennel and Cod with Morrocan Olives	Bone Broth Minestrone	6 oz chicken breast, Cauliflower Bisque
SNACK	½ Hass avocado, 2 tbsps mayonnaise, Cilantro Parmesan Crackers	1 oz Monterey Jack cheese, 5 black olives	Chipotle Lime Zucchini Crisps
DINNER	Mixed Asian Greens with Shredded Sesame Chicken	Italian Stuffed Cabbage	Smoky Habanero Chili, ½ Hass avocado
TOTAL NET CARBS	20.7g	20.8g	21.7g
TOTAL FV	13.3g	15.8g	14.8g

THURSDAY	FRIDAY	SATURDAY	SUNDAY
Creamy Avocado Smoothie	Power Mug Muffin with Cinnamon Butter	Birdies in a Basket	Salmon Eggs Benedict
1 oz Monterey Jack cheese, 5 black olives	Prosciutto-wrapped Shrimp with Kale Mayonnaise	Tuna-stuffed Deviled Eggs	2 stalks celery, 2 tbsps Ranch Dressing
6 oz white fish, Watercress Bacon Salad with Ranch Dressing	Wilted Brussels Sprout Salad with Warm Pancetta Dressing	Chilled Avocado Crab Gazpacho, Avocado Toast	Lemon Pepper Shrimp with Snow Peas
Asparagus with Burrata Cheese and Kale Pesto	Tuna-stuffed Deviled Eggs	1 oz Monterey Jack cheese, 5 black olives	Artichoke Dip–stuffed Mushrooms
Salsa Verde Chicken Soup, For dessert: Chocolate Chip Cookies	Chimichurri Steak Bites, Sautéed Spinach with Caramelized Shallots	Mixed Power Greens with Prosciutto-wrapped Chicken Tenders	Fried Sage Chicken and Zucchini, For dessert: Salted Caramel Cheesecake Bites
20.7g	20.2g	21.6g	20.8g
14g	13.5g	15.1g	13.5g

HOW TO GET STARTED ON
ATKINS 40

ATKINS 40 IS A RELATIVE newcomer to the Atkins family. It has less structure than Atkins 20 but a few more guidelines than Atkins 100, and it is quite popular and effective. If you would like to reduce your carb intake while eating a greater variety of food, this is the way to go, especially if you're motivated and ready to see how making these changes to your eating habits can have a positive impact on your overall wellness and energy levels.

As you may have guessed, on Atkins 40, you eat 40 grams of Net Carbs a day. Here's what else you need to know about this simple and effective way of eating:

- As with Atkins 20, 12 to 15 grams of Net Carbs a day come from that extensive list of tasty Foundation Vegetables.

- You can take your pick from the Acceptable Foods list in Appendix D to bring your total grams of Net Carbs up to 40.

- Eat three 4- to 6-ounce servings of protein a day.

- Consume two to four servings of added fat a day.

TIPS FOR ATKINS 40

- **Enjoy a variety of foods while continuing to limit some.** I need to emphasize that although you do get to eat a wide variety of foods on Atkins 40, there are still some that I suggest you limit or avoid, and I'm sure you can guess which they are:

  - Avoid or limit foods containing added sugars.

  - Avoid or limit refined carbs, such as white rice and anything containing white flour.

  - Avoid foods that might trigger cravings.

  - Avoid foods containing hidden sugars; I'll teach you how to watch your portions of these.

DID YOU KNOW

CRUNCHING THE CARB NUMBERS

To **make the math easy,** the foods on the Acceptable Foods list (Appendix D, page 300) are rounded up in **5- to 10-gram increments.**

ATKINS 40®

Each day, you'll enjoy a wide variety of delicious and filling foods. Allocate 40g Net Carbs throughout the day as follows:

3 Meals Per Day

10g 10g 10g

2 Snacks Per Day

5g 5g

Occasionally you can bump up a meal to 15g of Net Carbs.

FOUNDATION VEGETABLES
6 to 8 servings

15g
Net Carbs

PROTEIN
3 servings (4 – 6 oz. per serving)

0g
Net Carbs

ADDED FATS
3 servings (1 TBSP each)

0g
Net Carbs

OTHER CARBOHYDRATES
3 – 5 servings (5 net carbs per serving)

25g
Net Carbs

When you're 10 lbs from your goal weight add 10g of Net Carbs/week from this list

When your goal weight is achieved, you can expand your list of acceptable carbs. Refer to our Acceptable Foods list (page 300) to make sure you stay on track.

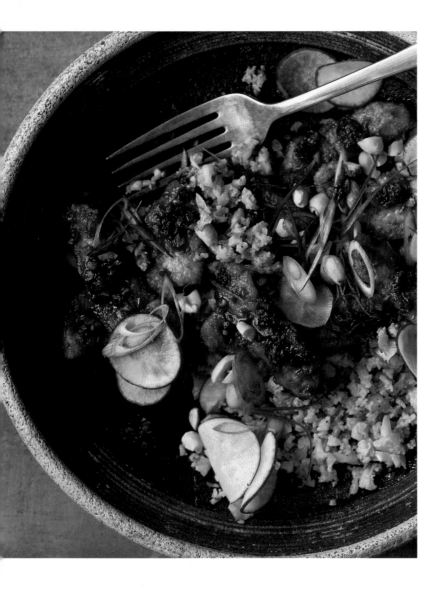

- **Speaking of portions . . .** You'll notice that some of the recommended portions of foods are smaller than others. That is because these foods are higher in carbohydrates and lower in fiber, increasing the potential Hidden Sugar Effect in your body. By eating smaller portions of these foods, you can make the most of the nutritional impact of the 40 grams of Net Carbs you consume each day.

- **Don't sweat a slip-up.** Even with the added flexibility that Atkins 40 gives you, it's still possible you may slip up now and again, which is perfectly natural. Don't beat yourself up, but don't use it as an excuse to forgo this nutritional approach entirely. Make sure your next meal is a low-carb one, and put a little extra effort into planning some other meals and snacks, enjoying being able to choose from a delicious and satisfying variety of Acceptable Foods.

See Appendix D for the complete Acceptable Foods list for Atkins 40 (page 300).

FINE-TUNING
ATKINS 40

*If you feel you are not making as much progress
on Atkins 40 as you would like, remember that this is a more
gradual way to reduce your carb intake while still
eating a wide variety of food.*

Ask yourself some questions: Are you feeling better? Do you have more energy? Have you noticed that you're no longer craving foods you used to? Are your clothes fitting better?

Keep up the good work! If you still think you need to make a few tweaks to speed up your progress, here are some tips that might help:

- Decrease the daily amount of Net Carbs you consume by 5 or 10 grams.
- Increase the amount of fat you eat, and decrease the amount of protein if you are consuming more than 4 to 6 ounces of protein per serving.

If you would like to **reduce your carb intake** while eating a greater **variety** of food, **Atkins 40** is the way to go.

- Find and eliminate hidden sugars in the form of processed foods that may contain sugar.
- Increase your activity level.
- Drink at least eight 8-ounce glasses of water daily.
- Look at which higher-carb foods you've consumed recently, and try eliminating or limiting them for a week.

ATKINS 40 is practically foolproof if you start out by following this meal plan, which features two weeks' worth of low-carb meals and snacks. As always, you can swap out the recipes in this meal plan for others in this book.

ATKINS 40 MEAL PLAN WEEK 1		MONDAY	TUESDAY	WEDNESDAY
	BREAKFAST	Antioxidant Berry Smoothie	Birdies in a Basket	Coconut Muesli Clusters, Greek yogurt
	SNACK	1 stalk celery, 2 tbsps cream cheese	1 wedge honeydew, 2 oz prosciutto	1 stalk celery, 1 tbsp Ranch Dressing
	LUNCH	Thai Tom Yum Soup, Crispy Brussels Sprouts with Sriracha Mayo Dipping Sauce	Green Goddess Salad with Lemon Tahini Dressing	Thai Peanut Buddha Bowl
	SNACK	Bruschetta Duet	Fried Green Tomatoes with Ranch Dipping Sauce	Chipotle Lime Zucchini Crisps
	DINNER	Bolognese Skillet Lasagna	Spicy Korean Soup with Scallions, For dessert: Lime Coconut Rum Cupcakes	Broiler Miso Salmon, Turnip Fries
	TOTAL NET CARBS	39.6g	40.5g	40.9g
	TOTAL FV	15.8g	18.8g	20.1g

THURSDAY	FRIDAY	SATURDAY	SUNDAY
Broiler Huevos Rancheros, 1 wedge honeydew	Avocado Kale Berry Smoothie Bowl	Sunny-side Up Eggs with Cauliflower Hash Browns	Lemony Protein Pancakes, 5 large strawberries
½ cup sliced cucumbers, 1 oz Monterey Jack cheese	Basic Bone Broth, Cilantro Parmesan Crackers, 1 oz Monterey Jack cheese	Antioxidant Berry Smoothie	Chocolate Egg Cream, 12 walnut halves
6 oz turkey cutlets, Pear and Manchego Mesclun Salad with Caramelized Onions	Jalapeño Cheddar Broccoli Soup, Low-carb Flax Meal Bread	Kale Caesar Salad with Creamy Meyer Lemon Dressing	Cauliflower Mac & Cheese
Power Mug Muffin with Cinnamon Butter	1 carrot, 4 tbsps hummus	Avocado Toast	Artichoke Dip–stuffed Mushrooms
Mongolian Beef Wraps, Shishito Peppers with Hot Paprika Mayonnaise	Kung Pao Chicken with Cauliflower Rice	Superfast Stroganoff, For dessert: 2 Chocolate Chip Cookies	Shellfish Cioppino
40.1g	39.5g	39.9g	40.4g
15.9g	17.3g	18.5g	16.6g

	MONDAY	TUESDAY	WEDNESDAY
BREAKFAST	Power Mug Muffin with Cinnamon Butter	Cauliflower Rice Scrambles, 1 wedge honeydew	Carrot Spice Smoothie Bowl
SNACK	Antioxidant Berry Smoothie	Low-carb Flax Meal Bread, 1 tbsp almond butter, ⅓ cup sliced strawberries	½ cup sliced cucumbers, 1 oz Monterey Jack cheese
LUNCH	Salsa Verde Chicken Soup	Mixed Asian Greens with Shredded Sesame Chicken	Mongolian Beef Wraps
SNACK	1 carrot, 4 tbsps hummus	Artichoke Dip–stuffed Mushrooms	Avocado Toast
DINNER	Beef Bourguignon, 2 cups baby spinach, 5 large radishes, 2 tbsps blue cheese dressing	Roasted Fennel and Cod with Morrocan Olives	Chicken and Dumplings, Cheesy Scallion Cheddar Cauliflower Mash, For dessert: Double Chocolate Brownies
TOTAL NET CARBS	38.4g	38.8g	40g
TOTAL FV	16.5g	15.7g	14g

ATKINS 40 MEAL PLAN WEEK 2

THURSDAY	FRIDAY	SATURDAY	SUNDAY
Sunny-side Up Eggs with Cauliflower Hash Browns	Coconut Muesli Clusters, 4 oz Greek yogurt	Chai Cinnamon Waffles	Sweet or Savory Crepes (with raspberries)
4 oz Greek yogurt, 5 large strawberries	1 carrot, 4 tbsps hummus	1 wedge honeydew, 2 oz prosciutto	1 oz soft goat cheese, Cilantro Parmesan Crackers
Turmeric Carrot Ginger Soup, Low-carb Flax Meal Bread	Mushroom Spinach Egg Skillet	Lemon Pepper Shrimp with Snow Peas	Green Bean Chicken Skillet, 2 cups mixed greens, ¼ cup grated carrot, 2 tbsps Ranch Dressing
Baked Sriracha Hot Wings and Kale Chips	Chipotle Lime Zucchini Crisps	2 stalks celery, 1 tbsp Ranch Dressing	Portobello Pizza
Garlic Rosemary Pork Loin with Creamed Spinach, For dessert: Salted Caramel Cheesecake Bites	Smoky Habanero Chili, Brushetta Duet (tomato-mozzarella)	Fried Sage Chicken and Zucchini, Fried Green Tomatoes with Ranch Dipping Sauce	Parmesan Scallops, 1 cup mixed greens, 2 tbsps Mustard Vinaigrette
39.4g	38.7g	39.7g	40.7g
19g	16.5g	12.1g	21.9g

HOW TO GET STARTED ON
ATKINS 100

EVEN IF YOU HAVE THROWN in the towel on traditional "diets," with Atkins 100, it's all about small changes leading to big results. You have the opportunity to pay attention to what kinds of foods you are eating and how they affect you both physically and emotionally, because this is not a diet, it is simply a better, smarter way of eating and living.

With Atkins 100, you'll consume 100 grams of Net Carbs a day. It's that simple! Here's what else you'll do:

- You'll eat a minimum of 12 to 15 grams of Net Carbs a day of Foundation Vegetables.

- You'll eat three 4- to 6-ounce servings of protein a day.

- You'll eat two to four servings of added fat a day.

- You'll budget the remaining 85 grams of Net Carbs from the complete Acceptable Foods list on page 300 in Appendix D.

With **Atkins 100,** it's all about small changes leading to **big results.**

ATKINS 100 ACCEPTABLE FOODS LIST

Keep in mind that on Atkins 100, the Acceptable Foods list is simply a guideline to start you on your journey toward making smart, healthy choices since no food is really off limits. As a guideline, you can use the Acceptable Foods list on page 300.

ATKINS 100®

Each day, you'll enjoy a wide variety of delicious and filling foods. Allocate 100 net carbs throughout the day as follows:

3 Meals Per Day

25g 25g 25g

2 Snacks Per Day

 10 to 15g 10 to 15g

FOUNDATION VEGETABLES
6 to 8 servings

12-15g Net Carbs

PROTEIN
3 servings (4 – 6 oz. per serving)

0g Net Carbs

ADDED FATS
2-4 servings (1 TBSP each)

0g Net Carbs

OTHER CARBOHYDRATES
3 – 5 servings (5 net carbs per serving)

      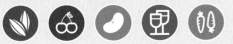

85g Net Carbs

When you're 10 lbs from your goal weight add 10g of Net Carbs/week from this list

When your goal weight is achieved, you can expand your list of acceptable carbs. Refer to our Acceptable Foods list (page 300) to make sure you stay on track.

Just as with Atkins 20 and Atkins 40, I'm giving you a two-week meal plan and Acceptable Foods list with low-carb meals and snacks, plus recipes from this book that you can mix and match.

	MONDAY	TUESDAY	WEDNESDAY
BREAKFAST	Coconut Muesli Clusters, 1 cup whole milk, ½ small banana	Sunny-side Up Eggs with Cauliflower Hash Browns, 1 wedge honeydew	Carrot Spice Smoothie Bowl, 2 mini oat bran muffins
SNACK	Cilantro Parmesan Crackers, 1 tbsp cream cheese	2 carrots, 4 tbsps black bean dip	1 large tomato, ½ cup cottage cheese
LUNCH	Turmeric Carrot Ginger Soup, 2 cups mixed greens, 1 large tomato, ¼ cup chickpeas, 2 tbsps Mustard Vinaigrette	Kale Caesar Salad with Creamy Meyer Lemon Dressing, 1 large slice whole wheat baguette	Smoky Habanero Chili, ½ Hass avocado, ½ cup black beans, ¼ cup crushed tortilla chips, 2 cups mixed greens, 2 tbsps Mustard Vinaigrette
SNACK	½ cup pineapple chunks, ½ cup cottage cheese	Chocolate Egg Cream, 1 oz cashews	1 small apple, 1 oz cheddar cheese
DINNER	5 oz steak, Turnip Fries, ¼ acorn squash, ⅓ cup wild rice	Fried Sage Chicken and Zucchini, Crispy Brussels Sprouts with Sriracha Mayo Dipping Sauce, ½ small baked potato	Roasted Fennel and Cod with Moroccan Olives
TOTAL NET CARBS	98.6g	101.2g	96.5g
TOTAL FV	23.9g	28.8g	19.5g

THURSDAY	FRIDAY	SATURDAY	SUNDAY
Broiler Huevos Rancheros, one 6-inch whole wheat tortilla	½ cup oatmeal, 1 cup whole milk, 1 wedge cantaloupe	Chai Cinnamon Waffles, 1 small banana, 10 pecan halves	Salmon Eggs Benedict, 1 whole wheat English muffin
½ cup sliced cucumbers, 1 oz Monterey Jack cheese	Sweet or Savory Crepes (with raspberries)	½ cup sliced cucumbers, 2 tbsps creamy Italian dressing	½ cup cherries, 4 oz Greek yogurt
Bone Broth Minestrone, 1 oz whole wheat pasta	Chimichurri Steak Bites, 2 cups baby spinach, ½ cup black beans, ½ cup sliced cucumbers, ¼ cup grated carrot, 2 tbsps Mustard Vinaigrette	Hot-and-Sour Soup, ½ cup cooked rice noodles	Green Goddess Salad with Lemon Tahini Dressing, 1 large slice whole wheat baguette
1 small banana, 1 oz almonds	2 oz string cheese, 4 whole wheat crackers	1 large tomato, ½ cup cottage cheese	Brie-stuffed Grilled Jalapeños
Chicken and Dumplings, ⅓ cup corn kernels, 2 cups baby spinach, 2 tbsps Mustard Vinaigrette	Garlic Rosemary Pork Loin with Creamed Spinach, ½ cup Brussels sprouts, ½ cup brown rice	Shellfish Cioppino, ½ medium sweet potato, For dessert: Apple Crumble	Green Bean Chicken Skillet, ½ cup brown rice, ¼ cup corn kernels
101.2g	99.9g	101.3g	100.1g
20.6g	12.7g	21.3g	13.1g

	MONDAY	TUESDAY	WEDNESDAY
BREAKFAST	Power Mug Muffin with Cinnamon Butter, 1 small banana	Birdies in a Basket, ½ red grapefruit	Coconut Muesli Clusters, 1 cup whole milk, ½ cup sliced mango
SNACK	1 large tomato, ½ cup cottage cheese	1 whole wheat English muffin, 2 tbsps cashew butter	½ cup sliced cucumbers, 2 tbsps creamy Italian dressing
LUNCH	6 oz chicken breast, Watercress Bacon Salad with Ranch Dressing, 1 large slice whole wheat baguette	Bolognese Skillet Lasagna, 2 cups mixed greens, ½ cup cooked sliced beets, ¼ cup quinoa, 2 tbsps Mustard Vinaigrette	4 oz salmon, Pear and Manchego Mesclun Salad with Caramelized Onions, 2 mini oat bran muffins
SNACK	2 carrots, 4 tbsps black bean dip	4 oz vegetable juice cocktail, ¼ cup edamame	½ cup red grapes, 12 whole almonds
DINNER	Spicy Korean Soup with Scallions, ½ cup cooked rice noodles	Clam Linguine, 1 large slice whole wheat baguette, 2 cups arugula, 2 tbsps French dressing	Chicken Parmesan Meatballs, 1 cup spaghetti squash, 2 cups mixed greens, 1 large tomato, ¼ cup chickpeas, 2 tbsps Mustard Vinaigrette
TOTAL NET CARBS	99.4g	100.3g	98.3g
TOTAL FV	20.9g	26.7g	22.1g

ATKINS 100 MEAL PLAN WEEK 2

THURSDAY	FRIDAY	SATURDAY	SUNDAY
Egg-filled Avocado with Prosciutto, 1 wedge honeydew, 1 whole wheat English muffin	Avocado Kale Berry Smoothie Bowl, 2 mini oat bran muffins	Cauliflower Rice Scrambles, 1 whole wheat tortilla, 2 tbsps salsa	Lemony Protein Pancakes, ½ cup blueberries
Portobello Pizza	2 carrots, 2 tbsps black bean dip	2 carrots, 2 tbsps hummus	5 whole wheat crackers, 2 oz goat cheese
Thai Tom Yum Soup, ½ cup brown rice	Superfast Stroganoff, 1 oz whole wheat pasta, ½ cup Brussels sprouts	Crispy Duck Spinach Salad with Warm and Tangy Turmeric Dressing, ¼ acorn squash, ⅓ cup lentils	Cauliflower Mac & Cheese, 2 cups mixed greens, 1 large tomato, ¼ cup chickpeas, 2 tbsps French dressing
½ cup pineapple chunks, ½ cup cottage cheese	1 small banana, 24 whole almonds	4 whole wheat crackers, 2 oz string cheese	4 oz Greek yogurt, ½ cup cherries
Roast Beef with Greek Yogurt Horseradish Sauce, ½ small baked potato, 2 cups mixed greens, 2 tbsps Mustard Vinaigrette	Mixed Power Greens with Prosciutto-wrapped Chicken Tenders, For dessert: Apple Crumble	Turmeric Orange Scallops, Turnip Fries, ¼ cup quinoa	Beef Bourguignon, 1 oz whole wheat pasta, 1 cup broccoli
99.2g	100g	98.7g	99.8g
12g	20.1g	19.8g	18.1g

HOW DO YOU
WANT TO DO ATKINS?

———•———

IN MY MANY YEARS OF clinical practice as a nutritionist and certainly in my role at Atkins, I've found that most people naturally fall into one of two categories foodwise: those who've discovered which foods they prefer and eat them regularly and those who thrive on variety and are always looking for ways to shake things up. Identifying which of the two groups you fall into can go a long way to making your experience on Atkins a positive one—complete with lasting results. So let's see which one you are.

ARE YOU A CREATURE OF HABIT?

Do you have your tried-and-true meals and snacks that you rotate through on a weekly basis? Maybe you're perfectly happy with scrambled eggs every morning, and you have some easy meals that you can mix and match for lunch and dinner. You're most likely a big fan of leftovers as a way to save money and time; what was delicious at dinner will certainly be lovely at lunch. You have your routine down, and trying out new recipes or foods may seem like a stretch to you.

If this sounds like you to a "T," you'll probably be more comfortable following a structured version of Atkins, such as Atkins 20, so that your choices are carefully laid out for you right from the beginning, with a specific direction for how you can progress. You'll be in control of what you're eating; you'll know what you can eat, how much of it, and how your body responds to it. All you have to do is stick with the Acceptable Foods list and meal plan, and you're good to go.

ARE YOU A VARIETY SEEKER?

Do you get bored eating the same foods day in and day out? Are you always trying to come up with new ideas for lunch and dinner? Do you like to try new recipes and sample new ingredients? Do you get caught up in reading about food, recipes, and cooking techniques, and do you turn to Instagram and Pinterest for a daily dose of food inspiration or envy? A day at a farmer's market seems like a vacation, and a new kitchen gadget may bring you just as much excitement as a new pair of shoes. Cooking is probably a creative hobby for you instead of just a duty. Meanwhile, your family has become accustomed to the new tastes and combinations you present to them.

If this sounds like you, variety is the spice of your life, and Atkins 100 may be the way to go.

ARE YOU SOMEWHERE IN THE MIDDLE?

When time is tight, you have your go-to breakfasts, lunches, and dinners down to a science, but when given the chance, you love to mix them up with new recipes and different flavors. Or you stick with a tight routine during the week, but on weekends you love to roll your sleeves up and get going in the kitchen.

If this sounds like you, Atkins 40 may be a great starting point.

HOW ABOUT ME?

I'm right in the middle. My weeks are pretty busy with travel and work, so I typically have an Atkins shake or smoothie not long after getting up and a second minibreakfast, usually yogurt, slivered almonds, and berries, after I get to the office. Once I'm at work, I find I am so busy I just don't want to have to deal with making a decision about what to have for lunch. My go-to choices are a big green salad with leftovers, or tofu, tuna, chicken, or another protein source. For dinner, my husband and I usually have a huge salad and top it with chicken, burgers, salmon, or sometimes a steak. We usually make enough for more than one meal, so we often have the same meal twice in a week. But on weekends, I do like to try something new; we might explore the menu options at a new restaurant or enjoy leg of lamb, one of our favorites. We always have at least one vegetable with the meal and a side salad. If I have time on a Sunday, I like to try out the occasional new recipe—I've really been enjoying testing the ones from this book! And I'll always make extra, so we have leftovers to eat on Monday. After more than two decades following the Atkins lifestyle, this way of eating has become as natural as breathing. I barely have to think about it—other than to get myself to the supermarket!

IT'S YOUR CHOICE!

With Atkins 20, 40, and 100, you have learned how satisfying a low-carb lifestyle can be. Just by learning a few simple "hacks" to guide your eating choices, you can avoid the sugars and hidden sugars that so many of us are unaware we are eating and that lead to blood sugar spikes and an energy-level roller coaster. You can learn to recognize your hunger cues, eat when you're actually hungry, and stop when you're full, because the foods you eat on Atkins and the recipes in this book are naturally filling and guaranteed to please your palate. Now comes the fun part as you discover how living a low-carb lifestyle is possible in every situation, whether you're eating out in a restaurant, hitting the fast-food drive-through, celebrating holidays, or going on vacation.

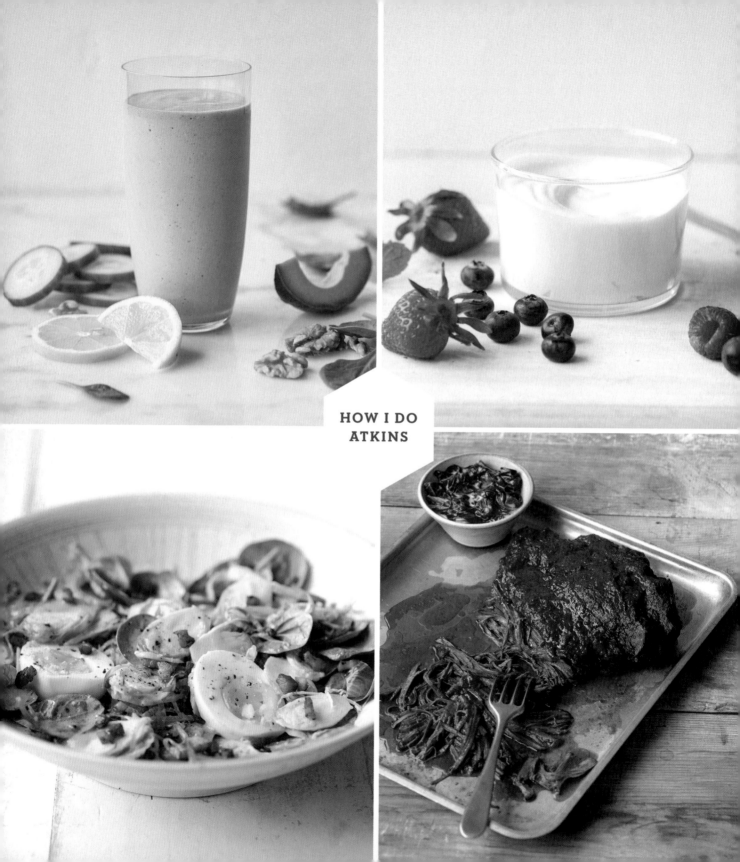

HOW I DO
ATKINS

MOVING BETWEEN ATKINS 20, ATKINS 40, AND ATKINS 100

The wonderful thing about eating right, not less,
is that depending on your goals and what's going on in your life,
you can move between the various levels of Atkins with ease.
Here are some scenarios to consider:

- If you're going on vacation and you're doing Atkins 20, you can move up to Atkins 40 so you can enjoy a wider variety of food while traveling. And if you're doing Atkins 40, you might consider moving up to Atkins 100.

- If the food choices on Atkins 40 are causing "carb creep," you might need the structure of Atkins 20 to help keep you honest and focused on your goals.

- Stressed out? Move up a level so you're still motivated to make healthy changes but have a few more options to choose from when time is tight and life is hectic.

- Are you still experiencing intense cravings and energy slumps, and do you feel that you really need to take control of the way you are eating? Buckle down and give Atkins 20 a try.

- Did you overdo it on vacation, and you're having a hard time getting back on track? Move down a level for the time being.

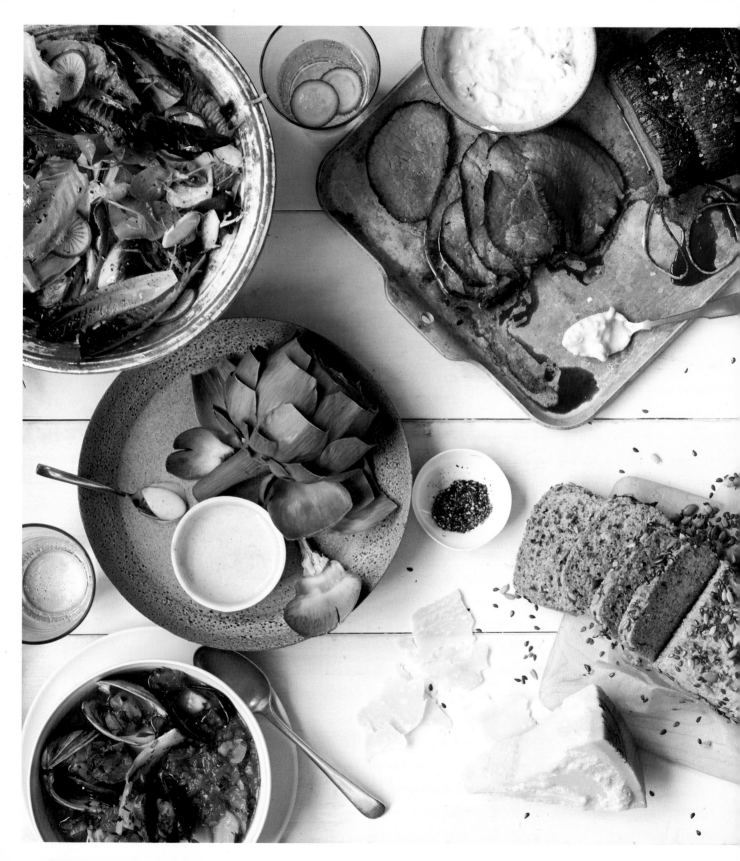

5

LIVING A
LOW-CARB AND LOW-SUGAR
LIFESTYLE

SMALL CHANGES = BIG RESULTS

Now that you know how your
LOW-CARB LIFESTYLE WORKS,

you can see how easy it is to incorporate small,
healthy changes into your life.

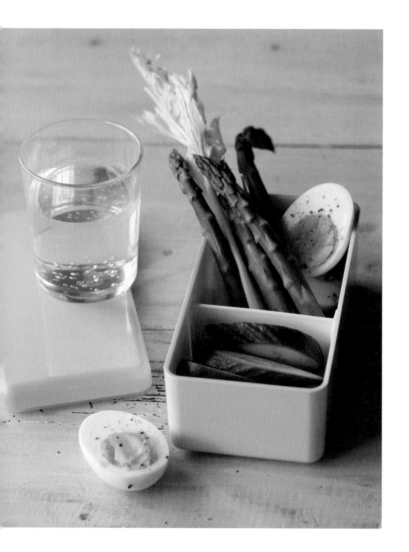

Instead of focusing on all the food you
think you can't eat, it's time to start
thinking about all the food you *can* eat
with Atkins, and how eating right, not
less, can change your life.

NOW YOU HAVE EVERYTHING YOU need
to start doing Atkins: a sparkling clean
kitchen stocked with naturally low-
carb foods, including colorful vegetables, dairy
products, fish, poultry, beef, and some pantry
essentials. Coming up, I'm going to show you
my smart carb swaps, easy low-carb snacks, my
favorite Atkins "hacks," and some valuable advice
for eating out in restaurants, traveling for work or
while on vacation, plus strategies for enjoying (not
just surviving) the holiday season so that you can
make this way of eating a lifestyle.

EAT YOUR VEGGIES!

INCORPORATING VEGETABLES INTO THE MAJORITY of your meals or snacks may seem like a challenge, but there are endless options for every part of the day. Soon you'll wonder why you haven't been eating this way all along! Here are some suggestions.

BREAKFAST

- Add spinach, scallions, and a little tomato to your eggs and top with slices of avocado.

- Make a low-carb breakfast wrap using turkey sausage, scrambled eggs, spinach, and avocado and wrap it all up in a romaine lettuce leaf or a low-carb tortilla.

- Whip up a breakfast hash by sautéing ground beef, ground turkey, or ground pork with scallions, red bell peppers, and cheese. You can top it with a fried or scrambled egg.

- Sautée ¼ cup chopped broccoli and ¼ cup chopped onion in 1 tablespoon real butter. Add two beaten eggs to the pan and stir over medium-high heat until the eggs are set. If you like, sprinkle 2 tablespoons shredded cheddar cheese over the eggs in the last 30 seconds of cooking.

- Add ¾ cup chopped tomato and ¾ cup chopped spinach or ¼ cup chopped onion and ½ cup chopped mushrooms to 2 scrambled eggs.

- For a breakfast on the run, grab a couple of hard-boiled eggs, a slice of cheese, and one of the following raw veggies to crunch in the car: 1¾ cups chopped cucumber, 1 cup string beans (green beans), 1½ cups chopped cauliflower, or 1 cup chopped green pepper.

LUNCH

- Combine deli meat, cheese, and mayo and roll up with a pickle or cucumber.

- Pile spinach, tomatoes, and mushrooms on a plate, drizzle with balsamic vinegar and olive oil, and top with sliced grilled chicken breast. Or start with 2½ cups shredded romaine lettuce and add any of the following: 2 cups chopped cucumber, ¾ cup chopped jicama, 2½ cups sliced mushrooms, 1 cup chopped green pepper, ¾ cup chopped red peppers, 2 cups sliced radishes, 1 cup chopped broccoli, 1½ cups chopped cauliflower, ¾ cup chopped tomatoes, 1½ cups sliced yellow squash. (If you want more than one added veggie in your salad, use half the measurement of one veggie, combined with half the measurement of another, such as ½ cup green pepper and 1 cup chopped cucumber.) Plus, you can add 4 to 6 ounces of sugar-free salad dressing.

- Try raw or cooked veggies, cooked in butter, topped with your favorite protein.
- Top a tomato with cooked ground beef seasoned with chili and cumin and Mexican-blend shredded cheese. Broil until the cheese is bubbling.

DINNER

- Experiment with your spinach salad; add various vegetables or dressings and top with grilled salmon, shrimp, or sliced steak.
- Stuff half of a bell pepper with turkey or pork sausage, cook at 350° degrees F for 45 minutes and top with grated cheese, no-sugar salsa, avocado, or even a fried or poached egg.
- Grill a steak, and serve with a side salad and mashed cauliflower or cauliflower rice.
- Whip up a stir-fry by sautéing your choice of meat or poultry, and adding sliced red bell pepper, broccoli florets, and mushrooms.
- Add butter or mayonnaise to hot cooked veggies for an instant flavor boost.

THE CURE FOR YOUR CARB CRAVINGS

Eating certain carbs may trigger cravings, hunger, and blood sugar swings, which all have the potential to derail your progress, but it's natural to yearn for those foods at times. Whether you have a sweet tooth or you're all about the salty crunch, the recipes in this book are the cure. Here are a few you can choose from when the cravings hit:

FOR SWEET-TOOTH CRAVINGS

- Lemony Protein Pancakes (page 135)
- Double Chocolate Brownies (page 282)
- Coconut Muesli Clusters (page 136)

FOR SWEET AND CREAMY CRAVINGS

- Almond Butter Smoothie Bowl (page 228)
- Salted Caramel Cheesecake Bites (page 281)
- Creamy Avocado Smoothie (page 130)

FOR SALTY CRUNCH CRAVINGS

- Crispy Brussels Sprouts with Sriracha Mayo Dipping Sauce (page 141)
- Baked Sriracha Hot Wings and Kale Chips (page 147)
- Turnip Fries (page 222)
- Chipotle Lime Zucchini Crisps (page 205)

FOR COMFORT FOOD CRAVINGS

- Cheesy Scallion Cheddar Cauliflower Mash (page 151)
- Cauliflower Mac & Cheese (page 267)
- Bolognese Skillet Lasagna (page 258)
- Cream of Heirloom Tomato Soup (page 175)

IT'S SNACK TIME

S NACKING IS AN IMPORTANT PART of Atkins. When you nosh on two tasty snacks a day between your three meals, you are able to keep your hunger in check and your blood sugar levels right where they should be. I've put together a variety of easy options that you can mix and match, depending on whether you're hungry for something salty or sweet or somewhere in between. You can check out some additional snack recipes in Chapter 7.

SNACKS WITH NO MORE THAN 3 GRAMS OF NET CARBS

- An ounce of string cheese
- Celery stuffed with cream cheese
- Cucumber "boats" filled with tuna salad
- Five green or black olives, perhaps stuffed with cheese
- Half a Hass avocado
- Beef or turkey jerky (cured without sugar)
- A deviled egg or hard-boiled egg
- A lettuce leaf wrapped around grated cheddar cheese
- Sliced ham rolled around a few raw or cooked green beans
- Two slices of tomato topped with chopped fresh basil and grated mozzarella and broiled for one minute
- Two cups of sugar-free gelatin topped with a dollop of whipped cream

SNACKS WITH NO MORE THAN 5 GRAMS OF NET CARBS

- A half cup of unsweetened whole milk yogurt mixed with 2 tablespoons no-added-sugar grated coconut and 1 packet sweetener
- Celery sticks stuffed with peanut butter or another nut or seed butter
- Cucumber "boats" filled with ricotta and sprinkled with seasoned salt
- Two chunks of melon wrapped in slices of ham or smoked salmon
- A "kebab" of two strawberries, two squares of Swiss cheese, and two cubes of jicama
- **Nutty Cheese Dip:** Blend 2 tablespoons cream cheese, 1 tablespoon grated sharp cheddar, a few drops of hot pepper sauce, a pinch of paprika, and 1 tablespoon chopped pecans. Serve with red pepper strips.

Low-Carb Product Buyers' Guide

For a list of recommended products for your low-carb lifestyle, see Appendix E (page 304). Follow these tips to make sure you're making smart choices when you're buying low-carb products:

• Look for 5 grams or less of total sugar

• Look for less than 15 grams of Net Carbs per serving

• Watch out for added sugars

• **Blue Cheese Dip:** Blend 2 tablespoons blue cheese into 3 tablespoons unsweetened plain whole milk yogurt. Serve with zucchini spears or another vegetable.

• Try a scoop of cottage cheese topped with 2 tablespoons no-sugar-added salsa.

• Mix 4 ounces tomato juice and 1 tablespoon sour cream in a bowl, and you've got a refreshing cold creamed soup. Top with chunks of avocado, if desired.

• Mash ¼ cup blueberries with 2 tablespoons mascarpone cheese and top with flaxseed meal.

• You can also enjoy a ¼ cup of blueberries while munching on a piece of string cheese.

SNACKS WITH NO MORE THAN 10 GRAMS OF NET CARBS

• Fruit other than berries, cherries, and melon, as long as they're eaten with some cheese, cream, plain whole milk or Greek yogurt, nuts, or protein

• A half cup red or purple grapes with a couple slices of turkey

• An apple with some almonds

• Hummus with vegetables or low-carb crispbreads

• Baba ghanoush (eggplant dip) with vegetables

• Homemade popcorn topped with butter, olive oil, or grated cheese

• Carrot sticks with aioli or ranch dip

• Soy chips

• Single-size container plain, unsweetened Greek yogurt mixed with half a scoop of low-sugar vanilla protein powder and topped with sliced strawberries

WHAT YOU NEED TO KNOW ABOUT COOKING WITH FATS

*Healthy fats add flavor to the foods
you eat and make your meals satisfying and delicious.
Here's what you need to know.*

Canola Oil

This heart-healthy oil, made from the seeds of the canola plant, is rich in omega-3 fatty acids, which lower blood pressure and heart rate.[1]

Use it for sautéing, baking, and marinating.

Olive Oil

Olive oil is a staple in many households and for cooking international cuisines. Opt for extra-virgin olive oil, which is made from the first pressing of olives and is high in heart-healthy antioxidants called polyphenols.

Use it for sautéing vegetables, or combine with balsamic vinegar for an easy salad dressing.

Peanut Oil

Made from unshelled peanuts, peanut oil contains heart-healthy phytosterols, plant fats associated with lower cholesterol levels and cancer prevention.

Good for deep-frying (due to its high smoke point), as well as for roasting and sautéing.

Grape Seed Oil

Grape seed oil, extracted from the seeds of grapes, is high in polyunsaturated fats and vitamin E.

Thanks to its high smoke point, you can use it for sautéing, stir-frying, or roasting.

Coconut Oil

Coconut oil is rich in a type of saturated fat that may help boost your level of "good" (HDL) cholesterol,[2] plus it is an excellent natural moisturizer for your skin and hair!

Use unrefined coconut oil for its subtle coconut flavor and in place of butter for baking. Use refined coconut oil for its neutral flavor in cooking or baking.

Nonhydrogenated Palm Shortening

Palm shortening comes from the tropical palm tree.

Use it for cooking or as a nondairy substitute for butter. Swap palm shortening for Crisco (or any other hydrogenated or partially hydrogenated fat) in moderation.

MY ATKINS "HACKS"

A hack is a trick or shortcut that makes your life easier. Since I have been living a low-carb lifestyle for going on twenty years and I'm constantly talking to folks who are doing the same, I've learned a number of hacks that help make Atkins pretty simple.

I DON'T ALWAYS DRINK PLAIN WATER. I carry a water bottle everywhere, and I like to boost the flavor with slices of cucumber, limes, or lemons. When I need a boost of carbonation, zero-calorie and zero-sugar sparkling spring water flavored with the essence of lime, berries, and other fruit flavors is a refreshing change.

I FOCUS ON FRESH FLAVORS. I love to add fresh herbs to my recipes. I'll make pesto out of basil and add cilantro or chives to egg dishes or any main dish. Dill goes great on fish (or as part of a lemon aioli you can dip steamed artichoke leaves in), and rosemary boosts the flavor of chicken, fish, lamb, and soups. I also enjoy frequenting farmer's markets during the warmer months and picking up an assortment of vegetables that are in season to add to my meals and snacks for the week.

I AM ALL ABOUT CONVENIENCE. When I don't have the time to spend a leisurely morning at the farmer's market or a relaxing evening at home preparing one of the recipes in this book, I have no problem hitting the deli and salad bar at the grocery store to fill up on sliced roasted meats, salad greens, marinated olives, and fresh mozzarella, plus fresh veggies to garnish my salad and complete my meal. I'll also grab prewashed salad greens and packages of riced cauliflower and spiralized zucchini in the produce section, a rotisserie chicken from the deli, and premade steak or chicken kebabs so that I can throw together delicious low-carb meals in minutes.

I EAT BREAKFAST FOR DINNER. Or dinner for breakfast. After a hectic day, sometimes a plate of scrambled eggs or an omelet filled with whatever veggies I have on hand is an easy and protein-packed evening meal. And if my meal of chicken, salmon, or steak is delicious tonight, the leftovers are sure to satisfy me tomorrow morning.

I'M NOT AFRAID TO GO "OFF THE MENU."
If I'm eating out, I have no problem politely
asking the server for my sauce or dressing
on the side, swapping a higher-carb side
for steamed vegetables with butter, or even
doubling up on two vegetable side dishes.

I EAT CARBS . . . in smaller portions. Though
I've shown you that even foods such as whole
wheat bagels and brown rice contain hidden
sugars—carbs that convert to sugar in your
blood—sometimes I just want a bagel. Instead
of chowing down on a full bagel (and watching
my energy levels and cravings go awry), I'll
toast ¼ of a whole wheat bagel, slather it with
some nut butter, and be perfectly satisfied.

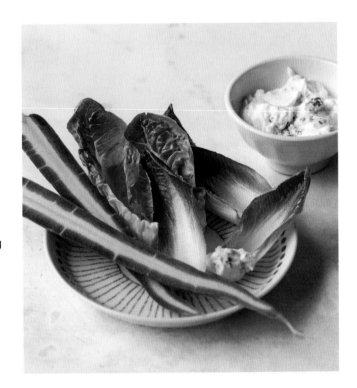

ATKINS, FAMILY-STYLE

———————— • ————————

JUST BECAUSE YOU HAVE DECIDED to explore a low-carb lifestyle does not mean you're relegated to eating bland, tasteless meals while the rest of your family feasts. Nothing could be further from the truth, plus the healthy choices you are making will have a positive impact on everyone around you. Here are some family-friendly options that will turn rushed family dinners into experiences you can all enjoy:

- **Burger bar:** Grill or cook a variety of burgers (beef, buffalo, turkey, chicken breast, or others; the choice is yours!), and lay out all the burger fixings so everyone can build his or her own burger. Skip the bun, and wrap your own burger in romaine lettuce leaves. Get creative with the fixings. In addition to tomato, lettuce, and onion, you can include sautéed onions and mushrooms, bacon, avocado slices, jalapeños for some spice, and even a fried egg.

- **Salad bar:** Start with shredded rotisserie chicken or sliced steak. Put out a variety of salad greens (romaine, spinach, and/or kale), and go crazy with the toppings. You can include sliced tomatoes and avocado, black or garbanzo beans, sliced mushrooms, broccoli florets, marinated artichoke hearts and sundried tomatoes, olives and shredded cheeses.

- **Taco bar:** Begin with shredded rotisserie chicken, ground beef, or both. Let everyone fill his or her tortilla with a choice of taco toppings: beans, lettuce, tomatoes, avocados, fajita veggies, onions, jalapeños, cheese, salsa, and sour cream. You can make your own taco with a low-carb tortilla or make a taco bowl instead, with lettuce as the foundation.

- **Chili bar:** This can be a cozy make-ahead meal when your family's evening schedule is a bit hectic. Start some chili in your slow cooker in the morning so it's ready to serve for dinner. Lay out shredded cheese, olives, jalapeños, and sour cream so all can garnish their chili as they please.

- **Make-your-own pizza:** Grab some ready-to-cook pizza crusts (look for a low-carb version, or try a cauliflower or portobello mushroom pizza "crust"), and let everyone pile on their choice of low-sugar (or homemade) tomato sauce, pepperoni, cooked and crumbled Italian sausage, ham, olives, sliced mushrooms, artichoke hearts, onions, bell pepper, sundried tomatoes, and shredded cheeses. Bake and enjoy!

LOW-CARB SWAPS FOR HIGH-CARB FAVORITES

You can have your (low-carb) cake and eat it, too,
not to mention pizza and pasta. Keep reading for delicious
low-carb swaps for some of your favorite foods.

Pizza

Did you think cheesy pizza was a thing of your high-carb past? You can still enjoy delicious low-carb pizza on Atkins, with the Portobello Pizza recipe (page 206).

French Fries

Crispy French fries fresh out of the fryer are hard to resist, but you can swap them out for baked alternatives that are lower in carbs, such as Turnip Fries (page 222) or sweet potato fries (stick with ¼ or ½ of a medium sweet potato).

Potato Chips

Skip the greasy fried potato chips. You can satisfy your salty and crunchy cravings with Chipotle Lime Zucchini Crisps (page 205).

Pasta and Noodles

Whether you're craving spaghetti and meatballs, lasagna, or a steaming bowl of ramen noodles, you can substitute zucchini "zoodles" for pasta and noodles to get your fix. Try our Thai Peanut Buddha Bowl recipe (page 230) and Bolognese Skillet Lasagna (page 258).

Brownies and Cookies

Good news! Swap out your traditional sugar- and flour-laden brownies and cookies for Double Chocolate Brownies (page 282) and Chocolate Chip Cookies (page 285). They feature the same rich chocolate taste, without the sugar.

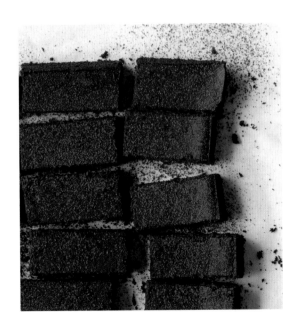

EATING OUT
WITH ATKINS

NO MATTER HOW YOU DECIDE to do Atkins, eating out can be a delicious and guilt-free experience, if you arm yourself with my tips. Our options have expanded over the years because of an added emphasis on where our food comes from and how it's prepared. Whether you're vegetarian, gluten-free, reducing carbs, or all of these, you'll find that many restaurants now cater to your way of eating.

Don't skip meals or arrive at a restaurant/ grocery store/holiday party starving. This is my mantra before you do almost any activity that involves food. Try having a boiled egg, a few slices of cheese, or a serving of almonds before you head out so that when you are faced with a basket of bread or a list of tempting happy hour appetizers, your appetite will remain in check.

Stay hydrated. Drink at least two glasses of water with your meal to help fill up.

Break out of your food rut. Whereas some people thrive on structure, others love the variety of being able to make different choices every day. If you prefer a clear-cut plan of action, review the menu online before you hit the restaurant and pick out one or two main dishes that fall into line with how you are doing Atkins. If you like to spice things up and need variety to help you stay on track, use this opportunity to be adventurous and pick a dish you've never had.

Skip the sides. Ask to have your dishes without the extras—rice, beans, potatoes, pasta—or ask for two sides of vegetables. Most restaurants will accommodate your request for a portion of vegetables or a side salad in lieu of such high-carb starches, and many restaurants now offer more nutrient-packed whole grains.

Go easy on the sauce. Ask for sauces on the side so you can decide whether and how much to consume. Instead of dousing your dish in sauce, dip a bite or two to get a hit of flavor.

Soup's on. I love soup, and it is a wonderful way to keep your appetite in check before your main course. Miso soup, many cream soups, vegetable purees, and clear broth with meat or vegetables are satisfying and delicious ways to jump-start your meal.

Splurge on steak. Do you want to treat yourself while still making healthy choices? You can't go wrong with a steak house—it is a decadent mecca of naturally low-carb choices. Shrimp cocktail? Check! Tender, juicy steak sizzling in butter? Check! Surf and turf? Check! Skip the mashed potatoes, and go for asparagus drizzled with hollandaise sauce, sautéed mushrooms, or creamed spinach.

Don't save room for dessert. Go ahead and fill up on everything else so that you are pleasantly satisfied, but not stuffed, by the end of the meal. If your dinner companions insist on dessert, just savor a small bite of theirs, or stick with fresh fruit or a cheese plate.

Don't beat yourself up. If you stray off course before your main course even arrives, remember that one bite or one meal is no reason to give up on your goal of eating right, not less.

YOUR FAST FOOD CHEAT SHEET

Although hitting the drive-through is not always optimal because it usually means you're in a rush (or you forgot your lunch), you can still make healthy choices if you stick with these tips.

- **AT THE BURGER JOINT:** Order your burger without the bun and a side salad instead of fries. Most fast-food burger places also offer chicken sandwiches. Once again, skip the bun, and go for grilled chicken instead of chicken that is battered or deep-fried. You'll usually find a few main dish salad selections that you can top with grilled (not fried) chicken. Watch out for the salad dressings, which may contain added sugar or corn syrup. Your best bet is usually vinaigrette, ranch, or blue cheese.

- **AT THE TACO PLACE:** You can usually find a taco salad or bowl on the menu. Try not to eat the deep-fried tortilla bowl that your salad comes in.

- **AT THE FRIED CHICKEN ESTABLISHMENT:** Typically, you can select grilled, roasted, or broiled chicken instead of fried chicken. Pass up the mashed potatoes dripping in gravy and the cheesy mac and cheese, and select sides such as steamed vegetables, creamed spinach, green beans (go with a ½-cup serving) or whole kernel corn (have a ¼- to ½-cup serving).

AROUND THE WORLD
WITH ATKINS

G**ET READY TO ENJOY A** world of international flavors, because no cuisine is off limits with Atkins. In this book I've even included suggestions for Atkins-friendly versions of traditional recipes from a few of these cuisines.

Italian

Italian food is not just about pizza and pasta; it varies by region, and you have your choice of seafood, shellfish, poultry, pork, and veal, tomatoes, garlic, olive oil, dark leafy greens, and whole grains, plus rich and creamy sauces. Herbs such as basil, flat-leaf parsley, rosemary, and oregano add flavor, and other important components of Italian cooking include salt, freshly cracked pepper, vinegar, anchovies, capers, olives, and sundried tomatoes. Here are some smart choices:

- Start with an antipasto platter (assorted meats, cheeses, olives, and marinated vegetables), caponata (an eggplant and caper salad), or a salad with shaved Parmesan cheese.

- Limit any seafood that's battered and fried (calamari, stuffed clams); order a seafood salad instead.

- You can have your fill of mixed grilled vegetables and grilled portobello mushrooms.

- Don't forget the soup course. Escarole soup features escarole, a lettucelike green, and meatballs or chicken. Stracciatella is an Italian version of egg drop soup made with eggs and spinach. While traditional minestrone is higher in carbs (it often contains pasta and beans), you can turn to page 164 to cook up our Atkins-friendly version, Bone Broth Minestrone.

DO YOUR RESEARCH

You can find the **menus for most restaurants** (including fast food and fast casual) online, with most listing a full **nutritional breakdown** so you can make **healthy choices** in advance.

- Focus on grilled dishes, and order veal or chicken piccata or scaloppini (made with lemon and capers) instead of veal, chicken, or eggplant Parmesan. Skip the pasta side dish, and ask if they can do broccoli or asparagus instead.

- You can satisfy your cravings for chicken Parmesan by making our Chicken Parmesan Meatballs on page 247.

Greek

Think of what's typically in a Greek salad: feta cheese, kalamata olives, tomatoes, cucumbers, and romaine, dressed with olive oil, oregano, lemon juice, and black pepper. Those foods are staples of Greek cuisine, in addition to many varieties of fresh fish, lamb, and beef. Here are some smart choices:

- Skip the skordalia (a garlicky dip made from potatoes) and try tzatziki, a sauce made from yogurt, cucumber, and garlic, or taramosalata, a creamy spread made from heart-healthy fish roe. Enjoy these dips with fresh vegetables and olives. You'll often find tzatziki drizzled on beef, pork, lamb, or chicken.

- Load up on cucumber salad, which is tossed with feta cheese, tomatoes, and vinaigrette. Skip the pita, and ask for cucumber and carrot sticks to dip in your tzatziki.

- Of course, there's always room for soup. You can try avgolemono, a chicken soup made with egg and lemon.

- Order beef, chicken, or lamb souvlaki. These skewers of grilled meat are naturally low in carbs and the perfect accompaniment to tzatziki sauce.

- Lamb is a Greek specialty, and there are many options to choose from: roast leg of lamb, grilled chops, and gyros.

- Choose grilled prawns, octopus, or swordfish seasoned with garlic and lemon juice instead of battered and fried calamari. You can also try seafood baked with yogurt and herbs, cooked in rich tomato sauce, added to soups, or served cold as a side dish.

- Though honey-drenched baklava sounds heavenly for dessert, if you're still hungry after your Greek feast, a cheese plate is your best bet.

Indian

Indian food is complex and full of flavors influenced by a range of cuisines from the Far East to Europe, with a variety of vegetarian options that often include rice, wheat, or legumes, including peanuts. There are also plenty of dishes with protein and fiber-rich vegetables. Here are some smart choices:

- Vegetable samosas are fried or baked pastries—they are tempting but a better choice is paneer, which is a homemade cheese similar to cottage cheese that is cooked in a variety of ways. Shahi paneer is paneer cooked in a creamy curried sauce, and palak paneer is paneer cooked in a spinach curry.

- Pakora is a battered and fried fritter; opt for roasted eggplant with onions and spices instead.

- Vindaloo is a spicy dish that often contains potatoes (to help cut the heat), while tandoori dishes do not. Tandoori dishes are very popular; you can choose from chicken, fish, shrimp, or lamb baked in a clay oven (called a tandoor) after marinating in yogurt, garlic, ginger, herbs, and spices.

- Lentil or mulligatawny soup may be high in carbs, but you can try a bowl of chicken shorba, which is made with chicken, garlic, ginger, cinnamon, cumin, and other spices.

- Instead of dal (made from lentils) or biryani (a rice dish), you can try korma, which is meat in a cream sauce, or any curried meat dish or meat or shrimp kebabs.

- Watch out for saag dishes, which are prepared with spinach and spices but might be heavily thickened with flour or another starch.

French

French cuisine encompasses all the regions of France, from the coastal areas to the mountains and everything in between. Though French cuisine may seem decadent, it is based on a combination of protein, healthy fats, and carbohydrates, and many traditional French sauces are perfectly acceptable if you're doing Atkins because they are made with butter or oil and thickened with egg yolks instead of flour. Here are some smart choices:

- French onion soup is traditionally topped with a large crouton of toasted bread under a layer of melted Gruyère cheese, but you can request it without the bread.

- You can also enjoy some classic chicken, lamb, and beef dishes without guilt. Coq au vin is chicken slowly simmered in a wine sauce. Just pass on the potatoes that may be included. Leg of lamb is roasted and rich in the flavors of garlic and rosemary, and boeuf bourguignon consists of cubes of beef slowly simmered in red wine, beef stock, onions, garlic, and herbs. You can try our version of this classic French dish on page 261.

- Rather than the bacon, onion, and egg pie known as an Alsatian tart, try a frisée salad with thin strips of bacon and a poached egg.

- Enjoy coquilles St. Jacques, scallops in a cream sauce topped with cheese, instead of lobster in puff pastry.

- For vichyssoise, the famous French cream of leek and potato soup, substitute mussels in a white wine sauce or the equally famous fish stew called bouillabaisse.

- Order entrecôte or tournedos bordelaise, steak in reduced shallot and red wine sauce, instead of croque monsieur, an egg-dipped, fried ham-and-cheese sandwich.

- Rather than veal Prince Orloff, which is roasted and stuffed with rice, onions, and mushrooms, have the veal Marengo, a stew with tomatoes and mushrooms.

- Instead of any potato dish, order buttered French green beans.

- If it's possible you still have room for dessert, you can't go wrong with a plate of French cheeses.

DATE NIGHT WITH ATKINS

*While there are plenty of low-carb options
to choose from when you're lingering over a romantic meal in a
restaurant, sometimes it's even more special when you
can enjoy date night in the comfort of your own home, especially
when you have your pick of the following mouthwatering
menus featuring recipes from this book.*

Vegetarian Delight

- Crispy Brussels Sprouts with Sriracha Mayo Dipping Sauce (page 141)
- Baby Kale and Blue Cheese Salad with Warm Hazelnut Dressing (page 189)
- Pear and Manchego Mesclun Salad with Caramelized Onions (page 195)
- Lime Coconut Rum Cupcakes (page 278)

Seafood Lovers

- Shishito Peppers with Hot Paprika Mayonnaise (page 157)
- Old Bay Shrimp Salad (page 182)
- Shellfish Cioppino (page 262)
- Lime Coconut Rum Cupcakes (page 278)

Farm to Table

- Cauliflower Bisque (page 167)
- Fried Green Tomatoes with Ranch Dipping Sauce (page 153)
- Crispy Duck Spinach Salad with Warm and Tangy Turmeric Dressing (page 185)
- Apple Crumble (page 286)

Paris Is for Lovers

- Steamed Artichoke with Homemade Lemon Mayonnaise (page 219)
- Turnip Fries (page 222)
- Beef Bourguignon (page 261)
- Salted Caramel Cheesecake Bites (page 281)

Surf and Salmon

- Garlic Butter Lobster Salad (page 198)
- Parmesan Scallops (page 242)
- Broiler Miso Salmon (page 235)
- Apple Crumble (page 286)

Mexican

There's more to this cuisine than tacos and burritos. You're probably quite familiar with the "Americanized" version of Mexican food, which often features enchiladas and tamales, and gets its spice from jalapeños. Head to New Mexico, where the flavors are influenced by Hatch green chilies, whereas California's take on Mexican cuisine predominantly features seafood and fresh vegetables. But Mexican cuisine is actually much more complex, with variations based on regions in Mexico, with some European, especially Spanish, influence and the flavors of garlic, chilies, cilantro, and cumin. Here are some smart choices:

- Start with guacamole, which is mashed avocado often flavored with onions, tomato, cilantro, lime, and jalapeños. Plus, Atkins-friendly avocado is rich in fiber, heart-healthy monounsaturated fat, and other nutrients. Instead of chips, ask for jicama sticks (a naturally sweet, crunchy root vegetable).

- Ceviche is a traditional Latin American dish made from raw fish marinated in lime or lemon juice, onion, and chili. This fresh, light appetizer is low in carbs or other raw vegetables.

- Sopa de albondigas (meatball and vegetable soup) is a much better swap for quesadillas.

- Enchiladas verdes are tortillas filled with spiced chicken and smothered in a tangy green sauce of tomatillos and cilantro. Just ask for yours minus the tortillas.

- Fajitas can still be a favorite when you pile your plate with sizzling carne asada (marinated skirt steak), chicken, or shrimp, sliced onions, and bell peppers and skip the tortillas and beans; but keep all the fixings of guacamole, sour cream, and pico de gallo.

- You can't go wrong with grilled fish, pollo asada (grilled chicken), camarones al ajili (shrimp in garlic sauce), or chicken or turkey mole. (Mole is a dark, rich sauce made from ground cocoa beans.)

Japanese

Since Japan is an island nation, its cuisine naturally emphasizes seafood. It's known for perfectly balanced flavors and a beautiful presentation, with ingredients including sesame seeds and sesame oil, shoyu (Japanese soy sauce), mirin (sweet rice wine), dashi (broth made from dried fish flakes), ponzu (dipping sauce made from shoyu, rice wine vinegar, dashi, and seaweed), and wasabi, which is similiar to horseradish. When you think of Japanese food, you probably think of sushi, which is loaded with heart-healthy fats. The challenge? Watch out for the rice that accompanies it. Fortunately, Japanese cuisine offers some other protein sources as well. Here are some smart choices:

- Start your meal with miso soup, which is a rich, light but flavorful soup made with fermented soybean paste (miso) and dashi broth. You'll often find it served with a few cubes of tofu and perhaps some seaweed, along with a garnish of green onions.

- You won't get a traditional salad at a Japanese restaurant. Vegetables are almost always served crisp, and with the exception of tempura, which you'll want to avoid because of the batter, vegetables are usually grilled or briefly blanched. Try burdock (a relative of the artichoke), daikon (a delicious radish), lotus root, Japanese eggplant, and edamame, which are steamed soybeans. Also sample the pickled vegetables, including seaweed, which are most often served as a snack or appetizer and are lower in carbs than other appetizers such as gyoza (fried dumplings).

- If you substitute sashimi for sushi, you won't be disappointed. Sashimi is artfully sliced raw fish, minus the white rice. Chances are it will be the very best the chef has available, because there's nothing to disguise any flaws in appearance and flavor.

- Shabu-shabu is thin slices of beef and vegetables that you cook at the table in a hot broth. It's a smarter choice than sukiyaki, which is seasoned with sugar.

- See if the menu offers any low-carb sushi rolls, which come wrapped in cucumber and avocado, minus the rice. Or ask if they can make you one.

Thai

Thai cuisine encompasses a delicate medley of flavors, including sour, sweet, salty, bitter, and spicy. Fresh herbs such as lemongrass and cilantro add brightness, and tropical influences come from coconut oil, coconut milk, tamarind, and lime. There is an emphasis on seafood, and noodle and rice dishes are popular, as well as smaller portions of meat. Here are some smart choices.

- You've probably heard of pad Thai, a noodle-based dish with shrimp or chicken, green onions, eggs, dried tofu, bean sprouts, and chopped peanuts. The distinctive flavors of this dish can also be found in many without noodles: Naua yang nam tok, similar to a main dish salad, is sliced steak marinated in lime juice and mixed with chilies, onion, tomato, cucumber, coriander leaves, and lettuce. If you're feeling adventurous, you can try yum pla muk, sliced squid. Similar dishes are made with pork, beef, or other forms of protein and dressed with a fish sauce along with salt, lemon or lime juice, garlic or shallots, and chilies.

- Thai cuisine features some delicious soups that are naturally lower in carbs. Try tom yum goong, a hot-and-sour shrimp soup with straw mushrooms, seasoned with lime juice, lemongrass, and hot peppers; or gai tom kha, made with chicken slices in coconut milk. Our version of tom yum soup is on page 174.

- Instead of curries (which often contain potatoes), go with sautéed scallops and shrimp with mushrooms, zucchini, and chili paste.

- Skip the fried rice in favor of sautéed mixed vegetables.

Korean

Korean food has some Japanese and Chinese elements, and fish, crab, shrimp, clams, oysters, and squid make up a large part of the typical diet. Some seafood is dried, pickled, or used to make a paste. Fresh fish is usually grilled or stewed in a sauce. Vegetables (both raw and pickled) are a big part of Korean cuisine. The defining flavors of Korean foods are garlic, ginger, soy sauce, rice vinegar, sesame oil, and pastes made from fermented soybeans or chilies, which can provide considerable fire. Traditional Korean meals include soup and an assortment of tiny dishes featuring dried and pickled vegetables and seafood. Here are some smart choices:

- You can't go wrong with kimchi, one of Korea's best-known specialties, which is made by fermenting cabbage in pepper, garlic, ginger, and scallions. This spicy side dish is naturally low in carbs while having a high nutritional value and fiber content. Plus, fermented foods such as kimchi and sauerkraut have been shown to help improve digestion and boost the immune system.[3]

- Skip the rice noodle dishes and try bulgogi, a savory dish of grilled marinated beef that you dip in a little sauce and wrap in a lettuce leaf. Samgyeopsal is grilled slices of pork belly meat wrapped in lettuce along with grilled slices of garlic and onion and shredded green onions and kimchi. Some sauces are higher in sugar, so keep an eye on those.

- Some soups are full of noodles, but twoenjangguk, a Korean version of miso soup, is made from fermented soybean paste and baby clams. If you want to whip up a Korean-inspired soup at home, check out our Spicy Korean Soup with Scallions on page 168, which is a low-carb version of yukgaejong, a spicy shredded beef soup with vegetables, although in this case, we have swapped the beef for chicken.

- You can enjoy many of Korea's tofu dishes, and don't forget to try the variety of tiny vegetable- and seafood-based dishes that are traditionally a part of many meals.

Chinese

Four regions of China influence Chinese cuisine. Cantonese cuisine is probably the Chinese food you are most familiar with: light delicate sauces, roasted meats, and steamed and stir-fried vegetables. Szechuan is best known for its extremely hot dishes such as kung pao chicken and double-cooked spicy pork. Hunan dishes are known for thick, rich sauces as well as complex and sometimes biting flavors, such as pepper chicken. Shandong cuisine emphasizes fresh ingredients and delicate flavors, sometimes brightened by the addition of garlic and scallions. The one thing all these regions have in common is that rice is a part of every meal. Here are some smart choices:

- Beware of the buffet. You'll want to avoid sweet-and-sour dishes amd anything breaded or battered. You can have any meat with sauce on the side and pile on the vegetables. If you miss Mongolian beef, which is typically doused in a sauce containing sugar, you can find our Atkins-friendly version on page 236.

- For an appetizer, try egg drop soup instead of fried wontons or an egg roll. The soup should be clear and thin, rather than thickened with cornstarch.

- Instead of shrimp, pork, beef, or chicken fried rice, have a sizzling shrimp platter.

- Substitute steamed tofu with vegetables or beef with Chinese mushrooms for any of the noodle-based dishes. If it comes with a sauce, request that it be served on the side.

- Rather than any of the sweet-and-sour dishes, try stir-fried pork with garlic sauce (sauce on the side, of course).

NAVIGATING THE WORLD OF FAST CASUAL FOOD

In today's world of fast casual restaurants, you can literally watch your meal made in front of you, choosing fresh ingredients as you go. If you've been paying attention up to this point, you should have an idea of all the choices available to you so you can enjoy a dish naturally low in carbs.

- **AT THE FAST CASUAL BURRITO RESTAURANT:** Go for a burrito bowl or salad, add the meat of your choice, pile on the fajita vegetables and salad greens, stick with a "garnish" of beans or rice, and pump up the flavor with your choice of salsas, guacamole, sour cream, and cheese.

- **AT THE FAST CASUAL NOODLE RESTAURANT:** Very often you can replace your serving of noodles with extra veggies, or you can choose freshly made soup and a side salad or a main dish salad.

- **AT THE FAST CASUAL SANDWICH RESTAURANT:** You can fill up on soup and salad or skip the bread and turn a traditional sandwich into a salad.

- **AT THE FAST CASUAL BURGER RESTAURANT:** Savor that juicy burger, skip the bun, and wrap it in lettuce. I've even seen fast casual burger restaurants that offer options such as portobello burgers and grilled fresh fish. Keep your eye on the fries, although some places may offer veggie frites—strips of veggies that are flash-fried. Yes, they are still fried, but they are a better choice than French fries, which spend much more time in the deep fryer.

CELEBRATING (NOT JUST SURVIVING)
THE HOLIDAYS

THERE IS NO REASON TO dread any holiday when it comes to embracing Atkins' nutritional approach of eating right, not less. If you stick with your routine of planning your low-carb meals and snacks (three meals and two snacks a day), it's easy to make smart choices, especially during times when temptations seem to be everywhere. When your hunger is under control, you'll be less likely to cave in under the pressure of unexpected holiday treats, and you will be able to maintain your blood sugar levels so you don't suffer energy dips, especially when you need the extra energy to finish all those holiday errands. Many holidays (with the exception of Halloween) feature foods that are naturally low in carbs. Let's take a look.

- **Thanksgiving:** Fill your plate with turkey or ham, and then focus on vegetable side dishes. Take advantage of any leftover turkey or ham and feast on roll-ups or add the meat to eggs, salads, or soups.

- **Hanukkah:** You can enjoy brisket and try out latkes made from shredded zucchini instead of potatoes. Once again, take advantage of any brisket leftovers.

- **Christmas:** If you're Italian, you may partake in the Feast of the Seven Fishes, which is your chance to indulge in heart-healthy fish. This holiday also involves dishes featuring turkey, ham, beef, or lamb.

- **St. Patrick's Day:** The traditional main dish of this holiday, corned beef and cabbage, is low in carbs. Just stick with a light version of green beer.

- **Easter:** You can eat ham and all the hard-cooked Easter eggs you would like, while taking advantage of spring vegetables such as asparagus, which you can smother in a rich hollandaise sauce. Turn the leftover hard-cooked eggs into deviled eggs for a yummy low-carb snack.

- **Fourth of July:** Skip the buns on your burgers and brats, and enjoy all the fresh vegetables that are in season this time of year, including tomatoes, cucumbers, summer squash, and even corn on the cob in moderation.

It doesn't matter if you're the host or the guest at a holiday celebration, because you can enjoy this special time without the guilt if you stick with these suggestions:

Eat before you eat. Before you hit a holiday lunch or dinner, a party, or an office celebration, fortify yourself with a filling Atkins-friendly snack (I've included some snacks on pages 87–88 in this chapter) before you go. Or you could have a small low-carb meal, such as a chef salad topped with grilled chicken. The combination of a small amount of carbs with either fat or protein will stabilize your blood sugar so you don't arrive famished. That way, you'll have the physical backup to your mental fortitude so you can pass up holiday foods that are not on your low-carb meal plan while still partaking in the festivities.

Give it away. If you receive personal or business gifts that are high in carbs—cookies, chocolate, fruitcake, flavored popcorn, and the like—regift them to your child's school or a homeless shelter. If such gifts arrive at your office, simply put them in a public area such as the coffee break room. I guarantee that they will disappear fast.

Keep snacks on hand. If your workplace is awash in holiday goodies, it's all the more important that you stick with your low-carb snacks to keep your appetite under control. If possible, avoid the parts of the office where bowls of candy and plates of cookies are set out. You might even want to talk to the office manager or whoever is responsible for this holiday custom and suggest some healthy alternatives such as fresh fruit and nuts.

Master the buffet. Buffets are actually full of Atkins-friendly options. Stick to the roast turkey, ham, roast beef, salmon filet, or other protein dishes, as well as tossed salads and Foundation Vegetables. Depending on if you are doing Atkins 20, 40, or 100, you can have modest portions of sweet potatoes, carrots, or other starchy veggies—or even some whole grain bread. At sit-down meals, there's no rule against simply not serving yourself a food you want to stay away from. If the cook insists, take a small portion, have a tiny taste, and leave it at that.

Stay on track. No matter how "good" you are when it comes to holiday temptations, the reality is that you'll probably take in a few extra carbs. The best way to deal with that is to get up the next morning and get back on track. The worst thing you can do is wallow in guilt and decide that you've blown it and need to wait until after the holidays to get back to your eating routine.

This is a time to enjoy family and friends and, yes, some favorite foods. If there isn't an Atkins-friendly alternative, enjoy a little bit of the real thing, and make sure your next meal or snack is low carb. I typically follow the 90/10 eating rule during the holidays: I make sure that 90 percent of the food I eat is on my low-carb plan and give myself 10 percent wriggle room to indulge. Finally, my mantra is to eat until I'm satisfied, not stuffed. A true sign of success is keeping your goals in sight while celebrating (not just surviving) the holidays.

ON THE ROAD
WITH ATKINS

WHETHER YOU'RE TRAVELING FOR BUSINESS, road-tripping with the family, or enjoying a well-deserved vacation, here is a road map for navigating every twist and turn.

Plan ahead. Dining out at every meal can do damage to both your wallet and your waistline. If you're vacationing with the family, rent or stay in homes or hotels that have kitchens or kitchenettes. If you're on an extended business trip, book a hotel room with a kitchenette or at least a refrigerator and microwave. Make a quick grocery run as soon as you arrive at your destination so you have options for breakfasts, lunches, and snacks. Forget fast food and hit the salad bar at the grocery store if you need a quick, convenient meal.

Pack a snack. Whether you're flying or driving, make sure you have low-carb snacks on hand such as jerky, trail mix, nuts, olives, turkey or ham roll-ups, and cut-up veggies and hummus.

Don't clean your plate. Stop eating when you're full, or split a salad and entrée. If you are staying in a place with a refrigerator, take your leftovers and have them for a snack or lunch the next day.

Make your splurge worth it. Save up for the delicious treats you won't be able to find at home. Cut out a snack in favor of the treat, and make sure you have your next low-carb meals and snacks planned out so your one splurge doesn't turn into a free-for-all. Or eat all your planned low-carb snacks and meals, and just indulge in a bite or two of the treat.

Stay hydrated. Bring bottled water, club soda, unsweetened tea, coffee, or herb tea if you're driving or "training" it, or request it on the plane.

Find nonfood distractions. Flight delay or hour five of a twelve-hour road trip? Instead of feeding your boredom with an overpriced coffee drink or bag of chips, take a walk around the airport terminal or stop the car and do some stretches or a quick nature walk around a point of interest. You could also catch up on your reading or get the family involved in the "license plate game."

THE NEWS ON BOOZE

A **cocktail** or two very often go
hand in hand with vacations, holidays, and business
dinners. Although that fruity tropical drink
with the umbrella looks mighty tempting, it's **packed
with sugar.** If you are going to have a drink,
choose wisely, and stick with **lower-calorie
drinks** such wine or light beer or drinks made
with **sugar-free mixers.**

Get active. Build your vacations around activities that
get your blood pumping. Research hikes in your area,
hit the beach for volleyball, rent bikes, and explore your
surroundings. Do you travel for business a lot? Pack your
workout clothes and hit the hotel gym or go for a walk or run
when you need to clear your head and boost your energy.

Do damage control. If you return from vacation a few
pounds heavier, that's okay. Cut roughly 10 grams of Net
Carbs a day from your intake until you return to your goal
weight.

Exercise Your Right to Exercise

Exercise is a great stress
reliever for me and helps me burn off
any extra holiday goodies
I may have consumed. During the
holidays, I always make a
plan to keep pace with my exercise
goals by scheduling fitness
time on my calendar, just as I would
a doctor's appointment or work
meeting. I also suggest
squeezing in some extra movement
every day, even if it's as simple
as taking the stairs instead of the
elevator, parking farther away in
the parking lot, or taking a brisk walk
around the block.

MAKING ATKINS
WORK AT WORK

———————— • ————————

THE WORKPLACE MAY SEEM LIKE a danger zone of carbs, with the lure of doughnuts at coffee breaks, fast-food lunches, and tempting treats in vending machines. But with some advance planning, you can make Atkins work at work.

Conquering Your Coffee Break

Eat breakfast. If you start the day with a breakfast of sufficient protein and healthy fats, it not only sets you up for a positive and productive day but keeps you from experiencing an energy dip and being ravenous by midmorning. That will be your secret to success if you are trying to limit your visits to the break room vending machine, which is often full of sugary soft drinks, cookies, candy, and other sneaky sources of hidden sugars, or the coffee cart, which might feature a trifecta of doughnuts, muffins, and pastries. Even nonbreakfast foods are good alternatives. There's nothing wrong with kicking off your morning with leftover chicken and salad from the night before or scrambling up that leftover chicken with some eggs, spinach, and cheese.

See Chapter 6 for a variety of breakfast recipes, including smoothies you can whip up in minutes and sip on the go if time is tight.

Curb your caffeine intake. If you have already had your morning coffee, decaffeinated coffee, tea, or herbal tea are better bets so you don't experience the midmorning jitters. Keep a water bottle at your desk, and drink from it frequently.

Sneak in a snack. Good, convenient choices include wrapped individual cheese portions, or bring in homemade snacks such as hard-cooked eggs, ham roll-ups, or celery sticks filled with cream cheese, as well as nuts, seeds, and some fruits. When it's your turn to bring in the doughnuts, it's your chance to introduce your coworkers to delicious and hearty Power Mug Muffins with Cinnamon Butter on page 133. They may never ask for doughnuts again!

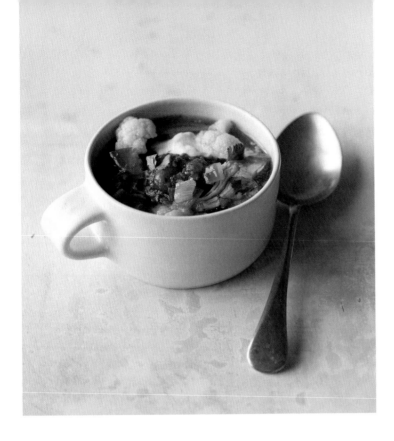

Lunch and Learn

Master the cafeteria. Skip the fried foods, sandwiches, and desserts. Instead, scrutinize the hot entrées, the salad bar, and the grill section for smart choices. Ask to substitute extra veggies for sides such as French fries.

Bring your own lunch. This is a surefire strategy for success. If a refrigerator is not available, pack your homemade lunch in an insulated bag or small cooler. Transport tuna fish, chicken, or egg salad in a plastic container; green salads can travel in a zip-top plastic bag with dressing on the side. Baked chicken legs, slices of roast beef, or turkey and steamed shrimp are also highly portable. And it's time to learn to love leftovers: prepare extra servings of your evening meal, so you can heat up a delicious lunch the next day.

OVERCOME OVERTIME

Overtime carbs at the office may be the hardest of all to avoid, especially if you weren't able to plan ahead by packing dinner or an **extra snack.** As your workday stretches out, your **stress** level rises—as does your desire for something sweet or crunchy. Keep an **emergency stash** of snacks so that healthy choices are at your fingertips before you get too ravenous. When your coworkers are sending out for dinnertime food, go ahead and join in, making the **best choices** you can from the available menu.

DEAR DIARY: SETTING THE STAGE FOR
SUCCESS WITH ATKINS

I'VE ALWAYS THOUGHT THAT A food journal is a valuable tool when it comes to helping you stay on track with Atkins (and also jump-starting your journey with Atkins, as I have mentioned earlier), and now there is research to confirm this approach. According to a study by the Fred Hutchinson Cancer Research Center and published in the *Journal of the Academy of Nutrition and Dietetics*, women who kept a food journal lost more weight than those who didn't.[4]

Whether you are tracking your daily food (and Net Carbs) intake on a sticky note or in a hard-copy journal, the Atkins app, or another food journal app, this type of accountability will help you be more successful.

Maybe you've been doing Atkins for a while, and you've been making steady progress toward accomplishing your goals—until you're not. Tracking your daily food and Net Carbs intake will give you an honest picture of what you are eating. Your Net Carbs may have been gradually increasing due to "carb creep," and you haven't noticed it until you started writing it down. Seeing the hard facts on paper (or on the computer) will help you get right back on track.

A journal can also help you identify the trigger foods that have the potential of setting you off on a carb free-for-all. Maybe you've noticed that you are ravenous every day at 3 p.m. First, ask yourself why this is happening. Are you not bringing enough food each day? Does this seem to be the peak time for stress for you at work, or are you simply eating out of boredom? Once you figure this out, you can have an Atkins-friendly snack ready to eat before your hunger gets uncontrollable, or go for a walk or practice some deep breathing to distract yourself or ease your stress. A journal can help you time your meals, and help you track with accuracy how often and when you are eating. The moral of the story? Spend a few minutes each day with your food journal to set the stage for success with Atkins.

Atkins is all about the experience of eating and enjoying food and becoming empowered by making healthy choices.

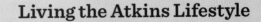

Living the Atkins Lifestyle

It's never been easier to eat healthfully,
especially when you're armed with this guidebook. Now
that you understand how Atkins works and why it makes
so much sense to eat this way, it's your choice
what level of Atkins you would like to start with. Or just
try out a few of the mouthwatering recipes coming
up, and see how this way of eating makes you feel. The
bottom line is that Atkins is all about the experience
of eating and enjoying food and becoming empowered
about making healthy choices. Turn the page, because
now it's time to start cooking!

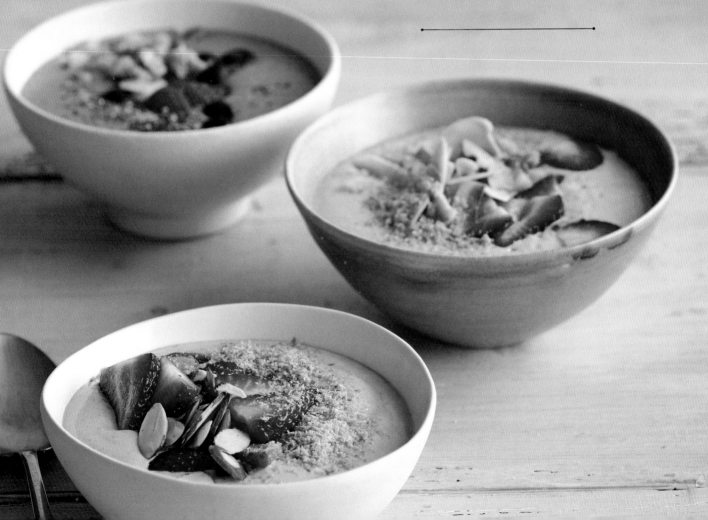

PART TWO

LET'S
GET
COOKING

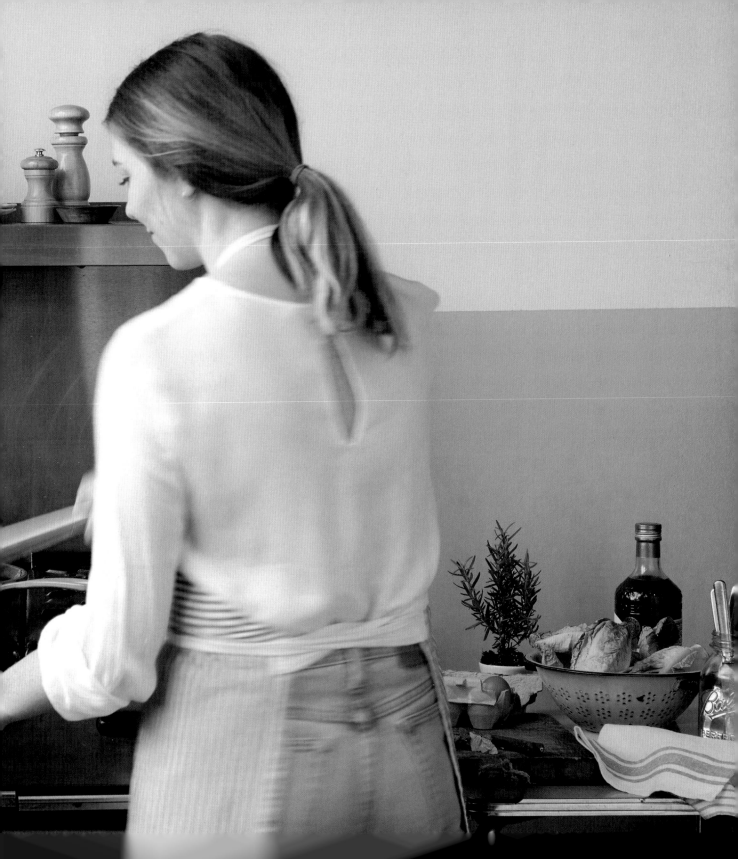

6

BREAKFAST

EGGS AND MORE,

plus brunch basics

FOR LEISURELY MORNINGS

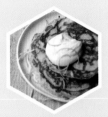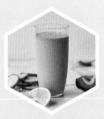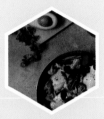

Breakfast does a body good! When you start the
day off on the right foot with a meal that features a good source of protein,
healthy fats, and carbohydrates rich in fiber and nutrients,
you set the stage for a full day of satisfying, smart choices. These hearty,
savory, and sweet breakfast recipes are deliciously easy to make,
whether you're grabbing a bite on the go or have time to relax with family
and friends while savoring a meal worth lingering over.

RECIPES

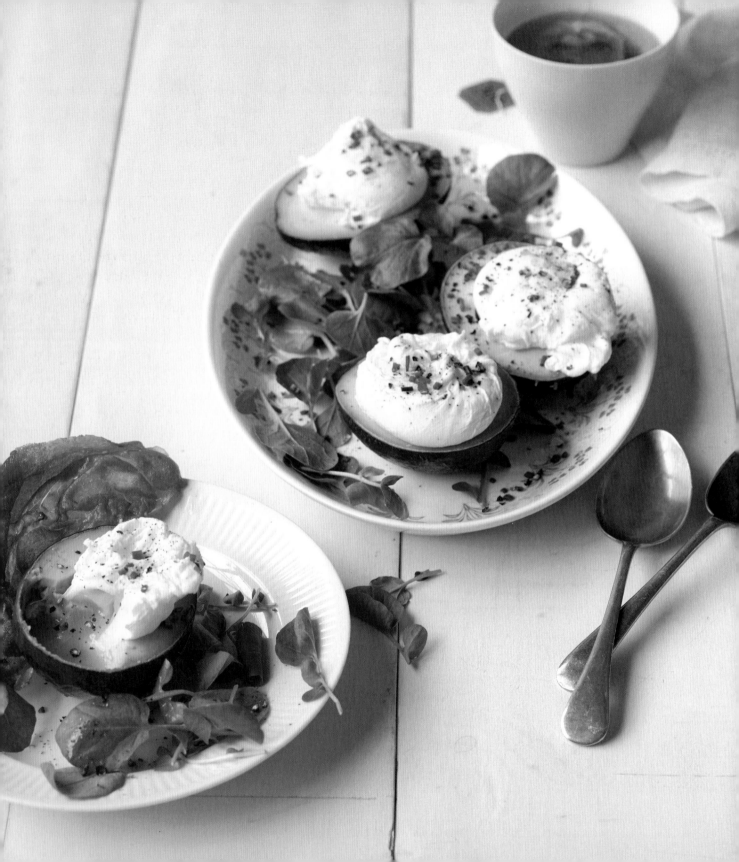

EGG-FILLED
AVOCADO
with Prosciutto

4.1g
NET CARBS

SERVES
4

422
CALORIES

This novel approach to "sunny-side up eggs with bacon" features softly poached eggs in avocado halves, served with a side of crisp prosciutto. Avocado with an "egg surprise inside" is a great way to introduce both adults and kids to eating the healthier fats found in vitamin E–rich avocados, which also happen to be packed with fiber. For picture-perfect eggs, use poaching cups to help the eggs keep a nice oval shape when simmering.

TIME	PER SERVING
Active: 10 minutes	*Total Carbs:* 16g *Fiber:* 11.9g
Total: 15 minutes	*Protein:* 18.5g *Fat:* 34g *FV* = 3.6

- 6 ounces watercress or baby spinach
- 2 tablespoons balsamic vinegar
- 8 large eggs
- 4 ripe Hass avocados, halved lengthwise and pitted
- Olive oil spray
- 8 slices (about 4 ounces) prosciutto

1 Place the watercress or baby spinach in a large bowl. Drizzle with the balsamic vinegar and toss well. Divide among four small plates.

2 In a large skillet, heat 2 inches of water over medium heat until bubbles cover the bottom and sides of the pan. Crack each egg into a separate small bowl (do not use eggs with broken yolks). When a few bubbles have broken the surface of the water, gently pour each egg into the pan, leaving room between them.

3 Cook the eggs, without stirring, until the whites are just set and the yolks are still runny, 2 to 3 minutes. Use a rubber spatula to gently release the eggs from the bottom of the pan, if necessary. Using a slotted spoon, remove the eggs from the water and drain on paper towels.

4 Place a poached egg into each avocado half. Coat a medium skillet with olive oil spray. Heat the skillet over medium heat and add the prosciutto. Cook until crispy, about 2 minutes per side. Transfer two avocado-filled egg halves to each plate, and serve immediately with two slices of prosciutto.

DID YOU KNOW
?

The abbreviation **FV** stands for **Foundation Vegetables** in each recipe.

SUNNY-SIDE UP
EGGS

with Cauliflower Hash Browns

7.4g   SERVES **4**   **271**

NET CARBS   CALORIES

This low-carb hash brown swap is made with an antioxidant-rich superfood, cauliflower, which is high in vitamin C (for immunity), folate (important for breast cancer protection), and vitamin K (for bone health). When shopping for cauliflower, avoid florets with black spots that resemble smudges, which is the result of oxidation (prolonged air exposure) that could mean spoilage or even mold.

TIME	PER SERVING
Active: **15 minutes**	*Total Carbs:* **11.4g**
	Fiber: **4.1g**
Total: **20 minutes**	*Protein:* **20g**
	Fat: **16.3g**
	FV = 6.3

1 small head cauliflower, cut into florets (about 5 cups) (see Tip)

4 slices bacon, chopped

1 green bell pepper, seeded and diced

½ onion, finely chopped

½ teaspoon seasoning salt (see Tip)

½ teaspoon freshly ground black pepper

4 teaspoons olive oil

8 large eggs

1   **To prepare the hash browns:** place the cauliflower florets in a food processor and roughly chop; you will need to do this in two batches. Warm the bacon in a large skillet over medium heat, and cook 4 to 5 minutes, stirring occasionally, until the bacon is well browned. Add the cauliflower, bell pepper, onion, salt, and pepper, cooking 5 to 6 minutes, stirring often, until the cauliflower is soft.

2   Add 2 teaspoons of the olive oil to another large skillet. Place over medium heat and add 4 eggs. Cook 1 to 2 minutes, until the edges of the eggs start to firm. Cover and reduce the heat to low. Cook 1 to 2 minutes, until the whites are cooked through but the yolks are still soft. Repeat with the remaining oil and eggs. Set out four plates, spoon equal portions of cauliflower hash browns on each plate, and top with 2 sunny-side up eggs. Serve immediately.

TIPS

To save time, "riced" cauliflower in the produce or frozen food section is ideal for this recipe and many others throughout the book.

Seasoning salts are a mixture of tasty spices blended with salt—a simple way to add more interest and flavor to recipes with just a shake. When shopping for seasoning salt, check the ingredients list to be sure it is free of added sugar, as brands vary.

SALMON
EGGS
BENEDICT

3.4g
NET CARBS

SERVES 4

383
CALORIES

This luscious brunch treat—hold the bread—has the same rich sauce that Benedict buffs love. Swapping heart-healthy smoked salmon for Canadian bacon gives you filling fats that are skin-healthy, too. An immersion blender, an inexpensive tool for faster and smarter prep, whips up the hollandaise sauce in a cinch.

TIME	PER SERVING
Active: 20 minutes	*Total Carbs:* **4.6g** *Fiber:* **1.2g**
Total: 30 minutes	*Protein:* **25.5g** *Fat:* **29.1g** *FV = 2.1*

Hollandaise Sauce

5 tablespoons unsalted butter, divided

¼ cup minced sweet onion or shallot

½ teaspoon salt

¼ teaspoon freshly ground black pepper

1 tablespoon white vinegar

1 large egg yolk

1 tablespoon lemon juice

Eggs

Olive oil spray

8 large eggs

8 ounces baby arugula or spinach

8 ounces smoked salmon, thinly sliced

¼ cup chopped fresh chives or cilantro

1 Prepare the hollandaise sauce: Melt 1 tablespoon butter in a small saucepan over medium heat. Add the onion or shallot, salt, and pepper, cooking 1 to 2 minutes, until the onion or shallot begins to soften. Stir in the vinegar; reduce heat to medium low, and cook until the vinegar is evaporated, 1 to 2 minutes. Reduce heat to low, and continue cooking, stirring frequently, until tender and translucent, about 4 minutes longer. Transfer the onion mixture to a tall blender cup or measuring cup. Set aside.

2 In the same saucepan in which you cooked the onion, melt the remaining butter over medium-low heat. Cool slightly, 4 to 5 minutes, on the countertop. Add the egg yolk and lemon juice to the blender cup, then add a few tablespoons of the melted butter, and use an immersion blender to blend until a thick yellow cloud forms. Add the remaining melted butter, and blend again until fully incorporated.

3 Prepare the eggs: coat a large skillet with olive oil spray. Place over medium heat and add 4 eggs. Cook 1 to 2 minutes, until the edges of the eggs start to firm. Cover and reduce the heat to low. Cook 1 to 2 minutes, until the whites are cooked through but the yolks are still soft. Repeat with the remaining eggs. Divide the greens among four plates, top with the smoked salmon, and place the eggs on top. Drizzle with the hollandaise sauce, sprinkle with the chives or cilantro, and serve.

CAULIFLOWER RICE
SCRAMBLES

5.1g
NET CARBS

SERVES 4

381
CALORIES

Your hearty appetite will breathe a sigh of relief when you feast your eyes on this well-portioned breakfast scramble. You can't go wrong with anything that features bacon, and jalapeños add a fresh and spicy kick.

1 small head cauliflower, cut into florets (about 5 cups)

8 slices bacon

2 jalapeños, seeded and diced

8 large eggs

1 cup shredded cheddar cheese

4 teaspoons hot sauce (optional)

1 Place the cauliflower florets in a food processor and chop roughly; you will need to do this in two batches.

2 Warm the bacon in a large skillet over medium heat, and cook 4 to 5 minutes, stirring occasionally, until the bacon is well browned. Transfer to a plate. Do not discard the bacon grease.

3 Add the cauliflower and jalapeños to the skillet, and cook 5 to 6 minutes, stirring often, until the cauliflower is soft.

4 Place the eggs and cheddar in a large bowl, and gently whisk. Add the eggs to the skillet and cook 3 to 4 minutes, stirring occasionally, until firm. Serve immediately with the bacon and hot sauce, if desired.

TIME	PER SERVING
Active: 10 minutes	*Total Carbs:* 8.4g
	Fiber: 3.3g
Total: 25 minutes	*Protein:* 28.1g
	Fat: 26.2g
	FV = 3.7

CHAI
CINNAMON
WAFFLES

10.3g
NET CARBS

SERVES
4

400
CALORIES

Chai spice mixes, used to make our American coffee shop caffè lattes so fragrant, actually hail from India and are part of a long tradition of using healing spices, including cinnamon, cardamom, black pepper, ground ginger, and nutmeg, in drinks and food. These waffles borrow the name and spices to turn plain waffles into something special. If you wish, garnish each serving with a few berries, but be sure to count their carbs!

TIME	PER SERVING
Active: 20 minutes	*Total Carbs:* 13.6g *Fiber:* 3.1g
Total: 30 minutes	*Protein:* 30.3g *Fat:* 25.8g *FV* = 0

- ½ cup heavy whipping cream, chilled
- 2 tablespoons unsalted butter
- 1 teaspoon vanilla extract
- 1 tablespoon stevia (see Tip)
- 1 teaspoon ground cinnamon
- 1 teaspoon freshly grated nutmeg
- 1 teaspoon ground ginger
- ½ teaspoon ground cardamom
- 1 cup Atkins Flour Mix (page 126)
- 1 teaspoon baking powder
- ¼ teaspoon salt
- 2 large eggs
- 1½ cups whole milk
- Olive oil spray
- ½ teaspoon ground cinnamon
- 4 teaspoons sugar-free caramel or vanilla syrup (optional)

TIP

Stevia, *a natural sugar substitute extracted from the stevia plant, can replace sugar in baking. It is calorie free, although it is 200 times as sweet as granulated table sugar, so a little goes a long way!*

1 Place the cream in a large bowl and beat with an electric mixer on high speed until light and fluffy. Refrigerate until ready to use.

2 Place the butter in a small saucepan and melt over low heat. Stir in the vanilla extract, stevia, cinnamon, nutmeg, ginger, and cardamom. Set aside to cool.

3 Place the Atkins Flour Mix in a large bowl along with the baking powder and salt, and stir well. Mix the eggs, milk, and butter mixture together, and add to the bowl with the flour mix. Stir until just combined.

4 Coat a waffle iron with olive oil spray. Heat the waffle iron according to the manufacturer's instructions. Add 1 cup of the waffle mix, and close the lid. Cook 3 to 4 minutes, until the waffle is cooked through. Repeat with the remaining batter. Serve immediately with the whipped cream, cinnamon, and sugar-free caramel or vanilla syrup, if desired.

BROILER
HUEVOS
RANCHEROS

9g
NET CARBS

SERVES 4

396
CALORIES

Huevos Rancheros, or "Rancher's Eggs" is the perfect brunch meal when breakfast time has passed you by, but you still crave eggs. Use chorizo, a spicy cured pork sausage flavored with chilies, or substitute cooked hot Italian pork sausage links instead.

TIME	PER SERVING
Active: 15 minutes	*Total Carbs:* 16.6g
	Fiber: 7.6g
Total: 20 minutes	*Protein:* 23.6g
	Fat: 27.2g
	FV = 7

Olive oil spray

2 cooked chorizo sausage links, (about 6 ounces) thinly sliced

1 bunch asparagus, trimmed and chopped

2 cups broccoli florets

2 cups cauliflower florets

8 large eggs

½ cup tomato salsa from a jar

1 ripe Hass avocado, cut into wedges

¼ cup sour cream

DID YOU KNOW ?

Don't confuse smoked **Spanish-style chorizo** links with the fresh, soft **Mexican version**, which is often sold in bulk (and also in links).

1 Set the oven to broil and coat a large skillet with olive oil spray. Place over medium heat and add the chorizo, browning for 3 to 4 minutes, stirring well, until it renders its fat. Add the asparagus, broccoli, and cauliflower, and cook 3 to 4 minutes, until the vegetables start to soften. Crack the eggs on top.

2 Place under the broiler on the middle oven rack, and cook 3 to 4 minutes until the whites of the eggs are cooked but the yolks are still soft. Serve immediately with the salsa, avocado, and sour cream.

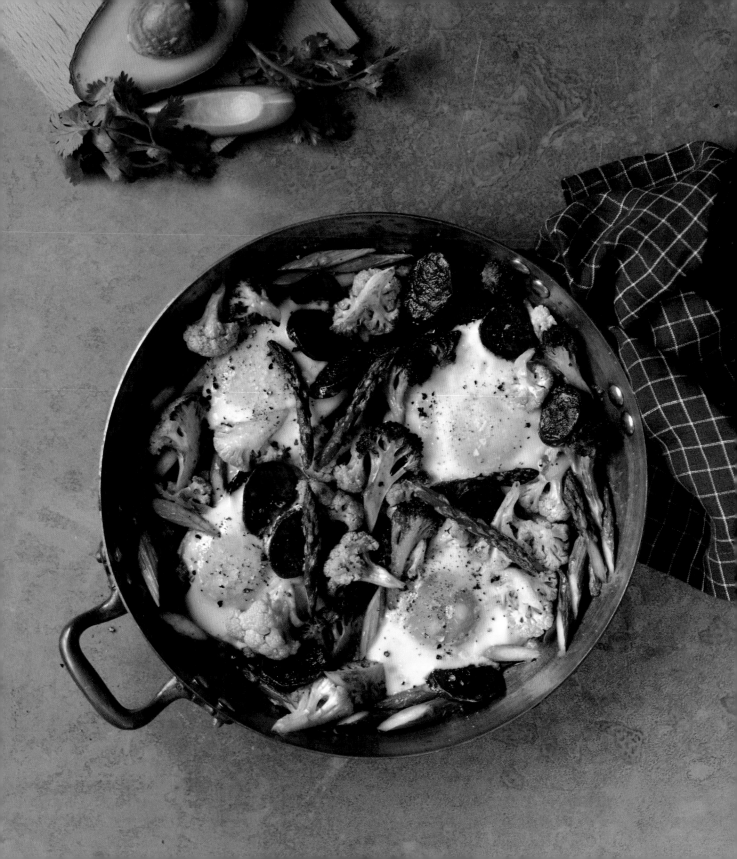

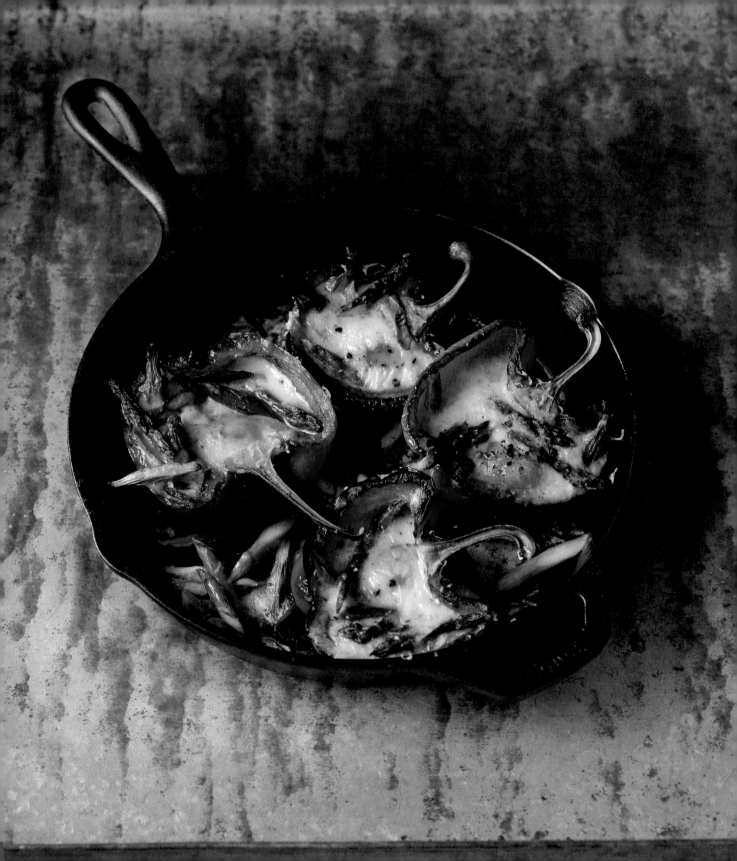

BIRDIES

IN A
BASKET

6g
NET CARBS

SERVES
4

362
CALORIES

The title of this recipe, also known as "eggs in a basket," has its roots in 1930s Hollywood, where actresses such as Betty Grable requested sunny-side up eggs cooked in toast. This version uses vitamin C—rich red bell pepper in place of the toast and adds even more veggie power with the addition of detoxifying asparagus, which is rich in fiber and folate.

1 tablespoon olive oil

½ bunch asparagus, trimmed and sliced

½ teaspoon seasoning salt

2 large red bell peppers

4 large eggs

2 cups shredded cheddar cheese

½ cup tomato salsa from a jar

1 Heat a large skillet over medium heat, and add the olive oil. Add the asparagus and seasoning salt; cook 3 to 4 minutes, until the asparagus softens. Transfer to a plate.

2 Preheat the oven to 350°F. Cut the peppers in half lengthwise, and discard the seeds. Place the peppers in the skillet, stem side down, and sear for 1 minute over medium heat. Flip and crack an egg into each pepper half. Top with the asparagus and sprinkle with the cheddar. Bake for 25 to 30 minutes, until the cheese is golden and the whites of the eggs are cooked through. Serve immediately with the salsa.

TIME	PER SERVING
Active: 10 minutes	*Total Carbs:* 8.8g *Fiber:* 2.8g
Total: 40 minutes	*Protein:* 21.6g *Fat:* 27.3g *FV* = 4.9

ATKINS
FLOUR
MIX

5g
NET CARBS

MAKES 3 CUPS

191
CALORIES

This versatile low-carb flour mix is an important component of many of the recipes in this book.

TIME	PER SERVING
Active: 10 minutes	*Total Carbs:* 8.2g
	Fiber: 3.2g
Total: 10 minutes	*Protein:* 31.3g
	Fat: 4.4g
	FV = 0

¼ cup wheat bran

1⅛ cups whole grain soy flour

⅔ cup vanilla whey protein powder

¼ cup golden flaxseed meal

⅔ cup vital wheat gluten flour

Combine all ingredients, and mix thoroughly. Use immediately, or store in an airtight container in the refrigerator for up to 1 month.

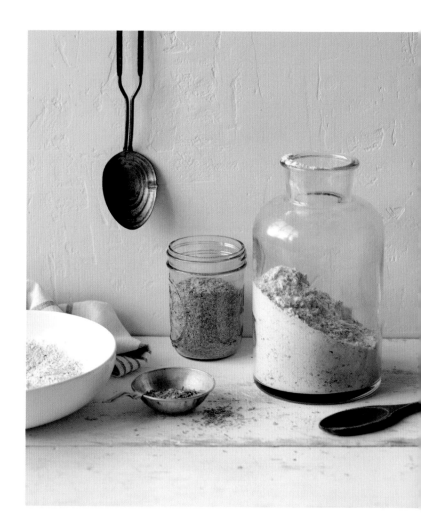

SWEET OR SAVORY
CREPES

SERVES
4

These delightfully thin pancakes are oh, so versatile and can be eaten with sweet or savory toppings. This recipe makes 12 crepes—make a double batch to freeze, and serve as the centerpiece of a fun brunch with eggs and a side salad. Crepes also make a great replacement for a standard high-carb wrap—just roll with a few slices of lean deli meat and cheese for a fast, portable lunch. Resting the crepe batter makes it easier to handle and stick less while cooking.

Crepes

4 large eggs

2 tablespoons heavy cream

1 cup Atkins Flour Mix (page 126)

¼ cup almond flour

¼ teaspoon salt

¾ cup water

For sweet crepes: add 1 teaspoon vanilla extract.

For savory crepes: add ½ teaspoon seasoning salt.

Olive oil spray

1 Prepare the crepe batter: Place the eggs, cream, Atkins Flour Mix, almond flour, salt, water, and vanilla extract or seasoning salt in a blender. Blend until smooth. Let rest in the fridge for 1 hour. Coat a griddle or small frying pan with olive oil spray. Place over medium-high heat. Add ¼ cup of the batter and cook 2 to 3 minutes, until the edges start to brown, then flip. Cook 1 minute more, until the crepe is firm, and transfer to a plate.

2 Repeat with the remaining batter, adding olive oil spray as needed.

RECIPE CONTINUES

SWEET CREPES	
TIME	PER SERVING
Active: 50 minutes	Net Carbs: 7.4g
	Total Carbs: 12.5g
Total: 1 hour, 50 minutes	Fiber: 5.1g
	Protein: 32.2g
	Fat: 22g
	Calories: 370
	FV = 0

SAVORY CREPES	
TIME	PER SERVING
Active: 50 minutes	Net Carbs: 5.6g
	Total Carbs: 8.8g
Total: 1 hour 50 minutes	Fiber: 3.2g
	Protein: 38.1g
	Fat: 19.5g
	Calories: 359
	FV = 0.1

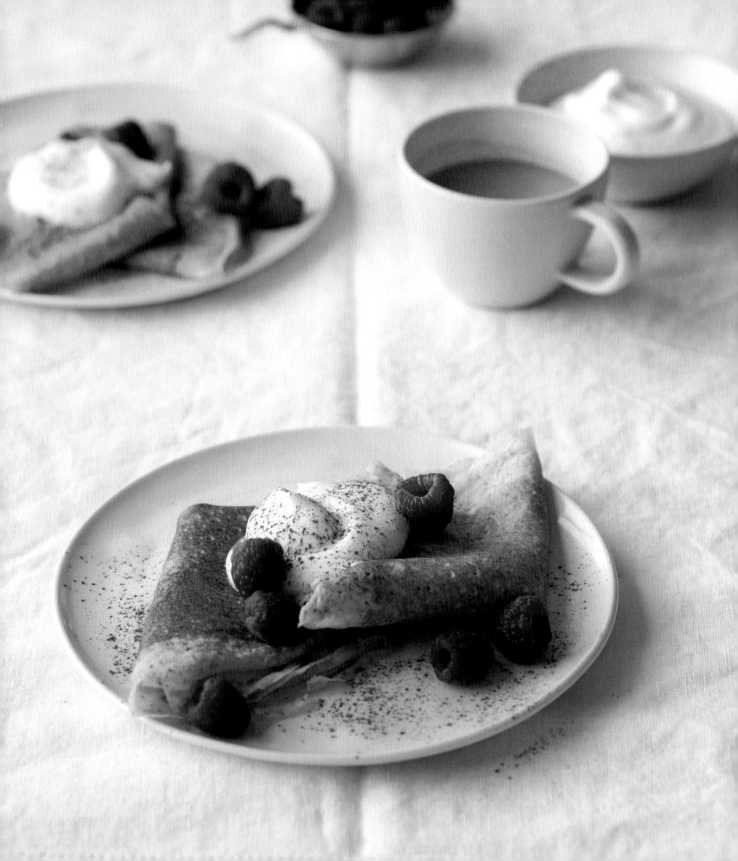

SWEET TOPPING

⅓ cup heavy cream, chilled

1 cup fresh raspberries

½ teaspoon ground
   cinnamon

Place the heavy cream in
a bowl and beat with an
electric mixer on high until
soft peaks form. For each
serving, fold 3 crepes into
quarters on a plate. Top each
with raspberries, a dollop
of whipped cream, and
cinnamon.

SAVORY TOPPING

Olive oil spray

4 large eggs

2 cups watercress

Spray a skillet with olive oil
spray and heat over medium
heat until hot. Break the
eggs and slip them into the
pan one at a time. Reduce
heat to low, and cook slowly
until the whites are set and
the yolks begin to thicken
but aren't hard. For each
serving, fold 3 crepes into
quarters on a plate. Top each
with a fried egg and an equal
portion of watercress.

CREAMY
AVOCADO
SMOOTHIE

5.3g NET CARBS — SERVES **2** — **308** CALORIES

Not a fan of overly "green"-tasting smoothies? This light, silky smoothie is the perfect way to get more greens into your morning, as avocado, a fruit packed with heart-healthy fats, mellows the flavor of spinach or kale. See Tip for more options for seasonal stir-ins.

1 cup baby spinach or kale

½ ripe Hass avocado

2 celery stalks

⅔ cup plain protein powder

1 tablespoon lemon juice

½ cucumber, peeled

14 walnut halves

½ cup water

8 ice cubes

Place the baby spinach or kale, avocado, celery, protein powder, lemon juice, cucumber, walnuts, water, and ice cubes in a blender. Blend until smooth, and serve immediately.

--- **TIP** ---

For a hint of freshness, add a pinch of mild chili powder in the winter or 2 tablespoons mint leaves (which add only .5 gram Net Carbs) in the summer.

TIME	PER SERVING
Active: 10 minutes	*Total Carbs:* 10.9g *Fiber:* 5.6g
Total: 10 minutes	*Protein:* 32.2g *Fat:* 16.2g *FV* = 2.6

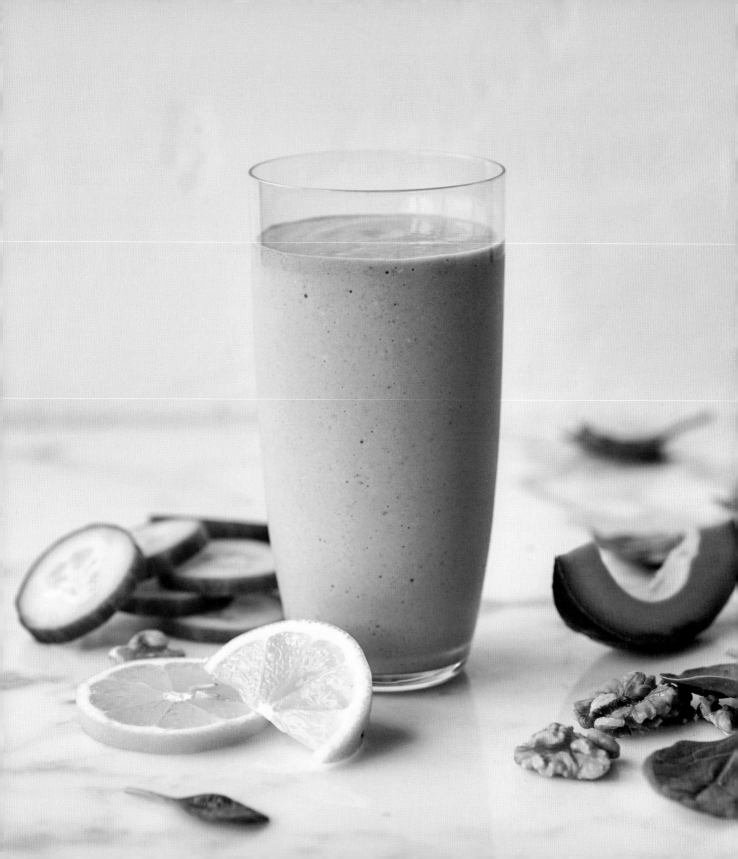

ANTIOXIDANT
BERRY
SMOOTHIE

7.1g
NET CARBS

SERVES
2

348
CALORIES

Berries are bursting with anthocyanins, colorful antioxidant pigments also responsible for their beautiful colors. This same antioxidant is being studied for a wide range of detox benefits for organs, from your heart to your liver and even your skin.[1]

TIME	PER SERVING
Active: 10 minutes	*Total Carbs:* **14.7g**
	Fiber: **7.7g**
Total: 10 minutes	*Protein:* **32.4g**
	Fat: **15.5g**
	FV = 0

½ cup mixed frozen berries (such as raspberries or blueberries)

¾ cup full-fat canned coconut milk

⅔ cup plain protein powder

2 tablespoons chia seeds

½ teaspoon ground cinnamon or cardamom

½ teaspoon ground turmeric

1 teaspoon vanilla extract

½ cup cold water

4 ice cubes

Place the berries, coconut milk, protein powder, chia seeds, cinnamon or cardamom, turmeric, vanilla extract, water, and ice cubes in a blender. Blend until smooth, and serve immediately.

TIPS

Protein powder is a good source of amino acids, which are the building blocks of muscle and may even be instrumental in weight loss and boosting your immunity. Most protein powders are made from two types of milk protein, although you can also find a blend of both.

- *Whey protein is one of the most popular of protein powders. It is fast acting, which means it is digested more quickly.*

- *Casein protein is a slow-acting protein powder, and is digested more slowly.*

In addition, there are nondairy, vegetarian sources of protein powder:

- *Soy protein is extracted from soybeans.*

- *Rice protein is isolated protein that comes from brown rice grains.*

- *Pea protein is concentrated protein extracted from split yellow peas.*

POWER
MUG MUFFIN

with Cinnamon Butter

3.9g
NET CARBS

SERVES
1

363
CALORIES

The power of this muffin comes from three superfoods: flax, almonds, and eggs, which deliver a lot of brain-boosting nutrients such as omega-3s, choline, and vitamin E. This faux "soufflé" blossoms before your eyes, making it a fun recipe for kids to make.

TIME	PER SERVING
Active: 10 minutes	*Total Carbs:* 11.3g
	Fiber: 7.4g
Total: 10 minutes	*Protein:* 12.6g
	Fat: 31.1g
	FV = 0

Cinnamon Butter

1 tablespoon unsalted butter, room temperature

½ teaspoon ground cinnamon

⅛ teaspoon salt

¼ teaspoon ground nutmeg

Muffin

2 tablespoons golden flaxseed meal

2 tablespoons almond flour

½ teaspoon baking powder

½ teaspoon stevia

1 teaspoon ground cinnamon

1 large egg

1 teaspoon unsalted butter, room temperature, or olive oil

1 Prepare the cinnamon butter: Place the butter, cinnamon, salt, and nutmeg in a small bowl, and mix well with a spoon. Set aside.

2 Prepare the muffin: Mix the flaxseed meal, almond flour, baking powder, stevia, and cinnamon in a coffee mug or single-serving soufflé dish. Mix the egg and butter into the dry ingredients. Microwave for 1 minute on high, until firm. Serve immediately with the cinnamon butter.

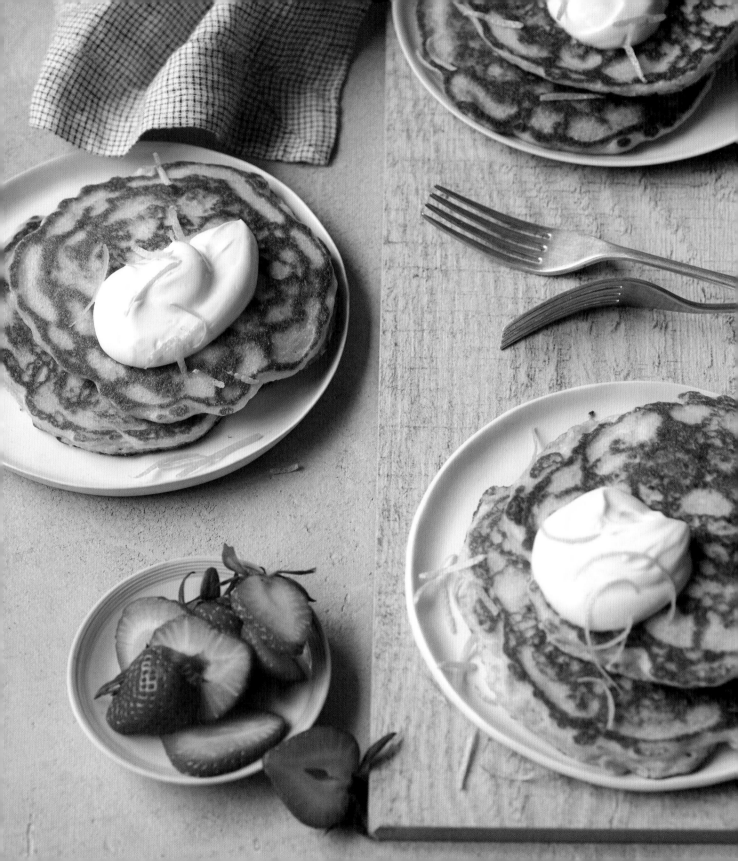

LEMONY
PROTEIN PANCAKES

5.5g
NET CARBS

SERVES
4

302
CALORIES

If you're a fan of lemon ricotta pancakes or cheese Danish, you'll flip for these higher-protein pancakes that will remind you a little of both, minus the blood sugar roller coaster. If you want to pump up the lemon flavor even more, look for Meyer lemons, a special breed of lemon in peak season from November through March.

½ cup Atkins Flour Mix (page 126)

⅓ cup almond meal

2 teaspoons baking powder

3 large eggs

½ cup cottage cheese

1 tablespoon finely grated lemon zest (from 1 lemon), plus thin strips of lemon zest for garnish

2 tablespoons lemon juice

3 tablespoons coconut oil

1 Place the Atkins Flour Mix, almond meal, and baking powder in a large bowl. Stir well. In a separate large bowl, whisk the eggs, then blend with the cottage cheese, lemon zest, and lemon juice until well incorporated. Add to the dry ingredients.

2 Melt the coconut oil over medium heat. Using a ¼-cup measuring cup, drop the batter onto the skillet or griddle. The batter will make about eight 4-inch pancakes. Cook 2 to 3 minutes, until the edges start to firm and bubbles begin to form in the middle of each pancake. Flip the pancakes, and cook another 1 to 2 minutes, until firm. Serve immediately.

TIME	PER SERVING
Active: 10 minutes	*Total Carbs:* 7.9g
	Fiber: 2.4g
	Protein: 21.5g
Total: 20 minutes	*Fat:* 21.8g
	FV = 0

COCONUT MUESLI CLUSTERS

3.9g
NET CARBS

SERVES
8

358
CALORIES

Cereal lovers don't have to go without with this clever mock muesli. The protein powder and egg coating help satisfy your hunger while giving this cereal a more cohesive texture and pleasing crunch—much better for you than the high-sugar honey typically used in muesli or granola. To switch up the flavor, replace the pecans with almonds and add ½ teaspoon almond extract.

TIME	PER SERVING
Active: 10 minutes	*Total Carbs:* 12.8g *Fiber:* 8.9g
Total: 20 minutes	*Protein:* 19.3g *Fat:* 27.3g *FV* = 0

Olive oil spray

1 cup plain protein powder

½ cup unsalted sunflower or pumpkin seeds

1 cup whole raw pecans

1 cup unsweetened whole flake shredded coconut

½ cup chia seeds or ground flaxseeds

1 tablespoon stevia

2 teaspoons cinnamon

½ teaspoon ground turmeric

1 tablespoon coconut oil

1 tablespoon peanut butter

1 teaspoon vanilla extract

2 large eggs

¼ cup water

1 Preheat oven to 350°F. Line a large baking sheet with parchment paper. Coat with the olive oil spray and set aside. In a large bowl, mix together the protein powder, sunflower or pumpkin seeds, pecans, coconut, chia seeds or flaxseeds, stevia, cinnamon, and turmeric.

2 In a large skillet, combine the coconut oil, peanut butter, and vanilla extract and melt completely, then stir in the nut mixture. Turn the heat off, and add the eggs and water, tossing well. Transfer to the prepared baking sheet, and spread the mixture in a layer about ½ inch thick over the baking sheet.

3 Bake for 10 to 15 minutes, until the mixture starts to brown and clumps together to make clusters. Cool completely on the baking sheet, then store in an airtight container, refrigerated, for up to 1 week.

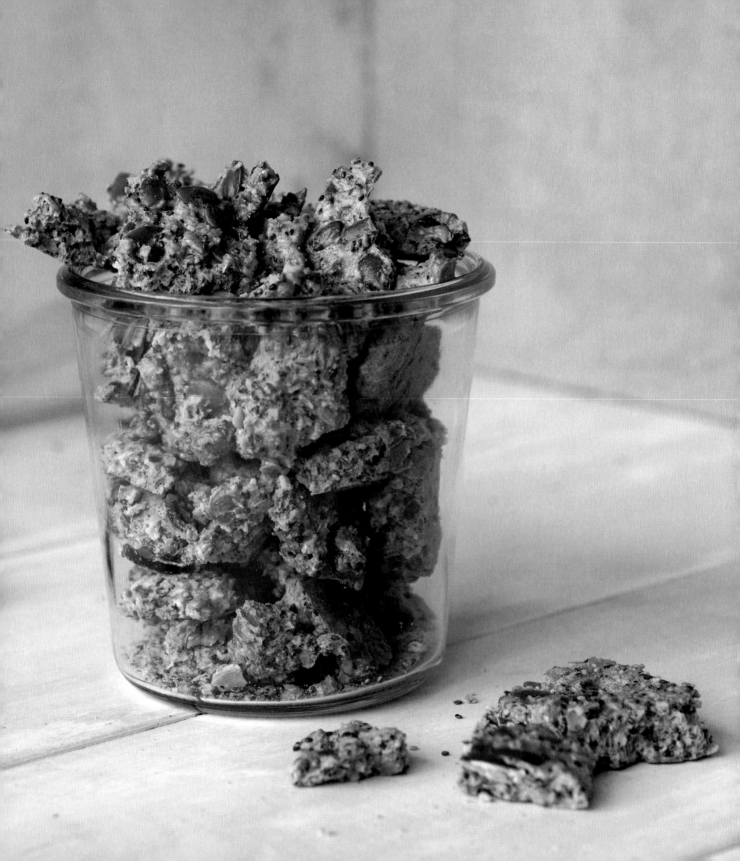

7

SNACKS AND SIDES

SATISFYING SNACKS

AND WINNING SIDE DISHES

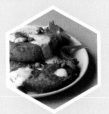 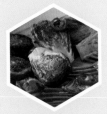 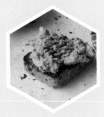

On Atkins, we recommend eating two snacks a day
to keep your hunger nicely in check, and what better way than with these
salty, savory, spicy, crunchy, cheesy, and creamy snacks that will
satisfy any craving. And the side dishes? They could very well become
the star of any meal! You'll be able to mix and match these recipes
with a variety of other recipes throughout this book.

RECIPES

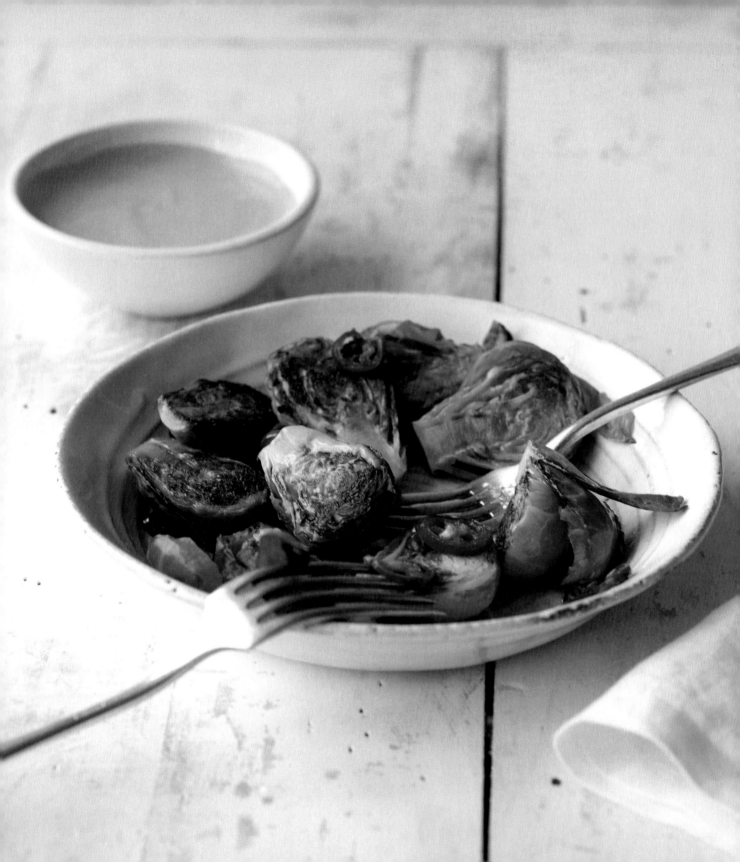

CRISPY
BRUSSELS SPROUTS

with Sriracha Mayo Dipping Sauce

7.5g
NET CARBS

SERVES
4

207
CALORIES

If you're seeking more flavor in your veggie sides, searing is the ticket to taste! Searing Brussels sprouts in hot oil, as you would meat, helps to caramelize them quickly for a slightly sweet flavor that is well balanced by the hot chilies and spicy dipping sauce. For best results, dry the sprouts in a paper towel or dish towel before you cook them.

TIME	PER SERVING
Active: 10 minutes	*Total Carbs:* 12g
	Fiber: 4.4g
Total: 20 minutes	*Protein:* 3.9g
	Fat: 17.1g
	FV = 6

Brussels sprouts

- 1 tablespoon grape seed or coconut oil
- 1 pound Brussels sprouts, dry, trimmed, and halved
- 2 serrano or jalapeño chilies, seeded and sliced
- ½ teaspoon salt or smoked salt
- ¼ teaspoon freshly ground black pepper

Sriracha mayo

- ⅓ cup mayonnaise
- 2 tablespoons sriracha hot sauce

1 Warm the oil in a large skillet over medium-high heat. Add the Brussels sprouts to the skillet, cut sides down, and cook about 3 minutes, until nicely browned. Add the chilies and sprinkle with the salt and pepper. Reduce the heat to medium low and cook until sprouts are browned all over and tender, about 8 minutes more.

2 While the Brussels sprouts are cooking, prepare the mayonnaise: Place the mayonnaise and sriracha in a small bowl, and stir well to combine. Transfer the Brussels sprouts to a platter, and serve immediately with the mayonnaise.

AVOCADO
TOAST

5g
NET CARBS

SERVES 8

318
CALORIES

It's no wonder the snack staple of rich avocado mash on crisp toast has been shared around the world for more than two decades. Creamy avocados are filled with healthy fats and fiber. They help you feel fuller longer while satisfying your "creamy" comfort food craving. The versatile "toast" is easy to make and can serve as the base for many snacks, including our bruschetta recipe on page 215.

1 large egg

1 tablespoon olive oil

¼ cup water

1½ cups almond flour

½ cup grated Parmesan cheese

½ teaspoon baking powder

½ teaspoon stevia

¾ teaspoon chopped fresh oregano

¼ teaspoon crushed red pepper flakes

Olive oil spray

4 ripe Hass avocados

4 tablespoons lemon juice

1 teaspoon seasoning salt

1 Preheat the oven to 375°F. Whisk together the egg, olive oil, and water in a small bowl. Set aside.

2 In a large bowl, combine the almond flour, Parmesan cheese, baking powder, stevia, oregano, and red pepper flakes, and stir to blend. Add the wet ingredients to the dry ingredients, stirring to form a sticky dough.

3 Coat a half sheet pan with olive oil spray. Smooth the dough onto the prepared pan with a spatula, into a 16-by-8-inch rectangle. Bake for 20 to 25 minutes, until golden and crisp around the edges. Allow the toast to cool, about 20 minutes.

4 While the dough is baking and cooling, prepare the avocados: Place the avocados in a large bowl with the lemon juice and seasoning salt, and mash well. Cut the toast into eight squares, and top with the avocado. Serve immediately.

TIME	PER SERVING
Active: 10 minutes	*Total Carbs:* 13.1g
	Fiber: 8.2g
Total: 40 minutes	*Protein:* 18.9g
	Fat: 28g
	FV = 1.6

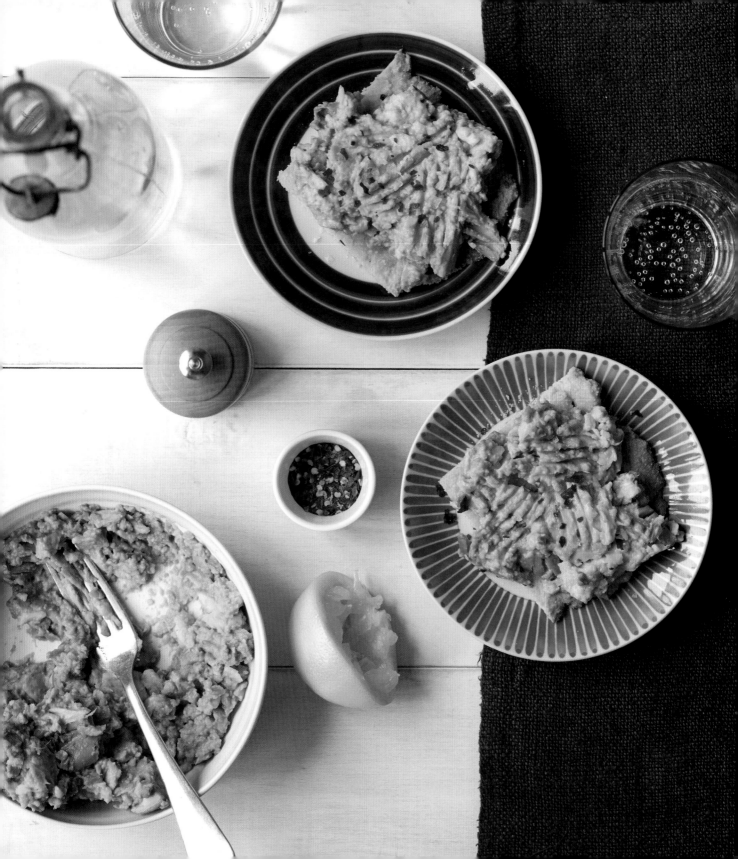

PROSCIUTTO-WRAPPED
SHRIMP

with Kale Mayonnaise

6.9g
NET CARBS

SERVES
4

474
CALORIES

Prosciutto is a lean Italian cured ham that crisps like bacon when sautéed. In this recipe, it makes a flavorful, high-protein wrap for shrimp that also helps to keep in moisture. Kale mayonnaise adds filling fat, plus all the goodness of kale, a superfood rich in a long list of detoxifying nutrients, including vitamins A, C, K, and more.

Kale mayonnaise

4 cups kale, chopped

½ cup mayonnaise

1 teaspoon paprika

½ teaspoon freshly ground black pepper

Shrimp

10 slices prosciutto (about .5 ounce)

20 extra jumbo shrimp, peeled and deveined, with tail segment attached

Olive oil spray

1 Prepare the kale mayonnaise: Place the kale in a food processor and process until minced. Add the mayonnaise, paprika, and pepper; pulse to combine. Set aside.

2 Prepare the shrimp: Cut each prosciutto slice in half lengthwise. Wrap each half slice around a shrimp and transfer to a plate. Coat a skillet with olive oil spray. Brown 3 to 4 minutes, turning occasionally, until the prosciutto is crisp and the shrimp is cooked through. Serve 5 shrimp per person with 2 tablespoons of the kale mayonnaise.

TIME	PER SERVING
Active: 10 minutes	*Total Carbs:* 8.4g
	Fiber: 1.6g
Total: 20 minutes	*Protein:* 20.1g
	Fat: 28.4g
	FV = 5.4

HOT
CRAB DIP

1g
NET CARBS

SERVES
4

298
CALORIES

Creamy, satisfying hot crab dip is a seafood restaurant staple that seems upscale, but this dish is incredibly easy to make. You can serve it with raw veggies, such as 1 celery stalk cut into matchsticks or ⅓ cup cucumber slices per person (for an extra 1 gram Net Carbs per serving) or our Cilantro Parmesan Crackers on page 155 (for an extra 3 grams Net Carbs per serving).

8 ounces pasteurized cooked crabmeat, picked over for shells and cartilage

½ cup mayonnaise

½ cup grated cheddar cheese

1 tablespoon lemon juice

2 garlic cloves

Preheat the oven to 400°F. Place the crabmeat, mayonnaise, cheddar, lemon juice, and garlic in a food processor, and pulse until the mixture is creamy. Transfer to an oven-safe baking dish, and bake for 20 to 25 minutes, until the mixture is hot and bubbly. Serve immediately.

TIME	PER SERVING
Active: 10 minutes	*Total Carbs:* 1g
	Fiber: 0.1g
Total: 40 minutes	*Protein:* 15g
	Fat: 25.7g
	FV = 0

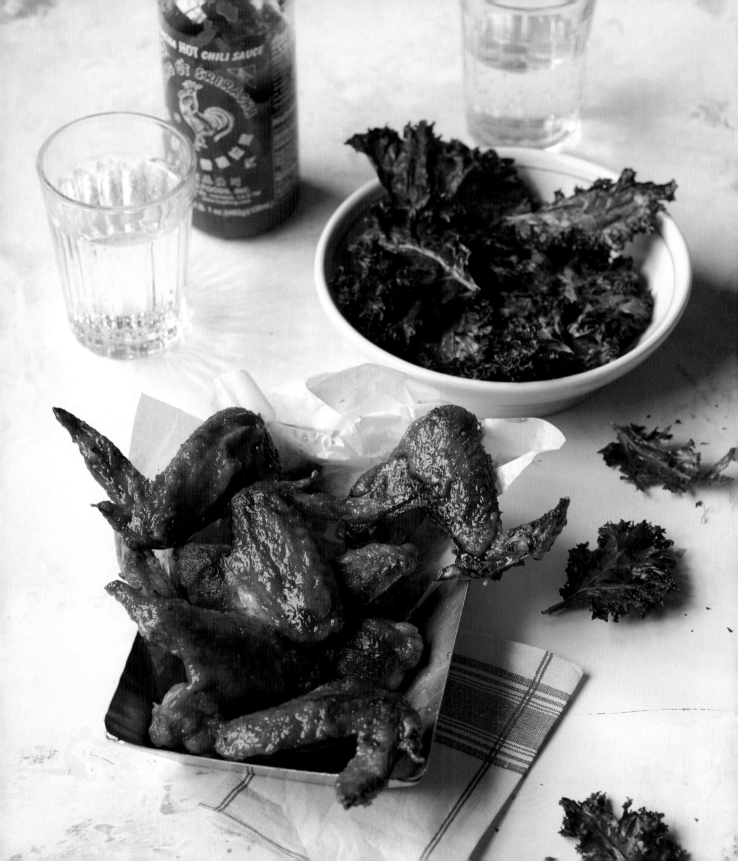

BAKED SRIRACHA
HOT WINGS
AND KALE CHIPS

5.9g
NET CARBS

SERVES
4

281
CALORIES

In this recipe, we take the American bar classic to a healthier level. Skip the breading and crisp the skin by rendering the fat in a skillet, then baking the wings at high heat. A quick toss in a sauce made of spicy sriracha butter adds richness plus heat. The kale chips crisp up quickly alongside the wings and are a great source of vitamins A, B, and C, iron, and potassium.

TIME	PER SERVING
Active: 15 minutes	*Total Carbs:* 6.7g *Fiber:* 0.8g
Total: 40 minutes	*Protein:* 17.3g *Fat:* 20.5g *FV* = 2.8

¼ cup sriracha hot sauce

3 tablespoons unsalted butter

½ teaspoon garlic salt

½ teaspoon freshly ground black pepper, divided

Olive oil spray

1 pound chicken wings

5 ounces kale, stems removed

½ teaspoon salt

1 Preheat the oven to 400°F. Cover a large baking sheet with aluminum foil.

2 Prepare the wing sauce: Place the sriracha, butter, garlic salt, and ¼ teaspoon of the black pepper in a large saucepan. Bring to a simmer over low heat, stirring continuously, until the butter melts. Turn the heat off and set aside.

3 Coat a large skillet with olive oil spray. Add the wings and cook 5 to 6 minutes, turning occasionally, until they brown. Transfer to the prepared baking sheet, and bake 12 to 15 minutes, until the chicken is cooked through and no longer pink at the bone.

4 While the chicken wings are cooking, prepare the kale chips: Remove the stems from the kale and discard. Tear the kale into 4-inch-wide pieces and arrange on another baking sheet. Spray the tops with olive oil spray. Flip the kale, and coat the other side with olive oil spray. Transfer to the oven, and bake 5 to 8 minutes, until crisp.

5 When the chicken is cooked, remove it from the oven and toss in the sauce. Season the kale chips with the salt and remaining black pepper. Serve the chicken immediately with the kale chips.

ASPARAGUS WITH BURRATA CHEESE

AND KALE PESTO

2g NET CARBS

SERVES 6

174 CALORIES

Move over, mozzarella, burrata has a smooth, elastic exterior and a creamy, buttery interior. Served over asparagus, burrata cheese creates an instant creamy sauce, made even more indulgent when topped with pesto. It's a good thing that this recipe serves six, because it is sure to be a crowd pleaser.

TIME	PER SERVING
Active: 10 minutes	*Total Carbs:* 4.1g
	Fiber: 2.1g
Total: 25 minutes	*Protein:* 8.8g
	Fat: 16.3g
	FV = 1.9

1 pound asparagus, trimmed

Olive oil spray

½ teaspoon seasoning salt, divided

¼ teaspoon freshly ground black pepper

1 cup kale leaves

1 cup packed basil leaves

3 tablespoons olive oil

2 garlic cloves, minced

2 to 3 tablespoons cold water

8 ounces burrata cheese

DID YOU KNOW ?

Burrata is a ball of mozzarella cheese with a **creamy,** runny (think poached egg) center. You'll find it packed in water with the other fresh mozzarella products at the market and at Italian delicatessens.

1 Place the asparagus on a plate and coat with olive oil spray. Sprinkle with half the seasoning salt and the black pepper. Heat a grill or large skillet over medium-high heat, and add the asparagus. Cook for 5 to 6 minutes, turning often, until the asparagus is tender. Transfer to a platter.

2 Add the kale and basil to a food processor, pulsing seven to eight times, until finely chopped. Add the olive oil, garlic, remaining ¼ teaspoon salt, and water; blend until smooth and creamy.

3 Cut the burrata into 6 wedges. Top a serving of asparagus with a wedge of burrata, including its creamy insides. Drizzle with the kale pesto and serve.

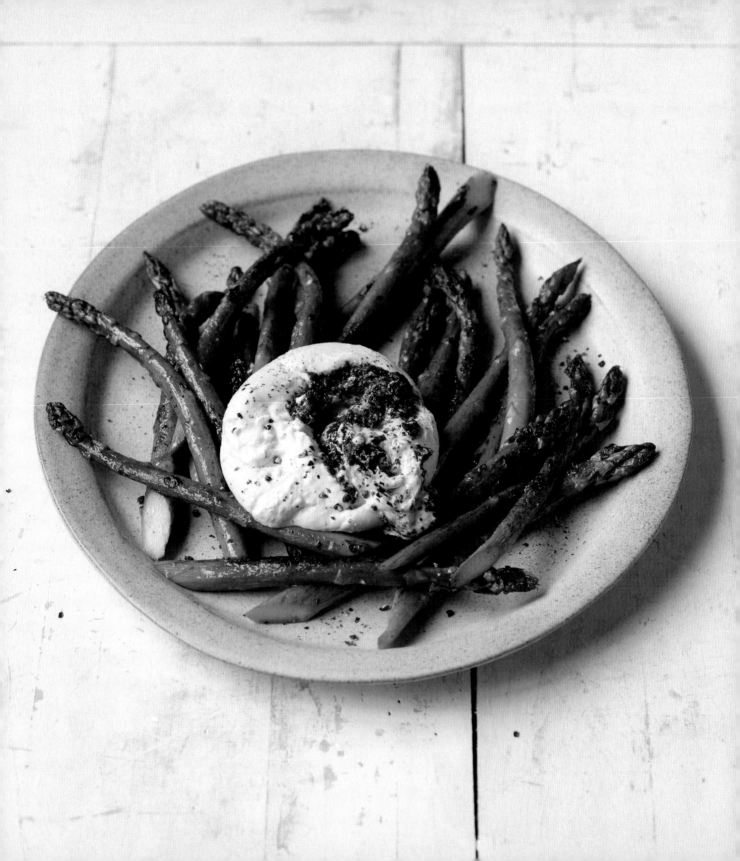

TUNA-STUFFED
DEVILED EGGS

1g
NET CARBS

SERVES
4

290
CALORIES

Deviled eggs received their name in the 1800s, when foods stuffed with a spicy flavoring such as Dijon mustard were termed *devilishly* hot. This version gets its "devil" from minced jalapeños, which also add a pleasant crunch and are rich in vitamin C. Add these Atkins-friendly eggs to your next party spread, potluck, or brunch.

TIME	PER SERVING
Active: 10 minutes	*Total Carbs:* 1.5g
	Fiber: 0.5g
Total: 30 minutes	*Protein:* 23.5g
	Fat: 20.4g
	FV = 0

8 large eggs

1 (6-ounce) can tuna, drained

¼ cup mayonnaise

1 jalapeño, seeded and minced

2 tablespoons capers, drained, rinsed, and chopped

1 teaspoon hot or sweet paprika or ground chili

1 Place the eggs in a medium saucepan, and cover with cold water. Place over high heat, and bring to a boil. Immediately turn the heat off and cover. Remove from the heat, and let cool for 1 minute. Place the eggs in a colander under cold running water for 1 to 2 minutes, until they are easy to handle. Peel them under cold running water, and transfer to a kitchen towel to dry.

2 Cut the eggs in half lengthwise and scoop out the yolks. Transfer the yolks to a small bowl along with the tuna, mayonnaise, jalapeño, and capers. Stir well until combined. Place the egg whites on a platter, center side up, and fill with the tuna mixture. Garnish with the ground paprika or chili, and serve immediately.

TIP

Hard-cooked eggs *make an "egg"cellent grab-and-go low-carb snack. All you have to do is the follow the instructions in this recipe for hard-cooking eggs.*

CHEESY

SCALLION CHEDDAR

CAULIFLOWER MASH

2.7g
NET CARBS

SERVES 6

78
CALORIES

Creamy comfort food such as mashed potatoes may seem like a high-carb treat of the past, but this cheesy cauliflower mash is just as satisfying in both flavor and texture. Pressing the cauliflower before whipping in a food processor is the secret to a mash that is light and fluffy.

TIME	PER SERVING
Active: 10 minutes	*Total Carbs:* **5g** *Fiber:* **2.2g** *Protein:* **4.1g**
Total: 15 minutes	*Fat:* **5.2g** *FV =* **2.6**

- **1 small head cauliflower, cut into florets (about 5 cups)**
- **½ cup grated cheddar cheese**
- **1 tablespoon unsalted butter**
- **1 teaspoon garlic salt**
- **¼ teaspoon ground turmeric**
- **2 scallions, thinly sliced**

1 Place a steamer basket in a large stockpot, add 2 cups of water, and bring to a boil over high heat. Add the cauliflower, and steam 10 to 12 minutes, until it is fork tender. (If you don't have a steamer basket, you can just add the cauliflower to the boiling water in the pot.) Drain the cauliflower in a colander, pressing down with a small pan lid, to drain the excess moisture.

2 Working in batches, transfer the cauliflower to a food processor and chop. Once all the cauliflower is chopped, put it all in the food processor along with the cheddar, butter, garlic salt, and turmeric. Process until smooth. Top with the scallions, and serve immediately.

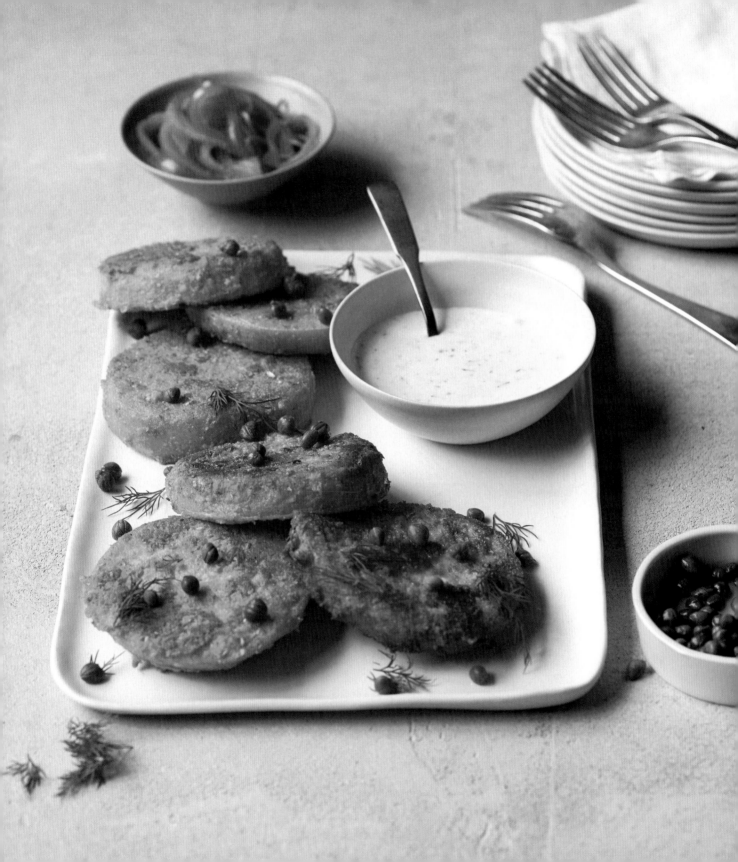

FRIED GREEN TOMATOES

with Ranch Dipping Sauce

6.8g
NET CARBS

SERVES
4

392
CALORIES

Fried green tomatoes are a southern comfort food that northerners will fall in love with at first bite. If you can't locate green tomatoes (underripe red tomatoes), search out less ripe brown tomatoes, such as Kumato. Capers make a tart garnish, if you happen to have them handy.

TIME	PER SERVING
Active: 20 minutes	*Total Carbs:* 9.7g
	Fiber: 2.7g
Total: 30 minutes	*Protein:* 15.1g
	Fat: 33.5g
	FV = 4.5

Ranch Dipping Sauce

½ cup mayonnaise

2 tablespoons coconut milk or heavy cream

1 teaspoon apple cider vinegar

½ teaspoon onion powder

½ teaspoon garlic salt

1 tablespoon chopped fresh dill or flat-leaf parsley

¼ teaspoon freshly ground black pepper

Fried Tomatoes

½ cup Atkins Flour Mix (page 126)

½ teaspoon garlic salt

½ teaspoon sweet paprika

½ teaspoon freshly ground black pepper

1 pound green tomatoes

1 large egg

3 tablespoons olive oil

1 **Prepare the ranch dipping sauce:** Combine the mayonnaise, coconut milk or heavy cream, vinegar, onion powder, garlic salt, dill or parsley, and black pepper in a small bowl and whisk well. Refrigerate until ready to use, or make ahead and refrigerate overnight.

2 **Prepare the fried tomatoes:** Place the Atkins Flour Mix, garlic salt, paprika, and pepper on a plate and toss with a spoon until well incorporated. Slice the tomatoes into four ½-inch-thick rounds. Place the egg in a shallow bowl and whisk. Dip the tomato slices into the egg, then dredge in the flour mixture and transfer to a plate.

3 Warm the oil in a large skillet and, working in batches, fry the tomatoes, 1 to 2 minutes per side, until crisp. Transfer to a paper towel–lined plate to drain. Transfer to a platter, and serve immediately with the ranch sauce.

SAUTÉED
SPINACH
with Caramelized Shallots

2.8g
NET CARBS

SERVES
6

62
CALORIES

Spinach and kale vie for the title of top superfood greens since they both contain high levels of many essential nutrients in just one small cup. Gentle sautéing doesn't destroy their nutrients, and it keeps the tender greens flavorful and fresh tasting, making this recipe an ideal companion for many of the heavier roasts and stews in this book. To prepare this recipe with either standard or Tuscan kale, substitute 1 pound of kale, stems removed, for the spinach.

TIME	PER SERVING
Active: 10 minutes	*2.8g*
	Total Carbs: **4.4g**
Total: 15 minutes	*Protein:* **2.4g**
	Fat: **4.5g**
	FV = 2.7

1 tablespoon unsalted butter

1 tablespoon olive oil

3 shallots, thinly sliced (about ⅓ cup)

¼ teaspoon salt

¼ teaspoon freshly ground black pepper

¼ teaspoon stevia, optional

Olive oil spray

1 pound baby spinach or baby kale

1 Warm the butter and olive oil in a small skillet over medium heat. Add the shallots, salt, black pepper, and stevia. Cook 10 to 12 minutes, stirring often, until the shallots are well browned, adding 1 to 2 tablespoons of water if the shallots stick. Transfer the shallots to a plate.

2 Coat the skillet with the olive oil spray and, working in batches, add the spinach; cook 1 to 2 minutes, until it is wilted and tender. Top with the shallots, and serve immediately.

CILANTRO
PARMESAN
CRACKERS

1.4g
NET CARBS

MAKES
3
DOZEN

80
CALORIES

Watch these get snapped up at your next gathering, because these aren't your average crackers—they're fragrant taste bombs, thanks to fresh cilantro mixed with Parmesan! See the tip for other savory flavor combinations and serve with Bourbon Pecan Pâté (page 212) or Hot Crab Dip (page 145).

TIME	PER SERVING
Active:	**(4 crackers)**
10 minutes	*Total Carbs:* **2.8g**
Total:	*Fiber:* **1.3g**
30 minutes	*Protein:* **3.7g**
	Fat: **6.7g**
	FV = 0

1 cup almond flour

1 large egg white

3 tablespoons grated Parmesan cheese

1 tablespoon finely chopped fresh cilantro

¼ teaspoon garlic salt

Olive oil spray

1 Place the almond flour, egg white, Parmesan, cilantro, and garlic salt in a medium bowl, and mix well with a spatula until a soft, slightly crumbly dough forms.

2 Coat two sheets of parchment paper with olive oil spray. Roll out the dough into a large rectangle about ⅛ inch thick between sheets of sprayed parchment paper. Slide onto a baking sheet and put in the freezer. Freeze for 15 minutes to make the dough easier to handle.

3 Preheat the oven to 325°F. Remove the top sheet of parchment and discard. Score the dough into 36 rectangles, about 2 by 1-inch each. Leaving the dough on the parchment paper–lined baking sheet, bake 15 to 20 minutes, until the crackers are golden and firm. Cool completely on the baking sheet. Break into crackers along the score marks. Serve or store in an airtight container at room temperature for up to 4 days.

TIP

Switch up your crackers with these other flavor combinations:

SWAP THIS	FOR THIS
Parmesan	*Pecorino, aged Gouda, or grated Asiago*
Cilantro	*Basil, parsley, chopped rosemary, or ½ teaspoon crushed red chili flakes*

HOMEMADE
RED
SAUERKRAUT

with Fennel and
Caraway Seeds

6.9g
NET CARBS

MAKES
5½
CUPS

44
CALORIES

Fermented foods such as sauerkraut are now all the rage in health circles, since we now know that eating cultured foods can help improve gut health. Other benefits include boosting your immunity and keeping your metabolism humming at optimal levels.[1] Another bonus: one batch of this fermented feast can last for up to 3 weeks.

TIME	PER SERVING (½ cup)
Active: 20 minutes	*Total Carbs:* 10g
	Fiber: 3.1g
Total: 3 days, 15 minutes	*Protein:* 2g
	Fat: 0.4 g
	FV = 6.9

1 (3-pound) red cabbage, coarsely shredded

1 tablespoon fennel seeds

1 tablespoon caraway seeds

¼ cup apple cider vinegar

2 teaspoons salt

½ teaspoon ground turmeric

1 Toss the cabbage, fennel and caraway seeds, vinegar, salt, and turmeric in a large glass bowl. Squeeze the mixture with clean hands for 4 to 5 minutes, to soften the shreds and to release some juices to form part of the pickling liquid.

2 Transfer the cabbage and its juice to a large glass jar or pitcher, and press it down so the liquid covers the top. Add additional water if the natural juices don't completely cover the surface of the cabbage (this will protect it from molding).

3 Cover with a clean dish towel and let rest on your countertop for 3 to 4 days maximum, until the mixture starts to bubble and reaches the desired tanginess, then transfer to airtight containers and store in the refrigerator for up to 3 weeks.

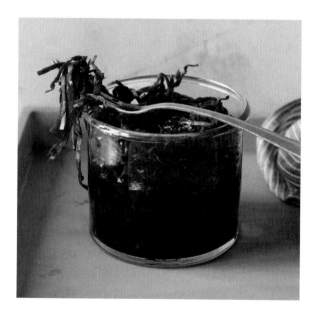

SHISHITO
PEPPERS

with Hot Paprika
Mayonnaise

2.7g
NET CARBS

SERVES
4

245
CALORIES

Shishito peppers are long, finger-shaped peppers that hail from East Asia but are typically served at Spanish tapas bars—upscale snack bars. Shishitos are generally mild, but one out of every ten is a spicy zinger! Search for them in gourmet markets and farmer's market stands that specialize in chilies, or substitute with little mild peppers called "ancient sweets" or "mini sweets," which also work well in this recipe.

TIME	PER SERVING
Active: 10 minutes	*Total Carbs:* **7.1g**
	Fiber: **4.4g**
	Protein: **2.2g**
Total: 15 minutes	*Fat:* **23.7g**
	FV = 2.3

4 quarts shishito peppers (about 48)

½ cup mayonnaise

Zest of 1 lemon, finely grated

1 tablespoon tomato paste

1 tablespoon hot or sweet paprika

1 tablespoon grape seed or coconut oil

1 Wash the shishito peppers and dry them well.

2 Prepare the paprika mayonnaise: Place the mayonnaise, lemon zest, tomato paste, and paprika in a small bowl, and stir well to combine.

3 Line a baking sheet with paper towels. Heat the oil in a large skillet over high heat, and add the peppers. Cook 2 to 3 minutes, stirring often, until the skins blister. Drain the peppers on the paper towels, and serve immediately with the mayonnaise.

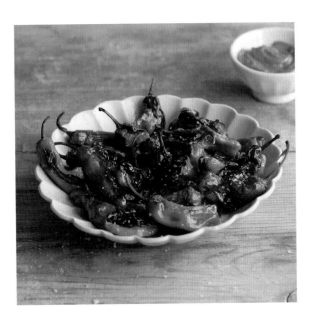

8

SOUPS AND STEWS

AND ANYTHING YOU CAN
SLURP UP IN A BOWL

◆

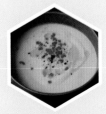 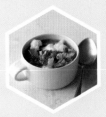 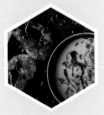

The international medley of flavors of these soups and stews will tantalize your taste buds. You can slurp on a smaller serving to ease your appetite before your main meal, or indulge in a steaming hot bowl as your main course, paired with a side salad.

RECIPES

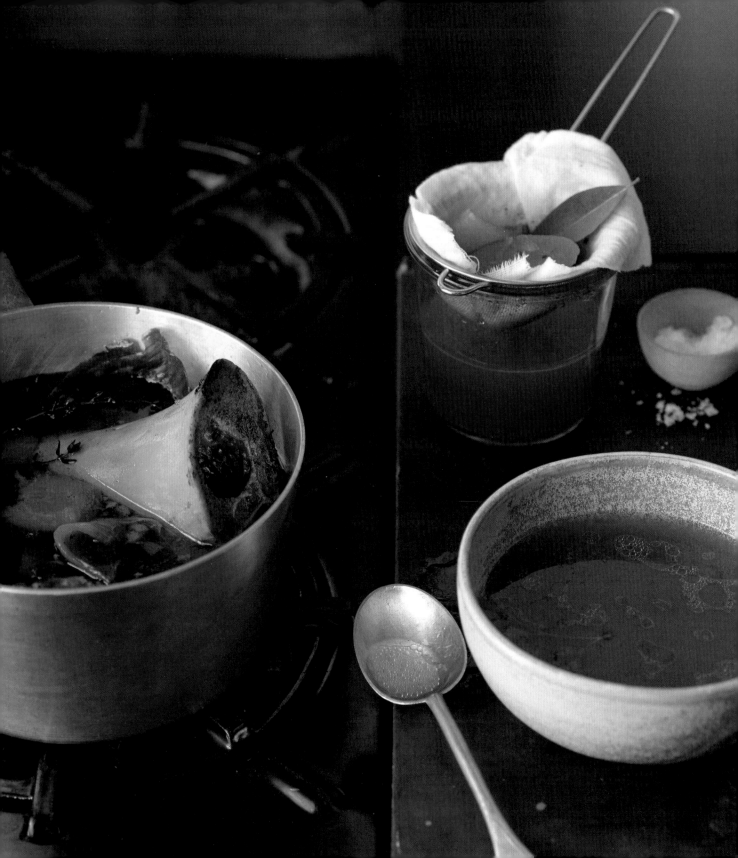

BASIC
BONE BROTH

0g NET CARBS **SERVES 8** **164** CALORIES

Bone broth has become a health staple and rightfully so. It's a low-cal drink with 0 gram Net Carbs that boasts a boost of protein, plus a rich, comforting flavor that helps cleanse your system. The high gelatin content can help soothe your stomach and aid with digestion. This slowly cooked broth is used in recipes throughout this book to enrich your dining experience. If you wish, use a slow cooker to simmer while you sleep (or are at work).

TIME	PER SERVING
Active: 20 minutes	*Total Carbs:* 0g
	Fiber: 0g
Total: 8 hours, 20 minutes	*Protein:* 12g
	Fat: 5g
	FV = 0

- 2 pounds beef shank bones with marrow (see Tip on next page)
- ½ teaspoon salt
- ¼ teaspoon freshly ground black pepper
- 1 tablespoon unsalted butter
- 2 carrots, chopped
- 1 onion, quartered
- 2 garlic cloves, chopped
- 2 tablespoons white distilled vinegar
- 2 bay leaves
- 1 sprig fresh thyme

1 Sprinkle the bones with the salt and pepper. Heat a large stockpot over medium heat, and add the butter. When the butter foams, add the bones and cook 3 to 4 minutes per side, turning occasionally, until the bones brown. Transfer the bones to a plate. Add the carrots, onion, and garlic. Cook 6 to 8 minutes, stirring often, until the vegetables brown. Return the bones to the pot, and fill the stockpot with water (about 12 cups), leaving at least a ½-inch space at the top of the pot.

RECIPE CONTINUES

Request beef shank bones *with marrow from the butcher at your local grocery store, as they are usually not sold in the prepackaged meat aisle.*

2 Add the vinegar, bay leaves, and thyme, and bring to a boil. As soon as the mixture boils, reduce to a simmer, cover, and cook 8 hours, adding additional water as needed to keep the water level high.

3 Remove and discard the bones. Strain the broth into a large bowl, discarding the solids. Cool completely and store in an airtight container in the refrigerator for up to 1 week or in the freezer for up to 6 months.

To prepare bone broth in a slow cooker: Place all the ingredients in an 8-quart slow cooker and cover with water. Set to low and cook 10 hours, until the marrow falls away from the bone. Discard the bones and strain. Discard the vegetables and marrow, and cool completely before storing in airtight containers in the refrigerator for up to 1 week or in the freezer for up to 6 months.

JALAPEÑO CHEDDAR
BROCCOLI SOUP

SERVES 4

Even if you are not a fan of spicy heat, this soup is surprisingly mild, since the seeds (where the spicy compound capsaicin resides) of the jalapeños are removed. The melted cheese on top will make you feel as though you're getting a bistro treat; however, it tastes just as good without the cheese.

3 tablespoons olive oil

1 head broccoli, cut into florets

6 jalapeños, seeded and diced

½ onion, chopped

1 teaspoon salt

½ teaspoon curry powder or ground turmeric

½ teaspoon freshly ground black pepper

2 tablespoons Atkins Flour Mix (page 126)

1 quart Basic Bone Broth (page 161), or unsalted chicken or beef broth

¼ cup heavy cream or canned coconut milk

1 tablespoon hot sauce

4 slices (4 ounces) cheddar cheese, optional

1 Warm the olive oil in a large stockpot over medium heat. Add the broccoli, jalapeños, onion, salt, curry powder or turmeric, and pepper; cook 5 to 6 minutes, stirring often, until the onion begins to brown. Sprinkle with the Atkins Flour Mix and cook 1 minute more, stirring often, until the flour coats the vegetables. Add the broth and cover.

2 Cook 10 to 15 minutes over medium heat, until the broccoli is fork tender. Using an immersion blender, blend until smooth. Stir in the heavy cream or coconut milk and hot sauce. Set the oven to broil. Transfer the soup to four oven-safe bowls and top each with one slice of cheese, if using. Place under the broiler for 2 to 3 minutes, until the cheese is melted and bubbly. Serve immediately.

WITH CHEESE	
TIME	**PER SERVING**
Active: 10 minutes	*Net Carbs:* 9.1g
	Total Carbs: 13.5g
	Fiber: 4.3g
Total: 30 minutes	*Protein:* 18.9g
	Fat: 27.4g
	Calories: 365
	FV = 6.8

WITHOUT CHEESE	
TIME	**PER SERVING**
Active: 10 minutes	*Net Carbs:* 8.8g
	Total Carbs: 13.1g
	Fiber: 4.3g
Total: 30 minutes	*Protein:* 11.8g
	Fat: 18g
	Calories: 251
	FV = 6.8

BONE BROTH
MINESTRONE

7.6g
NET CARBS

SERVES 4

280
CALORIES

Minestrone, a chunky vegetable soup from Italy, usually has high-carb ingredients such as white rice, pasta, and beans. This version features cauliflower instead and gets its rich savory flavor from your homemade bone broth and tangy Parmesan cheese. *Buon appetito!*

3 tablespoons unsalted butter

2 cups cauliflower florets, chopped

1 medium zucchini, cubed

½ onion, diced

4 garlic cloves, sliced

1 teaspoon Italian seasoning or chopped fresh oregano

1 teaspoon salt

½ teaspoon freshly ground black pepper

1 tablespoon tomato paste

1 quart Basic Bone Broth (page 161) or beef broth

1 cup baby kale leaves

½ cup packed fresh basil leaves

½ cup grated Parmesan cheese

1 Heat a large stockpot over medium heat and add the butter. When the butter foams, add the cauliflower, zucchini, onion, garlic, Italian seasoning or oregano, salt, and black pepper; cook 3 to 4 minutes, stirring often. Decrease the heat to low, and add the tomato paste. Cook 2 to 3 minutes, stirring often, until the paste becomes fragrant. Add the broth, and simmer on medium heat for 10 minutes, until the cauliflower is tender.

2 Add the kale and basil, and cook 3 minutes more, until the kale wilts. Spoon into four bowls, sprinkle with the Parmesan, and serve immediately.

TIME	PER SERVING
Active: 10 minutes	*Total Carbs:* 10.5g
	Fiber: 3g
Total: 40 minutes	*Protein:* 18.7g
	Fat: 19.3g
	FV = 7

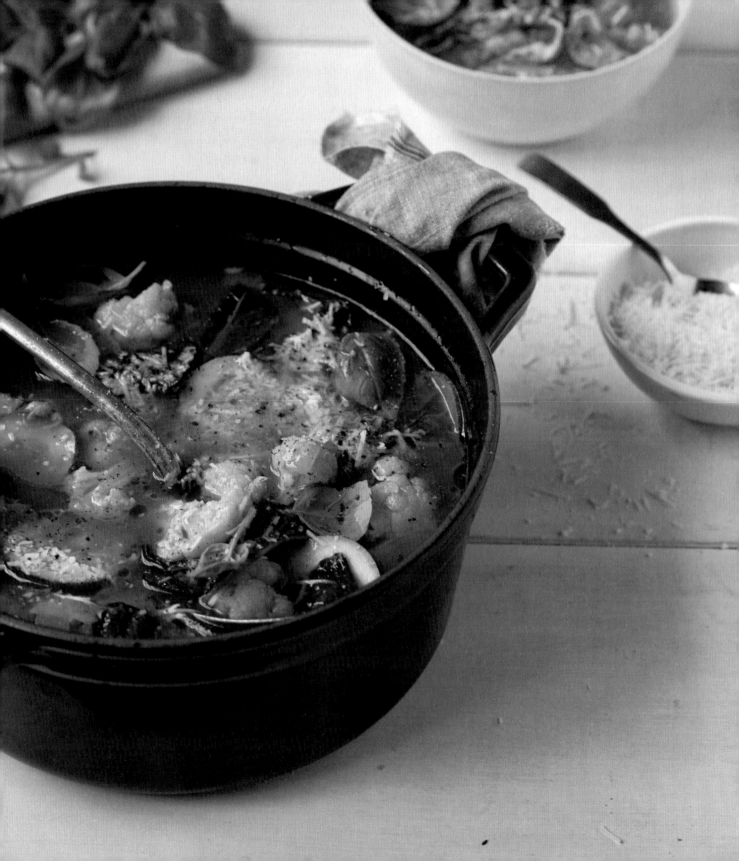

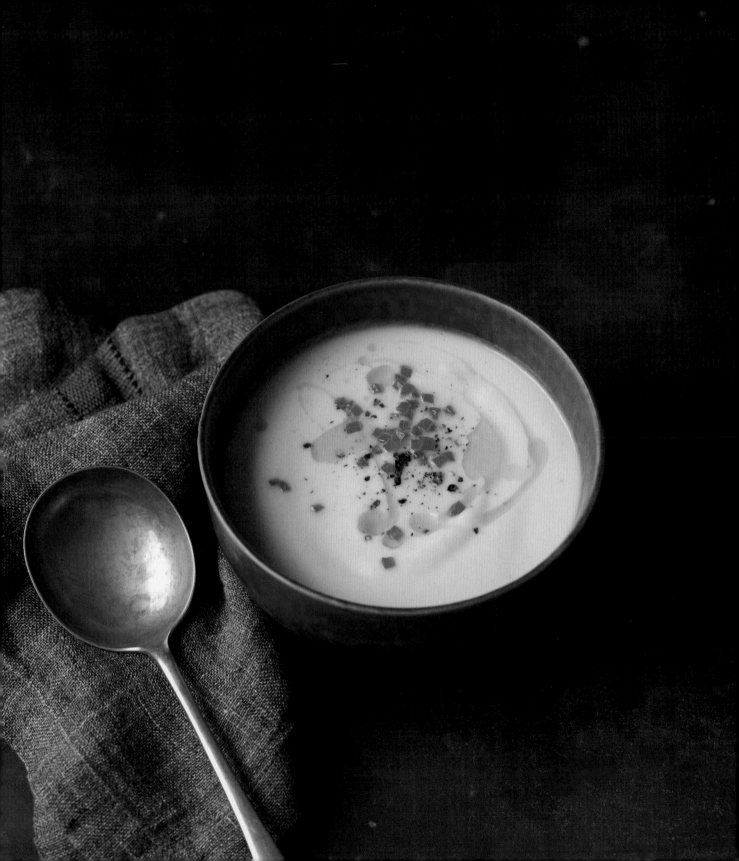

CAULIFLOWER
BISQUE

6.1g
NET CARBS

SERVES 4

339
CALORIES

Bisque is a smooth, creamy French soup that comes in many different flavors, from lobster to tomato and also cauliflower. Although this soup may appear to be a fine-dining treat, it's surprisingly easy to make and will satisfy any creamy craving.

TIME	PER SERVING
Active: 10 minutes	*Total Carbs:* 8.8g
	Fiber: 2.7g
Total: 30 minutes	*Protein:* 9.3g
	Fat: 27g
	FV = 5

3 tablespoons unsalted butter

1 small head cauliflower, cut into florets (about 5 cups)

4 garlic cloves, chopped

½ teaspoon salt

½ teaspoon freshly grated nutmeg

¼ teaspoon freshly ground black pepper

1 quart Basic Bone Broth (page 161) or unsalted chicken or vegetable broth

1 tablespoon lemon juice

½ cup heavy cream or canned coconut milk

4 teaspoons olive oil

½ red bell pepper, minced

1 Place the butter in a large stockpot, and warm over medium heat, about 1 minute, until the butter foams. Add the cauliflower, garlic, salt, nutmeg, and pepper; cook 5 to 6 minutes, stirring often, until the garlic begins to brown. Add the broth and lemon juice and cover.

2 Cook 15 to 20 minutes, until the cauliflower is fork tender. Using an immersion blender, blend until smooth. Stir in the heavy cream or coconut milk. Spoon into 4 bowls, garnish each serving with the olive oil and bell pepper, and serve immediately.

TIP

You can also puree creamy soups in a standing blender. Before you do so, be sure that the soup has cooled to room temperature. When hot soup is blended, it creates steam that will force the lid off the blender, so leave the lid ajar as a safety precaution. Reheat the soup as needed.

SPICY
KOREAN SOUP
with Scallions

4.7g
NET CARBS

SERVES 4

322
CALORIES

Yukgaejang, a spicy shredded beef soup with vegetables, is the inspiration for this beef soup with scallions. Depending on your carb intake, you can add 1 cup of spiralized zucchini noodles for an additional 3 grams of Net Carbs.

1 pound flank steak

½ teaspoon freshly ground black pepper

3 tablespoons sesame oil

10 ounces mushrooms, such as button, shiitake, or cremini

8 scallions, thinly sliced

4 garlic cloves, minced

1 to 2 teaspoons crushed red pepper flakes

¼ teaspoon salt

2 tablespoons soy sauce or tamari

2 tablespoons apple cider vinegar

1 quart beef broth or Basic Bone Broth (page 161)

1 Place the flank steak in a large stockpot, and cover with water. Add the pepper and bring to a boil over high heat. Reduce the heat to low and simmer for 2 hours, covered, until the meat is very tender. Drain, discarding the liquid, and let the beef cool. Use a fork to shred the meat. Wash and dry the stockpot.

2 Warm the oil in the stockpot over medium-low heat. Add the mushrooms, scallions, garlic, red pepper flakes, and salt, and cook for about 3 minutes, stirring often, until fragrant. Add the shredded beef, soy sauce or tamari, vinegar, and broth. Bring to a simmer and cook 4 to 5 minutes, until the mushrooms are tender. Serve immediately.

TIME	PER SERVING
Active: 15 minutes	*Total Carbs:* 6.4g
	Fiber: 1.7g
Total: 2 hours, 15 minutes	*Protein:* 29.7g
	Fat: 21.1g
	FV = 3.9

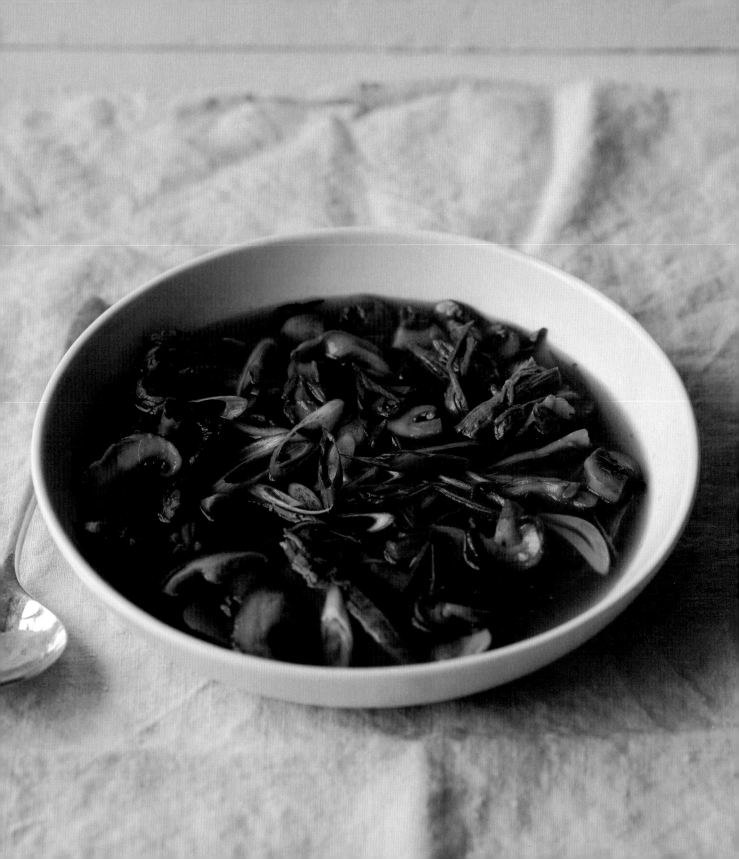

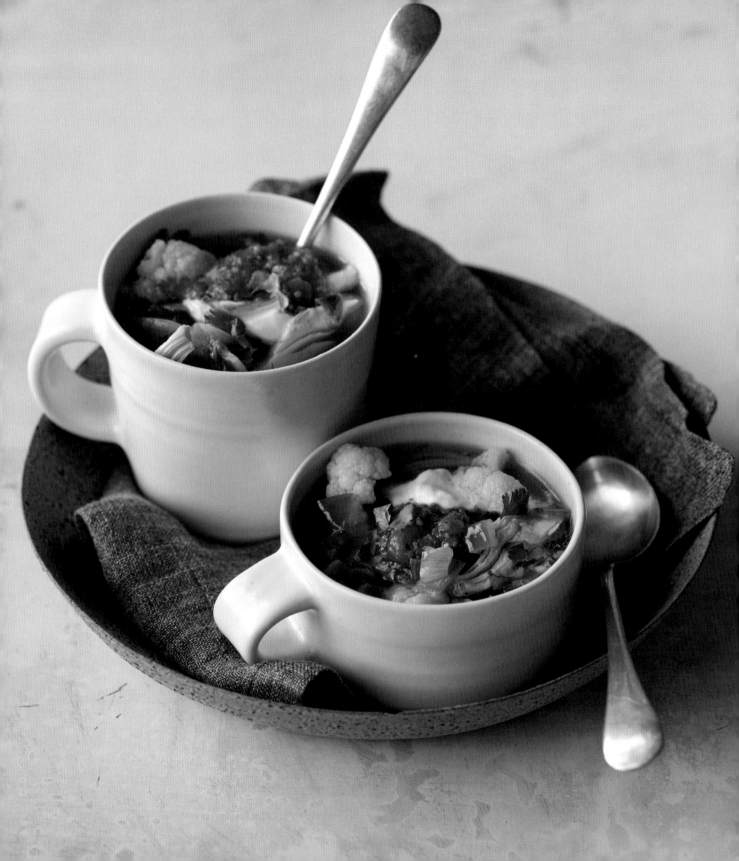

SALSA VERDE
CHICKEN SOUP

6.7g
NET CARBS

SERVES 4

340
CALORIES

Salsa verde, jarred or fresh, is a tangy green salsa made with tomatillos (husk tomatoes), onions, and plenty of cilantro. Hearty chicken, cauliflower, and sour cream turn this flavorful soup into a satisfying meal. Even if you are not a cilantro fan, you will enjoy cooked cilantro, since its flavor mellows quite a bit.

TIME	PER SERVING
Active: 10 minutes	*Total Carbs:* 8.6g
	Fiber: 2g
Total: 45 minutes	*Protein:* 33.5g
	Fat: 18.3g
	FV = 5

4 chicken breasts, on the bone, skin intact (about 1½ pounds)

½ teaspoon salt

½ teaspoon mild chili powder

¼ teaspoon freshly ground black pepper

2 tablespoons olive oil

½ red or white onion, minced

2 cups cauliflower florets

2 cups fresh cilantro leaves and stems, chopped and divided

4 garlic cloves

1 quart unsalted chicken broth

½ cup salsa verde from a jar

¼ cup sour cream

1 Sprinkle the chicken with the salt, chili powder, and pepper. Warm the oil in a large stockpot over medium heat. Add the chicken and cook 7 to 8 minutes, turning a few times, until the chicken is well browned. Transfer the chicken to a plate. Add the onion, cauliflower, half the cilantro, and the garlic, cooking 5 to 6 minutes more, until the vegetables soften.

2 Return the chicken to the stockpot, and cover with the broth. Bring to a simmer over medium heat and cook 20 to 25 minutes, until the chicken is cooked through. Transfer the chicken to a cutting board to cool. Discard the skin and bones, then shred the chicken. Return it to the soup, and top with the salsa verde and the remaining cilantro. Serve with the sour cream.

TURMERIC CARROT GINGER SOUP

9.6g
NET CARBS

SERVES 4

310
CALORIES

Turmeric is one of the top healing spices; in fact, this powerful anti-inflammatory spice has more than seven hundred medical studies behind it! Turmeric, a relative of the ginger root, has a tart flavor that works well with sweeter foods such as carrot and is a great way to perk up mild-tasting proteins such as shrimp.

TIME	PER SERVING
Active: 15 minutes	*Total Carbs:* 13.3g
	Fiber: 3.7g
Total: 25 minutes	*Protein:* 30g
	Fat: 15.2g
	FV = 7.4

- **4 tablespoons unsalted butter or olive oil, divided**
- **4 carrots, thinly sliced**
- **2 cups cauliflower florets**
- **4 garlic cloves, chopped**
- **½ teaspoon salt**
- **¼ teaspoon freshly ground black pepper**
- **1 small fresh turmeric root, chopped (about 2 teaspoons) or 1 teaspoon ground turmeric**
- **1 tablespoon peeled, grated ginger**
- **1 quart Basic Bone Broth (page 161) or chicken broth**
- **1 pound jumbo shrimp (21 to 25 count), with heads**
- **½ teaspoon hot or sweet paprika**

TIP

For a restaurant-worthy garnish, mix 2 tablespoons minced fresh cilantro with a few teaspoons of water and drizzle it into the soup.

1 Warm 3 tablespoons of the butter or olive oil in a large stockpot over medium heat. Add the carrots, cauliflower, garlic, salt, and pepper; cook 5 to 6 minutes, stirring often, until the vegetables start to brown. Add the turmeric and ginger and cook 1 minute more to blend the flavors.

2 Add the broth and cover, increasing the heat to medium high. As soon as the soup comes to a boil, reduce to low and cook 7 to 8 additional minutes, until the carrots and cauliflower are tender. Using an immersion blender, blend until smooth.

3 Warm the remaining 1 tablespoon butter or olive oil in a large skillet over medium heat. Add the shrimp, and sprinkle with the paprika and pepper. Cook 6 to 8 minutes, turning the shrimp often, until the shells are pink and the meat is no longer translucent inside. Divide the shrimp among four soup bowls, ladle the soup over the shrimp, and serve immediately.

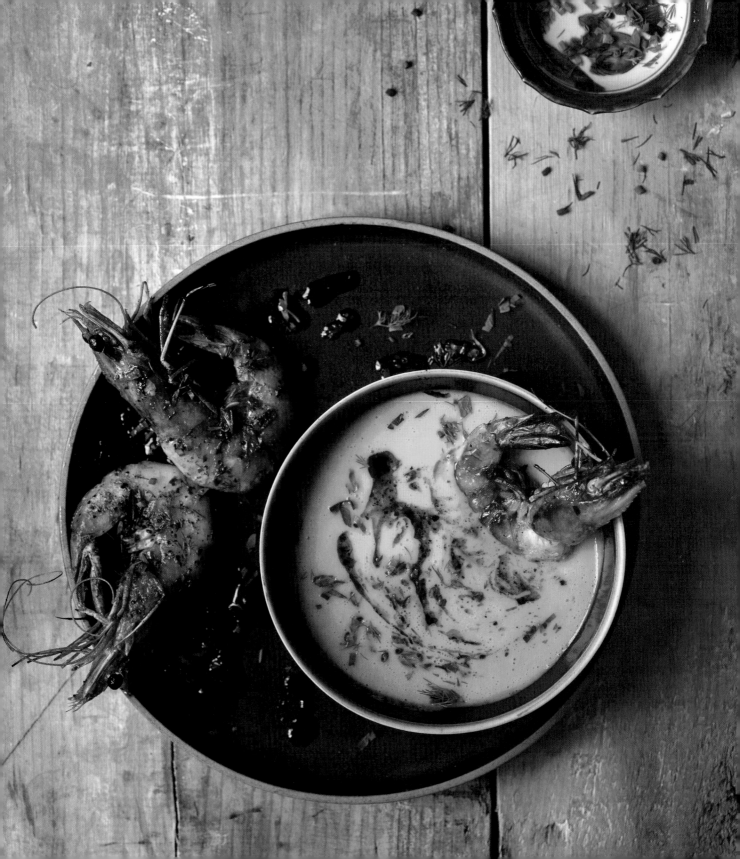

THAI
TOM YUM SOUP

6.8g
NET CARBS

SERVES
4

274
CALORIES

Thai tom yum soup has a sweet and hot flavor that any chili fan will enjoy, and it can easily be paired with your favorite protein. If you can't locate the tiny but pungent Thai chilies, look for serrano chilies or even a sliver of habanero to use instead. You can also take the hotness factor down a notch by cutting the amount of chilies and chili paste in half.

TIME	PER SERVING
Active: 10 minutes	*Total Carbs:* 7.3g
	Fiber: 0.5 gram
Total: 20 minutes	Protein: 29.9g
	Fat: 12.4g
	FV = 2.9

1 quart chicken broth

1 stalk lemongrass, chopped

1 (1-inch) piece ginger, peeled and minced

2 small red or green chilies, such as Thai bird chilies, halved

1 pound large shrimp (31 to 35 count), peeled and deveined, or 1 pound thinly sliced chicken

1 cup canned coconut milk

1 tablespoon red chili paste

1 tablespoon fish sauce

2 scallions, thinly sliced

½ cup fresh cilantro leaves and stems

1 Place the broth in a large stockpot along with the lemongrass, ginger, and chilies. Bring to a simmer over medium heat.

2 Add the shrimp or chicken, coconut milk, chili paste, fish sauce, scallions, and cilantro. Turn the heat off, cover, and let rest for 5 to 6 minutes, until the shrimp or chicken slices are cooked through. Remove and discard the lemongrass. Serve immediately.

CREAM OF
HEIRLOOM
TOMATO SOUP

5.8g NET CARBS

SERVES 4

364 CALORIES

Like the cauliflower bisque, this silky soup, made from freshly roasted farmer's market tomatoes, will hit the spot when you're in the mood for something creamy and seasonal. If you can't locate heirlooms, red tomatoes on the vine or beefsteak tomatoes work well, too.

TIME	PER SERVING
Active: 15 minutes	*Total Carbs:* 7.7g
	Fiber: 1.9g
Total: 30 minutes	*Protein:* 43.1g
	Fat: 16.9g
	FV = 4

1 pound heirloom tomatoes, chopped

1 tablespoon olive oil

2 tablespoons tomato paste

1 teaspoon Italian seasoning or herb salt

1 quart Basic Bone Broth (page 161) or unsalted chicken broth

¼ cup heavy cream

¼ cup grated Pecorino cheese

2 tablespoons Atkins Flour Mix (page 126)

1 pound shredded or cubed chicken (optional)

1 Preheat the oven to 400°F. Line a baking sheet with aluminum foil. Place the tomatoes on the baking sheet, and drizzle them with the olive oil, dot with the tomato paste, and sprinkle them with the Italian seasoning or herb salt. Roast for 20 to 25 minutes, until the tomato paste starts to brown. Transfer to a large stockpot, and add the broth. Bring to a simmer over medium heat and cook 2 to 3 minutes, until the tomatoes begin to break apart.

2 Turn the heat off, and add the cream and Pecorino cheese. Sprinkle the flour mix over the surface of the soup. Use an immersion blender and blend until smooth. Top with the chicken, if desired.

TUSCAN
KALE SOUP

8.1g NET CARBS   SERVES **4**   **260** CALORIES

Lacinato kale (also known as black, dinosaur, or Tuscan kale), with its bumpy dark skin, is delicious cooked in soups, since it has a heartier texture with a hint of spice that pairs well with sausage. If you're a spice fan, go for spicy Italian sausage and a dash of chili flakes.

TIME	PER SERVING
Active: 15 minutes	*Total Carbs:* 9.7g *Fiber:* 1.6g
Total: 45 minutes	*Protein:* 26.4g *Fat:* 13.3g *FV* = 5.2

Olive oil spray

5 sweet or hot Italian sausage links, chopped (3 ounces each)

2 cups chopped lacinato or Tuscan kale (see Tip, page 187)

2 celery stalks, thinly sliced

4 garlic cloves, minced

1 quart Basic Bone Broth (page 161), beef broth, or chicken broth

2 tablespoons tomato paste

½ teaspoon crushed red pepper flakes (optional)

½ cup grated Parmesan cheese

1   Coat a large stockpot with olive oil spray. Add the sausage, place over medium heat, and cook 8 to 9 minutes, stirring often, until the sausage browns and is cooked through. Add the kale, celery, and garlic, and cook 1 to 2 minutes more, coating with the rendered fat from the sausage. Add the broth, tomato paste, and red pepper flakes, if desired.

2   Bring to a simmer and cover. Cook 2 to 3 minutes, until the kale is cooked through. Sprinkle with the Parmesan, and serve immediately.

CHILLED
AVOCADO
CRAB
GAZPACHO

3.9g
NET CARBS

SERVES 4

168
CALORIES

Gazpacho, a Spanish chilled soup made from tomatoes, is typically served as an appetizer to cool you down on a blistering hot day. This filling version, based on fiber-rich avocado, is also great for summer dining when you're ready to beat the heat and get out of the kitchen.

TIME	PER SERVING
Active: 10 minutes	*Total Carbs:* 8.1g
	Fiber: 4.2g
Total: 10 minutes	*Protein:* 15.5g
	Fat: 8.6g
	FV = 3.4

- **2 cups unsalted chicken broth or Basic Bone Broth (page 161)**
- **1 ripe Hass avocado, cubed**
- **1 cucumber, peeled and chopped**
- **2 garlic cloves, peeled and cut in half**
- **1 green bell pepper, seeded and chopped**
- **½ cup packed fresh mint leaves**
- **2 tablespoons red wine vinegar**
- **½ teaspoon salt**
- **¼ teaspoon freshly ground black pepper**
- **8 ounces pasteurized crab meat, picked over for shells and cartilage**

Place the broth, avocado, cucumber, garlic, bell pepper, mint, vinegar, salt, and pepper in a blender, and process until smooth. Transfer to a large bowl, cover, and refrigerate until chilled, at least 2 hours and up to 8 hours. Dish into four bowls, top with the crab meat, and serve immediately.

ROPA VIEJA

SOUP

6.2g
NET CARBS

SERVES 4

322
CALORIES

Ropa Vieja is a national dish from Cuba; in Spanish, it means "old clothes," since the tender, shredded beef resembles twisted old fabric. This soup skips the rice and beans of the traditional version but still has the great flavors of oregano, green bell pepper, cilantro, and tomato. You can serve this soup with cauliflower rice (page 232) instead of rice and beans.

TIME	PER SERVING
Active: 15 minutes	*Total Carbs:* 8.3g
	Fiber: 2.1g
Total: 2 hours, 30 minutes	*Protein:* 27g
	Fat: 21g
	FV = 6

1 pound flank steak

3 tablespoons olive oil

1 green bell pepper, seeded and chopped

½ onion, chopped

½ cup fresh cilantro leaves and stems

4 garlic cloves, minced

1 teaspoon dried oregano

½ teaspoon ground cumin

½ teaspoon salt

¼ teaspoon freshly ground black pepper

1 quart Basic Bone Broth (page 161) or beef broth

2 tomatoes, chopped

1 tablespoon tomato paste

1 Place the steak in a large stockpot, and cover with water. Cook 2 hours, covered, until the meat is very tender. Drain and set the beef aside. Using a fork, shred the meat. Wash and dry the stockpot.

2 Place the olive oil in the stockpot over medium heat. Add the bell pepper, onion, cilantro, garlic, oregano, cumin, salt, and black pepper; cook 5 to 7 minutes, stirring occasionally, until the onion is soft. Add the broth, tomatoes, and tomato paste, along with the shredded beef. Bring to a simmer and cover. Cook 4 to 5 minutes more to allow the flavors to meld, then serve immediately.

HOT-AND-SOUR
SOUP

7.4g
NET CARBS

**SERVES
4**

318
CALORIES

Hot-and-sour soup, popular on Chinese take-out menus, combines Szechuan-based flavors such as spicy red chilies with savory vinegar and healing shiitake mushrooms. Hot-and-sour soup is typically made with pork—this one uses tender pork chop meat—but feel free to substitute the pork with equal portions of firm tofu or even peeled, deveined shrimp.

3 tablespoons sesame oil

4 pork chops (1 pound), thinly sliced against the grain, bone discarded

5 ounces shiitake mushrooms, stems discarded, caps sliced

½ red onion, thinly sliced

3 garlic cloves, minced

1 tablespoon peeled, minced ginger root

1 tablespoon crushed red pepper flakes

2 cups thinly sliced cabbage

1 quart Basic Bone Broth (page 161), beef broth, or unsalted chicken broth

2 tablespoons tamari or soy sauce

2 tablespoons white distilled vinegar

1 teaspoon stevia

1 Place the sesame oil in a large stockpot over medium heat. Add the pork, shiitakes, onion, garlic, ginger, and red pepper flakes; cook 4 to 5 minutes, stirring occasionally, until the pork starts to brown and the mushrooms are tender.

2 Add the cabbage, broth, tamari, vinegar, and stevia. Bring to a simmer, and cook 2 to 3 minutes more to allow the flavors to meld and the cabbage to soften. Serve immediately.

TIME	PER SERVING
Active: 15 minutes	*Total Carbs:* 9.5g *Fiber:* 2.1g *Protein:* 22.9g
Total: 30 minutes	*Fat:* 21g *FV* = 6.3

9
SALADS

FRESH VEGETABLES,

Leafy Greens, and

FLAVORFUL DRESSINGS

⬡

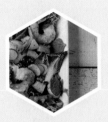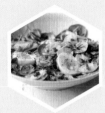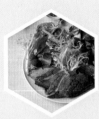

Salads are a staple of Atkins, because there are so many delicious and naturally low-carb variations of vegetables, leafy greens, fresh and creamy dressings, and meat, poultry, and fish that you can put together in no time at all. If you're ready to break out of your "same old" salad routine, these recipes are the key.

RECIPES

OLD BAY
SHRIMP
SALAD

3g
NET CARBS

SERVES
4

409
CALORIES

Old Bay seasoning, created in the 1930s in the Chesapeake Bay area, is the perfect flavoring for delicate seafood such as crab and shrimp, with its blend of many savory spices including celery salt, black pepper, bay leaf, and red pepper. This chilled shrimp salad is ideal picnic fare and a great low-carb swap for traditional potato salad.

TIME	PER SERVING
Active: 15 minutes	*Total Carbs:* 4.7g
	Fiber: 1.8g
Total: 30 minutes	*Protein:* 24.4g
	Fat: 32.2g
	FV = 1.9

1 pound frozen cooked baby shrimp, defrosted

1 cup cauliflower florets, chopped

2 celery stalks, thinly sliced

¾ cup mayonnaise

2 scallions, thinly sliced

1 tablespoon Old Bay seasoning or seasoning salt (see Tip)

1 head Bibb lettuce, broken into 12 leaves

Drain the baby shrimp on paper towels or a kitchen towel to be sure they are dry. Transfer to a large bowl along with the cauliflower, celery, mayonnaise, scallions, and Old Bay. Stir well. Set the leaves out and divide the salad between the 12 leaves and serve immediately.

TIP

If you want to sub out the Old Bay, *a blend of ¼ teaspoon each of sweet paprika, celery salt, garlic salt, and black pepper is an option.*

WATERCRESS
BACON
SALAD
with Ranch Dressing

4.4g
NET CARBS

SERVES 4

353
CALORIES

Spicy watercress is part of the superhealing cruciferous family, which also includes kale, broccoli, and cauliflower—some of the most nutrient-dense foods around. Watercress is most abundant in spring, and it adds the vitamins, fiber, and anti-inflammatory nutrients your body thrives on. Topped with tomatoes, bacon, and ranch dressing, this salad is jam-packed with flavor.

TIME	PER SERVING
Active: 15 minutes	*Total Carbs:* 9.6g
	Fiber: 5.2g
	Protein: 7.5g
Total: 30 minutes	*Fat:* 33.2g
	FV = 3.8

½ pound watercress

½ pound baby spinach

2 tomatoes, chopped

1 ripe Hass avocado, diced

4 slices cooked bacon, crumbled

Combine the watercress and spinach, tossing well. Divide among four plates and top with the tomatoes, avocado, and bacon. Serve immediately with the dressing.

RANCH DRESSING

½ cup mayonnaise

2 tablespoons canned coconut milk or heavy cream

1 teaspoon apple cider vinegar

½ teaspoon onion powder

½ teaspoon garlic salt

1 tablespoon chopped fresh dill or flat-leaf parsley

¼ teaspoon freshly ground black pepper

Place the mayonnaise, coconut milk or heavy cream, vinegar, onion powder, garlic salt, dill or parsley, and black pepper in a large bowl. Whisk well to combine. Serve over the salad.

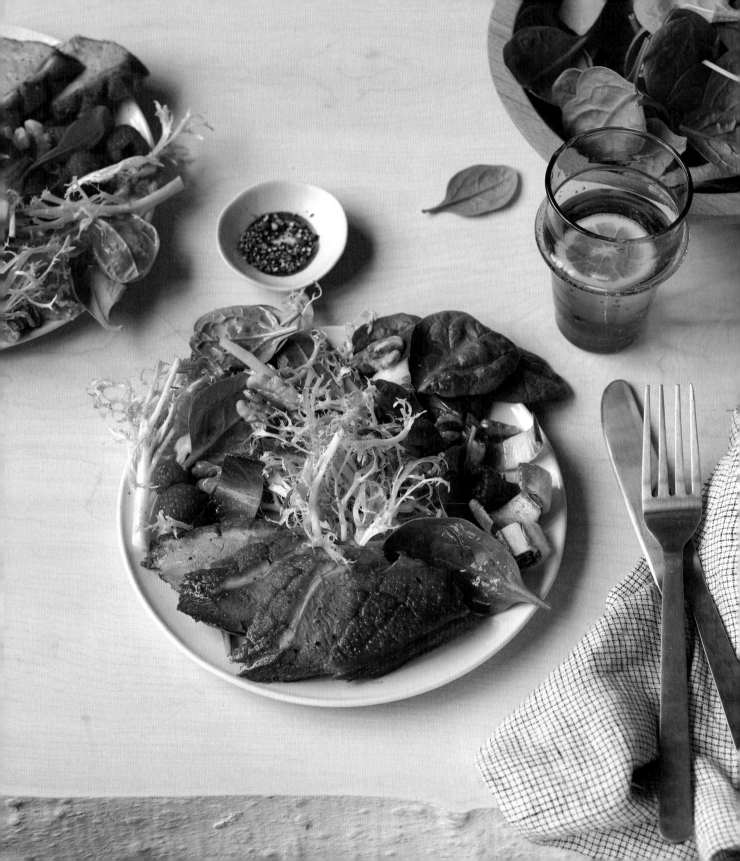

CRISPY DUCK
SPINACH SALAD

with Warm and Tangy Turmeric Dressing

3.5g
NET CARBS

SERVES 4

333
CALORIES

Don't be daunted by the idea of cooking duck, which has delicious red meat that any steak lover will appreciate. Duck is traditionally paired with something sweet, so high-antioxidant raspberries provide a hint of sweetness without sugar overload.

TIME	PER SERVING
Active: 15 minutes	*Total Carbs:* 9.2g
	Fiber: 5.7g
Total: 30 minutes	*Protein:* 33.3g
	Fat: 18.5g
	FV = 1

2 duck breasts, fat trimmed to ½ inch thick

¼ teaspoon salt

¼ teaspoon freshly ground black pepper

½ pound baby spinach

½ pound frisée or endive leaves, chopped

¼ cup walnuts

1 cup fresh raspberries

1 Score the fat side of the duck breast with a sharp knife. Sprinkle the duck with half the salt and black pepper. Place the duck breast, fat side down, in a large, cold skillet. Cook 7 to 8 minutes, until the fat is crisp. Flip and cook 4 to 5 minutes more, until the duck is no longer translucent red inside but still pink. Remove the duck from the skillet, reserving the fat. Let the duck rest for 5 minutes. Slice the duck across the grain. Make the dressing as directed.

2 Divide the spinach and frisée or endive among four plates, and drizzle with the dressing. Top with the sliced duck, walnuts, and raspberries. Serve immediately.

WARM AND TANGY TURMERIC DRESSING

¼ cup red wine vinegar

¼ teaspoon salt

¼ teaspoon freshly ground black pepper

½ teaspoon ground turmeric

½ teaspoon sweet paprika

Add the vinegar to the warm reserved fat in the skillet, along with the salt, pepper, turmeric, and paprika, whisking well.

TIP

Look for duck breasts *(magrets) at farmer's markets or in upscale grocery chains that handle specialty meats. Just trim away some of the "fat cap," or thick fat flap, that covers the breast meat of most commercial brands of duck, leaving the skin attached.*

TIP

If you have time, *refrigerate the duck breasts overnight, leaving the skin side uncovered, but the flesh protected with plastic wrap. This will air-dry and tighten the skin to release even more fat during cooking.*

KALE CAESAR SALAD

with Creamy Meyer Lemon Dressing

SERVES 4

Tired of the same old Caesar salad? This version uses the top superfood kale and Meyer lemon—a sweeter variety of lemon—to create a fresh take on an everyday classic. The Meyer lemon is a hybrid citrus fruit that isn't as sweet as an orange but is less tangy than a standard lemon. The secret to tender kale salad? Massage the leaves first.

1 (14-ounce) package extra-firm tofu, well drained

2 tablespoons Atkins Flour Mix (page 126)

½ teaspoon Old Bay seasoning or garlic salt

Olive oil spray

10 ounces kale, curly or lacinato (see Tip)

½ cup shaved Parmesan cheese

1 Place the tofu onto paper towels, and pat dry. Cut into 16 (1-inch) cubes. Place the Atkins Flour Mix and Old Bay seasoning or garlic salt on a plate. Mix well with your fingers or a fork. Dredge the tofu cubes in the flour mixture. Coat a large skillet with olive oil spray, and place over medium heat. Add the tofu cubes and cook 3 to 4 minutes, adding more olive oil spray as necessary, until the tofu is crisp.

2 Place the kale in a large bowl, and toss with the dressing. Divide among four plates and top each with the tofu croutons and Parmesan.

CREAMY MEYER LEMON DRESSING

¼ cup mayonnaise

¼ cup heavy cream or canned coconut milk

½ teaspoon garlic salt

½ teaspoon onion powder

½ teaspoon freshly ground black pepper

2 tablespoons fresh Meyer lemon or regular lemon juice

Place the mayonnaise, heavy cream, garlic salt, onion power, black pepper, and lemon juice in a small bowl. Whisk well and set aside.

WITH TOFU	
TIME	**PER SERVING**
Active: 15 minutes	*Net Carbs:* 9g
	Total Carbs: 12.2g
	Fiber: 3.2g
Total: 30 minutes	*Protein:* 19.5g
	Fat: 24.2g
	Calories: 340
	FV = 5.6

WITH CHICKEN	
TIME	**PER SERVING**
Active: 15 minutes	*Net Carbs* 7.8g
	Total Carbs: 9.7g
	Fiber: 1.9g
Total: 30 minutes	*Protein:* 20.1g
	Fat: 22g
	Calories: 310
	FV = 5.6

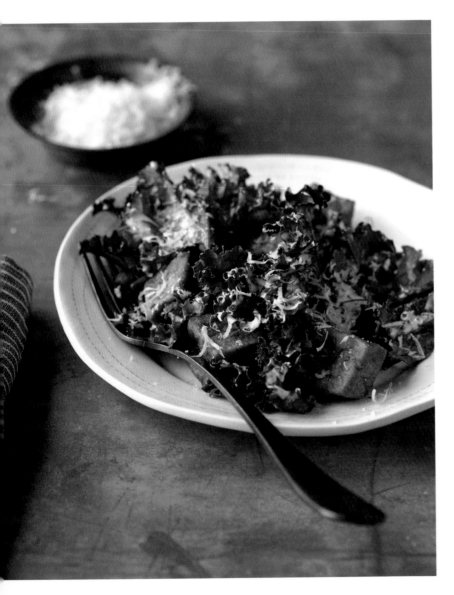

To prep tougher, larger leaves *for kale salads, remove the tough bottom stem and thick rib that runs up the center of the leaf. Tear the leaves into bite-sized pieces and squeeze them, about 1 minute, to tenderize the kale.*

You can serve this salad as a **healthy side,** *without the tofu croutons, or, as a protein swap in place of the tofu, toss with cooked shrimp, chicken, or slices of grilled flank steak.*

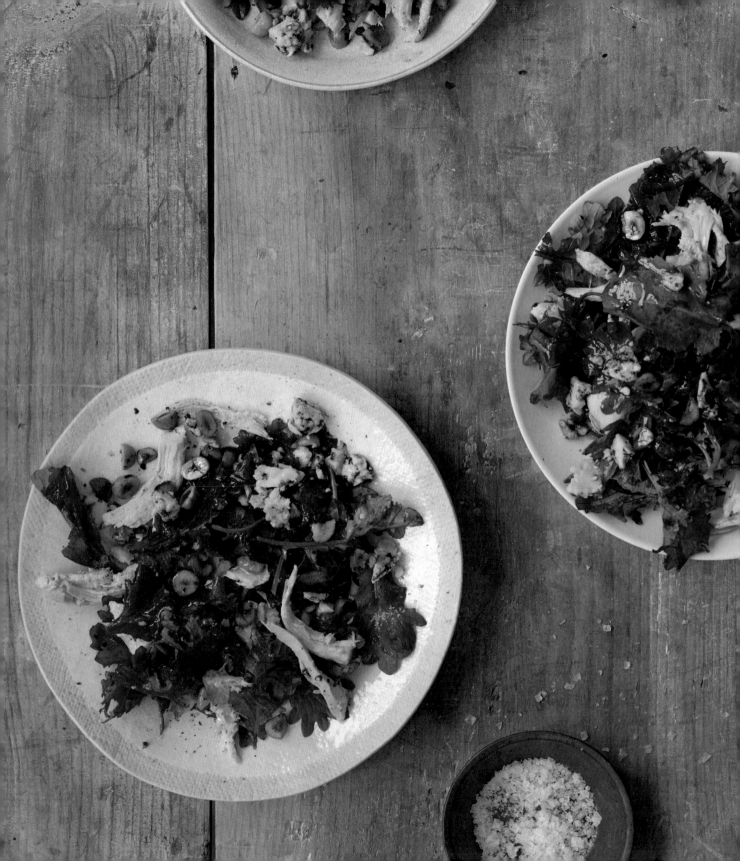

BABY KALE

AND BLUE CHEESE SALAD

with Warm Hazelnut Dressing

4.5g NET CARBS

SERVES **4**

362 CALORIES

You can enjoy this salad any time of year, but if you want to go seasonal, start your fall off with kale. Kale is best as the weather turns colder; it actually becomes sweeter when the first frost hits. Cooking hazelnuts in oil not only toasts them but also helps flavor this uniquely fragrant dressing.

TIME	PER SERVING
Active: 10 minutes	*Total Carbs:* 7.8g
	Fiber: 3.3g
Total: 10 minutes	*Protein:* 31.3g
	Fat: 22.3g
	FV = 3.8

10 ounces baby kale

¼ cup crumbled blue cheese

1 pound cooked shrimp or shredded chicken

Place the kale in a large bowl, pour the dressing over the greens, and toss well. Top with the blue cheese and shrimp or chicken, and serve immediately.

WARM HAZELNUT DRESSING

¼ cup olive oil

¼ cup skinned hazelnuts, chopped

4 large fresh sage leaves, chopped

½ teaspoon salt

¼ teaspoon freshly ground black pepper

¼ cup red wine vinegar

Warm the olive oil in a small skillet over medium heat. Add the hazelnuts, sage, salt, and pepper. Cook 1 to 2 minutes, until the sage is crisp. Turn the heat off, add the vinegar, and stir well.

WILTED
BRUSSELS SPROUT
SALAD

with Warm Pancetta
Dressing

4g
NET CARBS

SERVES
4

217
CALORIES

Think of Brussels sprouts as mini-cabbages with all the same great nutrition and antioxidants, including vitamin C, vitamins B$_1$ and B$_6$, and folate. They are delicious raw, especially with a hot dressing made from pancetta drippings , which take the place of the oil in standard dressings.

TIME	PER SERVING
Active: 15 minutes	*Total Carbs:* 8.1g
	Fiber: 3.1g
Total: 30 minutes	*Protein:* 13.5g
	Fat: 14.7g
	FV = 3.8

½ pound Brussels sprouts

5 ounces baby spinach or kale

4 hard-cooked eggs, quartered

4 ounces pancetta, diced

1 Shred the Brussels sprouts in a food processor with the shredder attachment. Divide the spinach and Brussels sprouts among four plates. Divide the eggs among the plates.

2 Place the pancetta in a small skillet over medium heat. Cook 4 to 5 minutes, stirring occasionally, until well browned, reserving the fat in the skillet. Make the dressing as directed. Divide the pancetta among the salad plates. Drizzle the dressing over the salad, and serve immediately.

WARM PANCETTA DRESSING

4 garlic cloves, minced

¼ cup apple cider vinegar

2 teaspoons Dijon mustard

Place the skillet with the fat from the pancetta that you cooked over low heat and add the garlic; cook 1 to 2 minutes, until fragrant. Turn the heat off, carefully add the vinegar and the mustard to the skillet, and stir well, scraping up any brown bits sticking inside the pan.

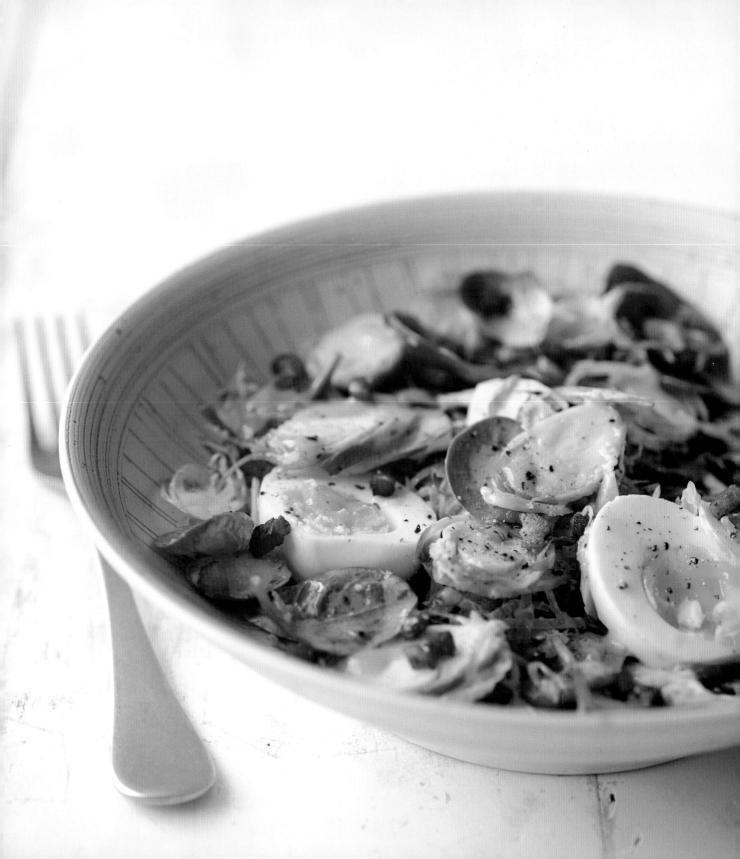

CHILLED ROMAINE
WEDGE
SALAD

with Gorgonzola Dressing

5.2g
NET CARBS

SERVES
4

367
CALORIES

Steak houses are famous for their iceberg wedge salads, which are delicious but offer few nutrients. This recipe uses vitamin A–rich romaine, a superfood, as its base, and teaches you a unique technique to make it just as crispy as a wedge of iceberg lettuce.

TIME	PER SERVING
Active: 15 minutes	*Total Carbs:* 8.7g
	Fiber: 3.6g
Total: 30 minutes	*Protein:* 21.3g
	Fat: 27.8g
	FV = 1.9

4 romaine lettuce hearts

4 slices cooked bacon, crumbled, or ½ cup cooked pancetta, chopped

½ pound cooked shrimp or chicken

Fill two large bowls with lukewarm water. Add the romaine hearts and soak 3 to 4 minutes while you prepare the dressing. Drain the romaine, wrap in paper towels, and chill in the fridge for at least 1 hour to crisp it up. Cut the romaine hearts in half and place two halves on each plate. Drizzle with the dressing and sprinkle with the pepper. Top with the bacon or pancetta and the shrimp or chicken.

GORGONZOLA DRESSING

½ cup full-fat Greek yogurt

½ cup mayonnaise

¼ cup Gorgonzola, cut into small pieces

2 tablespoons lemon juice

1 teaspoon onion powder

½ teaspoon garlic salt

¼ teaspoon freshly ground black pepper

¼ teaspoon sweet paprika

Place the yogurt, mayonnaise, Gorgonzola, lemon juice, onion powder, garlic salt, pepper, and paprika in a medium bowl along with 2 tablespoons warm water and whisk well. Refrigerate until ready to serve.

MIXED
POWER GREENS

with Prosciutto-wrapped Chicken Tenders

4.8g
NET CARBS

SERVES
4

295
CALORIES

Many farms are calling their salad mixes "power greens," since most of them are made up of superfood leafy greens such as beet, kale, red leaf, and romaine. If you can't find "power greens," you can still take advantage of the power of superfoods by using a mix of baby kale and spinach.

TIME	PER SERVING
Active: 15 minutes	*Total Carbs:* 9.3g
	Fiber: 4.6g
Total: 30 minutes	*Protein:* 33.5g
	Fat: 13.1g
	FV = 4.5

Olive oil spray

4 slices prosciutto (about 1 ounce)

8 chicken tenders (1 pound)

5 ounces mixed "power greens" or baby spinach

½ pound green beans or snow peas, trimmed and chopped

1 Preheat the oven to 400°F. Coat a baking sheet with olive oil spray. Cut the prosciutto slices in half diagonally, making a total of 8 pieces. Wrap each chicken tender in ½ slice of prosciutto and place on the baking sheet. Coat the tops of the tenders with olive oil spray, and bake 6 to 8 minutes, until the prosciutto is crisped and the chicken is cooked through and no longer pink in the center when sliced.

2 Divide the greens among four plates along with the green beans. Transfer the tenders to the salad, and drizzle with the dressing. Serve immediately.

MUSTARD VINAIGRETTE

3 tablespoons olive oil

2 tablespoons red wine or apple cider vinegar

1 teaspoon Dijon mustard

½ teaspoon garlic salt

¼ teaspoon freshly ground black pepper

Place the olive oil, vinegar, mustard, salt, and pepper in a small bowl and whisk well.

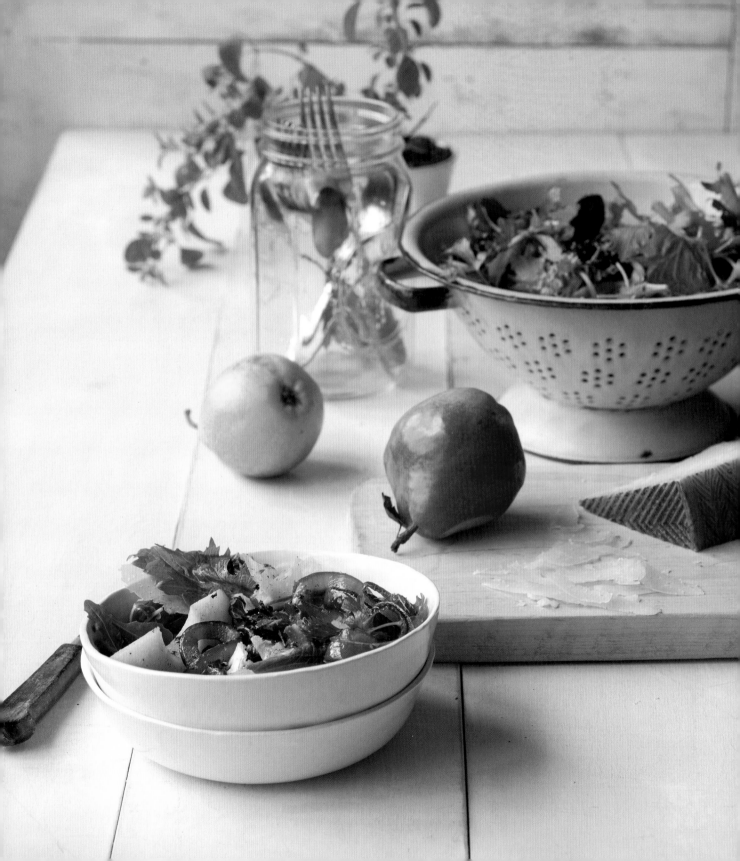

PEAR AND MANCHEGO
MESCLUN SALAD

with Caramelized Onions

7.8g
NET CARBS

SERVES
4

253
CALORIES

Juicy pear, salty Manchego, and sweet caramelized onions make a delectable salad topping, especially when drizzled with a sweet and tangy apple cider vinegar dressing. Manchego is an aged sheep's milk cheese from La Mancha, Spain, that you can find in most cheese shops, or you can use thinly sliced Romano or Parmesan in its place.

TIME	PER SERVING
Active: 15 minutes	*Total Carbs:* 11.5g
	Fiber: 3.6g
Total: 30 minutes	*Protein:* 8.9g
	Fat: 20.2g
	FV = 1.5

1 tablespoon olive oil

1 onion, thinly sliced

1 teaspoon stevia

8 ounces "power greens," mesclun, or spinach mixed with baby kale

¼ cup loosely packed fresh parsley leaves

½ pear, thinly sliced

¼ pound Manchego cheese, thinly sliced

1 Warm the olive oil in a medium skillet over medium heat. Add the onion and stevia; cook 8 to 10 minutes, stirring often, until golden brown. Add a few tablespoons of water to keep the onion from sticking as it cooks.

2 Divide the greens and parsley among four plates. Top with the pear slices, onion, and Manchego cheese. Drizzle with the dressing and serve immediately.

APPLE CIDER VINEGAR DRESSING

2 tablespoons olive oil

1 tablespoon apple cider vinegar

1 teaspoon Dijon mustard

½ teaspoon salt

¼ teaspoon freshly ground black pepper

Place the olive oil in a bowl along with the vinegar, mustard, salt, and pepper. Whisk well. Add one tablespoon of water and whisk again.

GREEN GODDESS
SALAD

with Lemon Tahini Dressing

7.7g
NET CARBS

SERVES
4

292
CALORIES

Tahini is a Middle Eastern sesame paste that you can find in the international aisle of your local grocery. Its texture makes an excellent smooth base for any salad dressing and sesame seeds are high in iron (for healthy blood and heart) and zinc, an immune system booster.

TIME	PER SERVING
Active: 15 minutes	*Total Carbs:* 14.9g
	Fiber: 7.2g
Total: 15 minutes	*Protein:* 28.6g
	Fat: 14.9g
	FV = 5.3

5 ounces mixed greens, "power greens," or baby spinach

1 ripe Hass avocado, diced

2 tomatoes, diced

½ cup pitted black olives

4 radishes, thinly sliced

½ pound alfalfa or other sprouts

1 pound cooked shrimp or shredded chicken

Divide the greens among four plates, and top with the avocado, tomatoes, olives, radishes, and sprouts. Drizzle with the dressing, then top with the shrimp or chicken. Serve immediately.

LEMON TAHINI DRESSING

2 tablespoons well-stirred tahini

¼ cup water

1 scallion, chopped

2 tablespoons fresh lemon juice

½ teaspoon garlic salt

¼ teaspoon stevia

Place the tahini, water, scallion, lemon juice, garlic salt, and stevia in a food processor, and process until smooth. Whisk well.

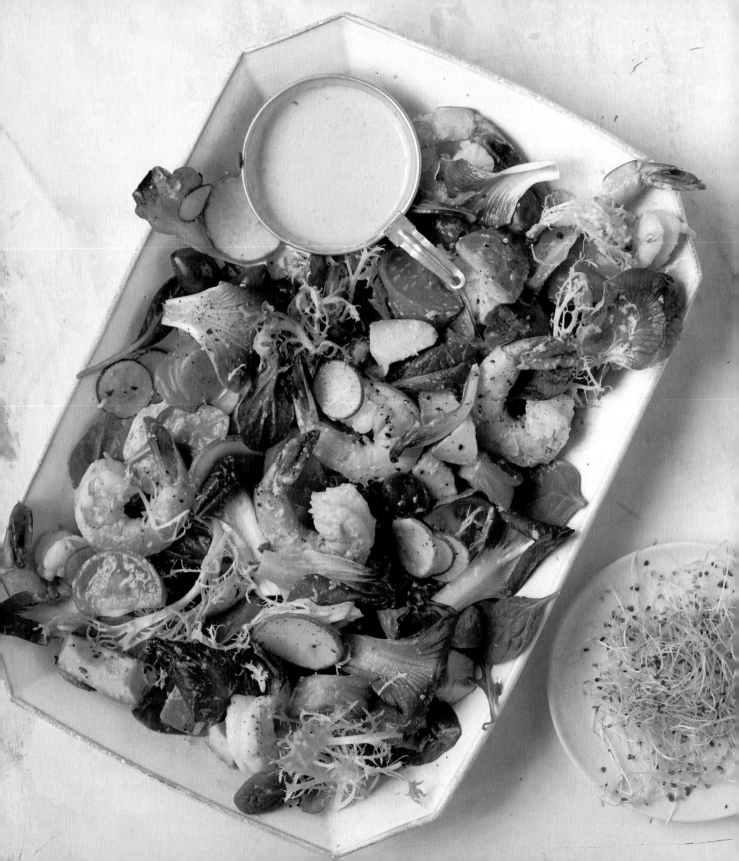

GARLIC BUTTER
LOBSTER
SALAD

5.3g NET CARBS

SERVES 4

215 CALORIES

Even if you're not an expert chef, this upscale dish is incredibly easy to make and will make you look like a champ in the kitchen. It's perfect for date night or any celebration. For added creaminess, top with 1 avocado, thinly sliced.

TIME	PER SERVING
Active: 15 minutes	*Total Carbs:* 9.4g
	Fiber: 4g
Total: 30 minutes	*Protein:* 25.1g
	Fat: 9.2g
	FV = 3.6

Zest of 1 lemon, finely grated

1 tablespoon lemon juice

1 tablespoon mayonnaise

½ teaspoon seasoning salt or garlic salt

2 cups chopped baby spinach or kale

2 celery stalks, minced

1 head butter lettuce, divided into 8 leaves

4 raw lobster tails (see Tip)

1 pound asparagus, cut into ½-inch pieces

2 tablespoons unsalted butter, room temperature

2 tablespoons finely chopped flat-leaf parsley

1 garlic clove, minced

4 radishes, thinly sliced

TIP

If you fear *snipping the lobster tails, most fishmongers will do it for you at the fish counter.*

1 Place the lemon zest and juice, mayonnaise, and seasoning salt or garlic salt in a large bowl, and whisk until well combined. Add the spinach or kale and celery, and toss well.

2 Prepare the lobster: Set the oven to broil. Using kitchen shears, snip through the hard top shell to expose the lobster meat. Transfer the tails to a baking sheet, and arrange the asparagus around the tails. Place the butter, parsley, and garlic in a small bowl, mashing the ingredients together. Spread the butter mixture over the exposed meat of the lobster, and place under the broiler on the middle oven rack.

3 Cook 8 to 9 minutes, until the meat is cooked through and the asparagus starts to brown. Transfer the asparagus to the bowl with the greens, and toss well. Remove the lobster meat from the shells and chop. Divide the lettuce leaves among four plates and top with the salad mixture and the lobster. Garnish with the radishes and serve immediately.

MIXED ASIAN GREENS

with Shredded Sesame Chicken

4.4g
NET CARBS

SERVES **4**

301
CALORIES

You'll adore this creamy Asian dressing, which sneaks in one of the top healing spices, turmeric. Turmeric may seem exotic, but even everyday spices and herbs are not only low in carbs but also make food more visually appealing and fresh tasting while adding health-promoting compounds, such as the curcumin found in turmeric.

TIME	PER SERVING
Active: 15 minutes	*Total Carbs:* 7.6g *Fiber:* 3.2g
Total: 30 minutes	*Protein:* 31.1g *Fat:* 17.1g *FV = 2.9*

1 pound boneless, skinless chicken breasts

2 jalapeños, seeded and diced

2 tablespoons soy sauce or tamari

1 tablespoon sesame oil

Cooking spray

½ pound Asian greens or mesclun

1 Place the chicken breasts in a bag with the jalapeños, soy sauce or tamari, and sesame oil. Marinate in the refrigerator for at least 6 hours or overnight. Coat a griddle or grill with cooking spray, and place over medium heat. Add the chicken and cook 10 to 12 minutes, turning occasionally, until the chicken is brown and no longer pink inside when sliced with a knife.

2 Transfer the cooked chicken to a cutting board to rest 5 minutes, and then slice. Divide the greens among four plates, top with the chicken, and drizzle with the dressing. Serve immediately.

CREAMY ASIAN DRESSING

¼ cup mayonnaise

2 tablespoons apple cider vinegar

2 tablespoons soy sauce or tamari

1 garlic clove, minced

1 teaspoon sesame oil

¼ teaspoon ground turmeric

1 tablespoon toasted sesame seeds

Place the mayonnaise, vinegar, soy sauce or tamari, garlic, sesame oil, turmeric, and sesame seeds in a small bowl, and whisk until smooth and creamy.

10
APPETIZERS

SAVORY BITES
AND SMALL PLATES

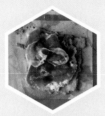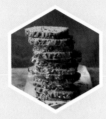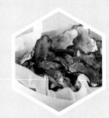

From fries to cheese-stuffed peppers, bruschetta,
personal-sized pizza, and more, the dishes in this chapter replicate
many appetizer favorites. The rich flavors and elegant
presentations (as well as the fact that they are naturally low in carbs)
are sure to impress your guests, but don't wait until you entertain
to treat yourself to these appealing appetizers.

RECIPES

LOW-CARB
FLAX MEAL
BREAD

2.3g **220**

NET CARBS   SERVES **8**   CALORIES

This low-carb artisan bread is so easy to make, it will become your weekly baking habit! It's powered by the superseed flax and is rich in fiber, plant-based omega-3s, and manganese (which is great for blood sugar control and skin health). Don't be deceived by the small amount of batter; it puffs up dramatically when it bakes and fills the house with the comforting aroma of freshly baked bread.

Olive oil spray

¾ cup 100% whole ground golden flaxseed meal

¾ cup almond flour

¾ cup grated Parmesan cheese

1 tablespoon dried herbs, such as Italian seasoning or rosemary

2 teaspoons baking powder

2 teaspoons stevia

1 teaspoon crushed red pepper flakes (optional)

5 large eggs

1 tablespoon olive oil

1 tablespoon whole flaxseeds

1 tablespoon sunflower seeds

1 tablespoon pumpkin seeds

1 Preheat the oven to 350°F. Coat a 1-pound loaf pan with olive oil spray. Mix the flaxseed meal, almond flour, Parmesan, dried herbs, baking powder, stevia, and red pepper flakes, if desired, in a large bowl, stirring well to combine.

2 Add the eggs and oil to the dry ingredients, using a wooden spoon to combine. Transfer to the prepared loaf pan, and sprinkle with the three seeds. Bake 35 to 40 minutes, until the loaf is firm to the touch and the crust starts to brown. Transfer to a wire rack to cool. Store, refrigerated, in an airtight container or aluminum foil for up to 5 days.

TIME	PER SERVING
Active: 15 minutes	*Total Carbs:* **6.6g**
	Fiber: **4.3g**
Total: 30 minutes	*Protein:* **12.5g**
	Fat: **16.5g**
	FV = 0

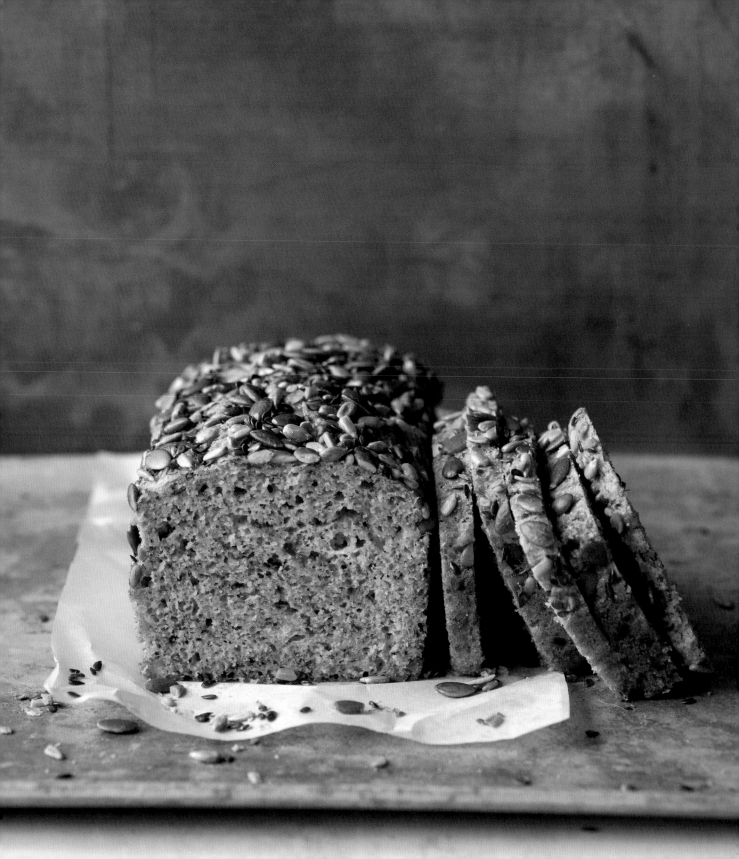

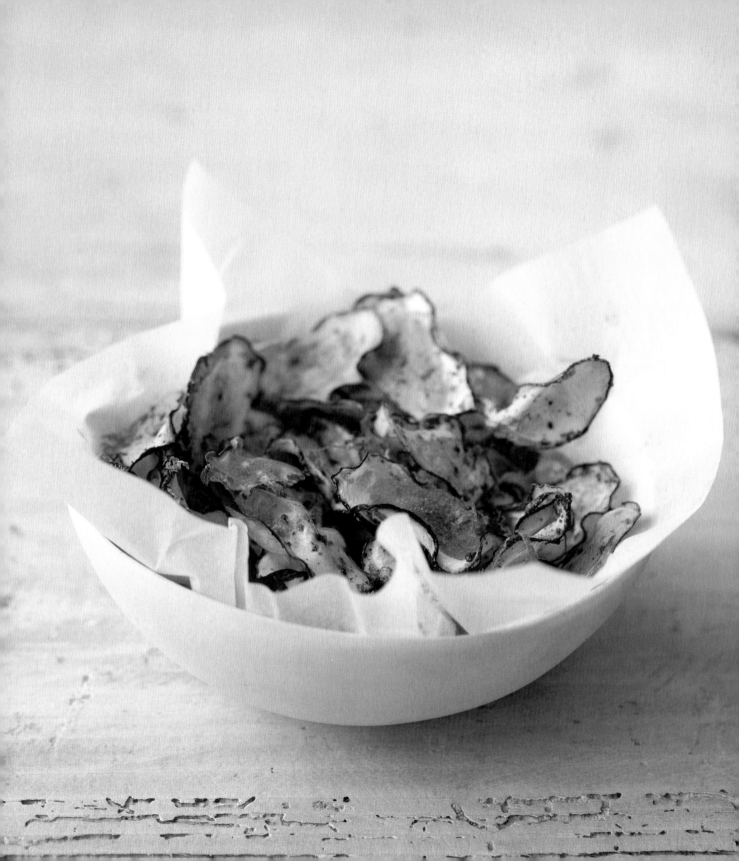

CHIPOTLE LIME
ZUCCHINI CRISPS

2.3g NET CARBS   SERVES **4**   **17** CALORIES

When baked at a low temperature, sliced zucchini transforms into lovely crisps that will cure your salty chip craving. Ground chipotle makes a tangy topping when paired with lime zest, but if you're not a spice lover, go for ground mild chili or paprika.

TIME	PER SERVING
Active: 15 minutes	*Total Carbs:* 3.6g
	Fiber: 1.3g
Total: 30 minutes	*Protein:* 1.3g
	Fat: 0.2g
	FV = 2.2

2 medium zucchini

Olive oil spray

1 teaspoon lime zest, finely grated

½ teaspoon ground chipotle

½ teaspoon garlic salt

¼ teaspoon freshly ground black pepper

1 Preheat the oven to 250°F. Using a Japanese mandoline, vegetable slicer, or large knife, slice the zucchini into ⅛-inch slices and transfer to a baking sheet. Coat with a layer of olive oil spray on both sides. Combine the lime zest, chipotle, garlic salt, and pepper in a small bowl, mix well, and sprinkle over the zucchini slices.

2 Set the slices on a baking sheet in a single layer and bake for 1 hour, 10 minutes, turning once. Cool on the baking sheet, then serve immediately or transfer to an airtight container and store at room temperature for up to 3 days.

PORTOBELLO
PIZZA

5g
NET CARBS

SERVES 4

179
CALORIES

A portobello mushroom makes a perfectly sized personal pizza. Not only are mushrooms a tasty low-carb base for pizza, they are rich in important nutrients such as niacin, which helps your body regulate cholesterol levels, and selenium, which helps keep your thyroid healthy and aids hair growth.

- Olive oil spray
- 4 large portobello mushrooms, stems removed
- ½ cup low-sugar marinara sauce
- ½ cup (2 ounces) shredded mozzarella cheese
- 16 slices pepperoni sausage or 1 chorizo link, thinly sliced

Preheat the oven to 375°F. Line a baking sheet with parchment paper. Coat with a layer of olive oil spray. Scrape out the dark gills from the mushrooms with a spoon, and discard the gills. Place the mushrooms stem side up, and top each with 2 tablespoons of the sauce. Sprinkle each with 2 tablespoons of the mozzarella and 4 slices of pepperoni or chorizo. Bake 20 to 25 minutes, until the cheese is bubbly and the mushrooms are soft. Serve immediately.

TIME	PER SERVING
Active: 10 minutes	*Total Carbs:* 7g
	Fiber: 1.9g
Total: 40 minutes	*Protein:* 10.7g
	Fat: 12.6g
	FV = 4.2

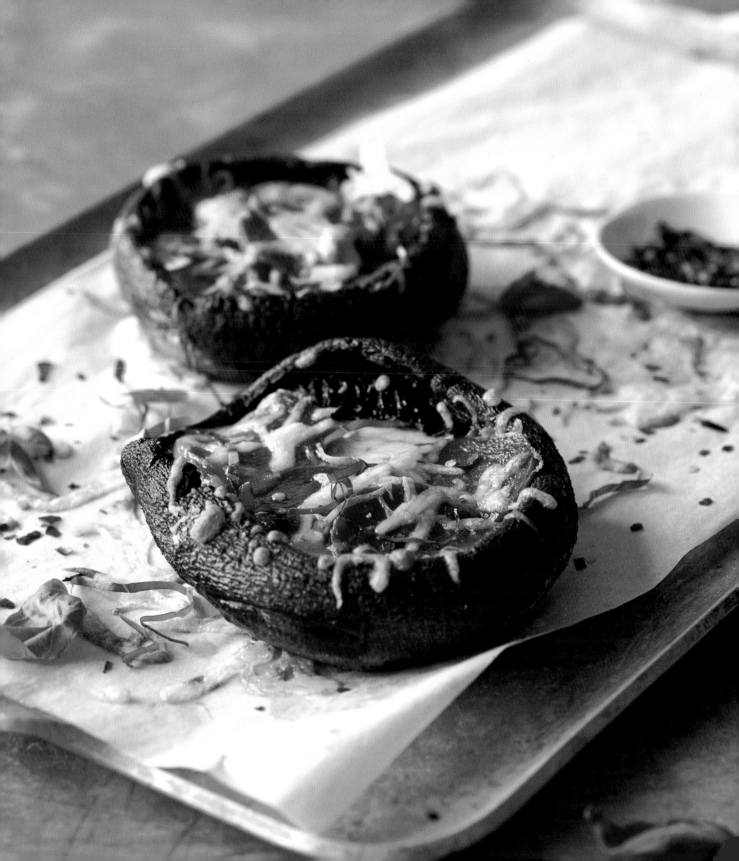

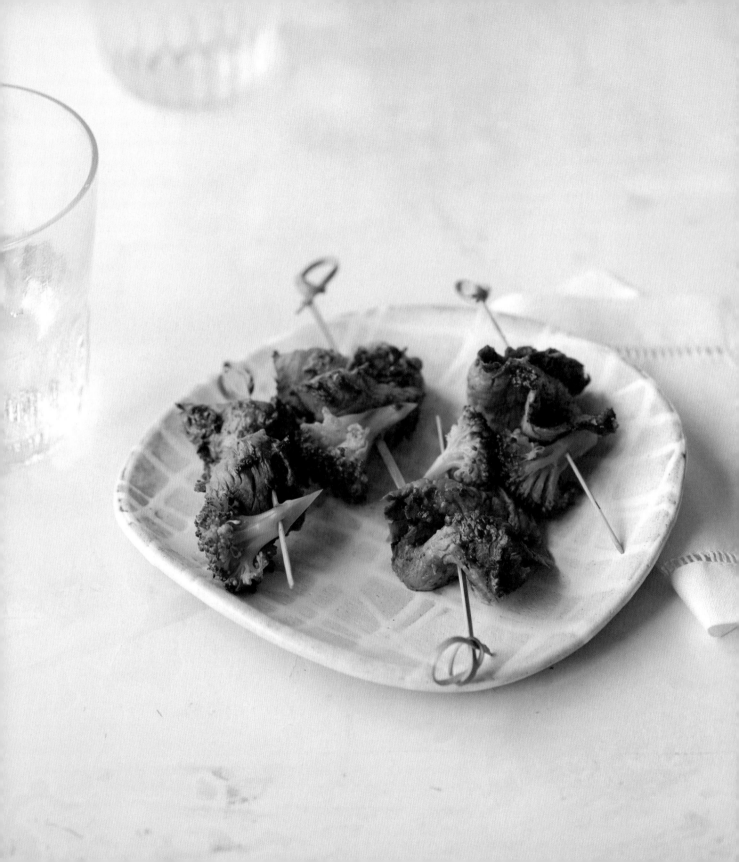

CHIMICHURRI
STEAK BITES

1.6g
NET CARBS

SERVES 4

208
CALORIES

Chimichurri is a tasty parsley-based green sauce and marinade that hails from Argentina, where the locals are experts at flavoring their renowned beef. The parsley and cilantro in this green sauce also happen to be high in antioxidants and antibacterial compounds; the two herbs also give the sauce flavor and color.

TIME	PER SERVING
Active: 15 minutes	*Total Carbs:* 2.6g
	Fiber: 1g
Total: 30 minutes	*Protein:* 18.3g
	Fat: 14.4g
	FV = 1.6

1 cup fresh flat-leaf parsley leaves

1 cup fresh cilantro leaves and stems

4 garlic cloves

¼ cup red wine vinegar

¼ cup olive oil

½ teaspoon salt

¼ teaspoon freshly ground black pepper

1½ pounds flank steak

Olive oil spray

½ head broccoli, cut into small florets (about 2 cups)

1 Place the parsley, cilantro, garlic, vinegar, olive oil, salt, and pepper in a blender, and process until a smooth sauce forms.

2 Place the steak in a large zip-top bag with half the sauce, and shake well to coat the steak. Transfer to the fridge, and marinate at least 1 hour or overnight. Refrigerate the remaining sauce, as well. Bring the steak to room temperature before grilling (about 1 hour) to enhance juiciness.

3 Coat a large stovetop grill with olive oil spray, place over high heat, and cook 15 to 20 minutes, turning occasionally, until the steak is no longer red in the center but still pink. Transfer to a cutting board, and let rest 5 minutes before slicing against the grain. Spear the slices on toothpicks, and top each with a broccoli floret. Serve immediately with the remaining sauce.

CLAM
LINGUINE

4.6g NET CARBS

SERVES 4

271 CALORIES

Tender, freshly cooked clams smothered in a white Alfredo sauce are a feast fit for a king or queen and also perfect on a regular weeknight, since this meal comes together in minutes. If you don't own a spiralizer or veggie noodle maker, many grocery chains sell zucchini noodles already cut. To complete the meal, serve with a side Caesar salad, such as the Kale Caesar Salad with Creamy Meyer Lemon Dressing on page 186.

TIME	PER SERVING
Active: **15 minutes**	*Total Carbs:* **5.8g**
Total: **30 minutes**	*Fiber:* **1.2g**
	Protein: **10g**
	Fat: **23.9g**
	FV = **2.2**

1 tablespoon unsalted butter

¾ cup heavy cream

¼ cup grated Parmesan cheese

⅓ cup grated Romano cheese

½ teaspoon freshly ground black pepper

⅛ teaspoon freshly ground nutmeg

Olive oil spray

1 pound clams, such as Manila, well washed under cold running water

2 zucchini, cut into long noodle shapes

1 Make the cheese sauce: Melt the butter in a medium saucepan over medium heat. Add the cream and simmer until reduced to ½ cup, about 3 minutes. Remove from heat. Stir in the Parmesan, Romano, pepper, and nutmeg until the cheeses have melted and the sauce is smooth.

2 Coat a large skillet with the olive oil spray and place over high heat. Add the clams and cover; cook 4 to 5 minutes, until the clams open. Add the zucchini noodles and cook an additional 4 to 5 minutes, until the noodles are tender. Drain off any excess liquid, and toss with the cheese sauce. Serve immediately.

MANCHEGO
MINI MUFFINS

2.1g
NET CARBS

SERVES
12

202
CALORIES

If you're missing your cornbread, this tasty muffin will hit the spot with a similar texture but far more protein. Manchego, a tangy Spanish cheese, is a perfect pairing with peppers, but feel free to mix it up with grated Asiago or even grated aged Gouda.

TIME	PER SERVING
Active: 10 minutes	*Total Carbs:* 3.4g
	Fiber: 1.4g
Total: 40 minutes	*Protein:* 13.5g
	Fat: 15.4g
	FV = 0.1

- ½ cup unsalted butter, cut into pieces
- Olive oil spray
- 1 cup Atkins Flour Mix (page 126)
- 1 teaspoon baking powder
- 1 teaspoon ground mustard
- ½ teaspoon garlic salt
- ¼ teaspoon ground cayenne or mild chili powder
- 4 large eggs, whisked
- 1½ cup grated Manchego or Asiago cheese
- 2 jalapeños, seeded and minced

1 Preheat the oven to 375°F. Place the butter in a small skillet and melt over low heat, 1 to 2 minutes. Set aside to cool. Coat a 24-count mini muffin tin with olive oil spray.

2 Place the Atkins Flour Mix, baking powder, mustard, garlic salt, and cayenne or chili powder in a large bowl, and whisk well to combine. Make a well in the center of the flour mixture, and add the eggs, melted butter, cheese, and jalapeños. Stir to combine. Divide the batter evenly among the muffin cups.

3 Bake until the muffins are golden around the edges and have puffed, 18 to 20 minutes. Cool in the muffin tin on wire racks for 10 to 15 minutes. Serve immediately, or store in an airtight container, refrigerated, for up to 3 days.

BOURBON PECAN PÂTÉ

1.4g NET CARBS SERVES **4** **264** CALORIES

Rich-tasting bourbon gives a hint of sweet aroma without adding carbs to this creamy, dreamy pâté. Chicken livers are incredibly high in energizing ingredients such as several B vitamins (to sooth your nerves) and iron (for energy and red blood cell production). Serve this upscale, uplifting dish with low-carb crackers and sliced cucumbers and celery.

TIME	PER SERVING
Active: 15 minutes	*Total Carbs:* 2.3g
	Fiber: 0.8g
Total: 30 minutes	*Protein:* 20.4g
	Fat: 15.3g
	FV = 1

1 pound chicken livers

1 teaspoon salt

½ teaspoon freshly ground black pepper

2 tablespoons unsalted butter

4 garlic cloves, chopped

¼ cup chopped fresh parsley

¼ cup bourbon, beef broth, Basic Bone Broth (page 161), or unsalted chicken broth

¼ cup chopped pecans

2 teaspoons fresh thyme leaves

1 Place the chicken livers in a large colander, and rinse under cold running water. Drain them well, then transfer to a cutting board. Cut away and discard any of the white sinew that holds the livers together and discard. Dry the livers well with paper towels. Sprinkle them with the salt and pepper.

2 Warm the butter in a large skillet over medium-high heat and add the livers, garlic, and parsley. Cook 10 to 12 minutes, turning once or twice, until the livers are cooked but still slightly pink (not red) in the center when sliced. Turn the heat to low, and carefully add the bourbon, stirring the mixture to scrape up any brown bits sticking to the pan, about 1 minute.

3 Turn the heat off, and cool 10 to 15 minutes. Transfer to a food processor, and blend until smooth. Transfer to a 4-cup airtight container, and sprinkle with the pecans and thyme leaves. Chill at least one hour before serving. Refrigerate any leftover pâté for up to 1 week.

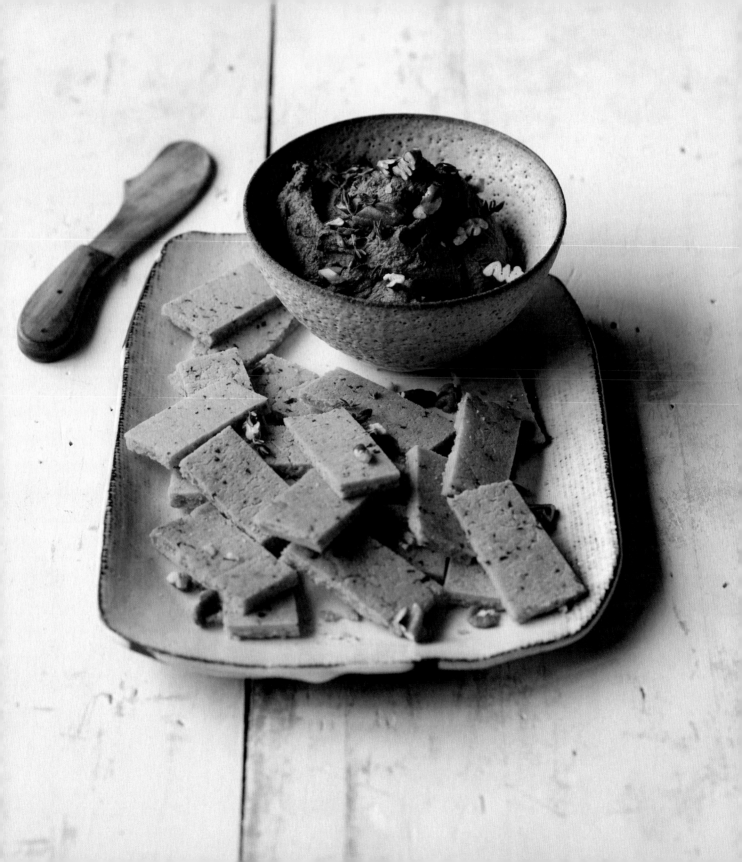

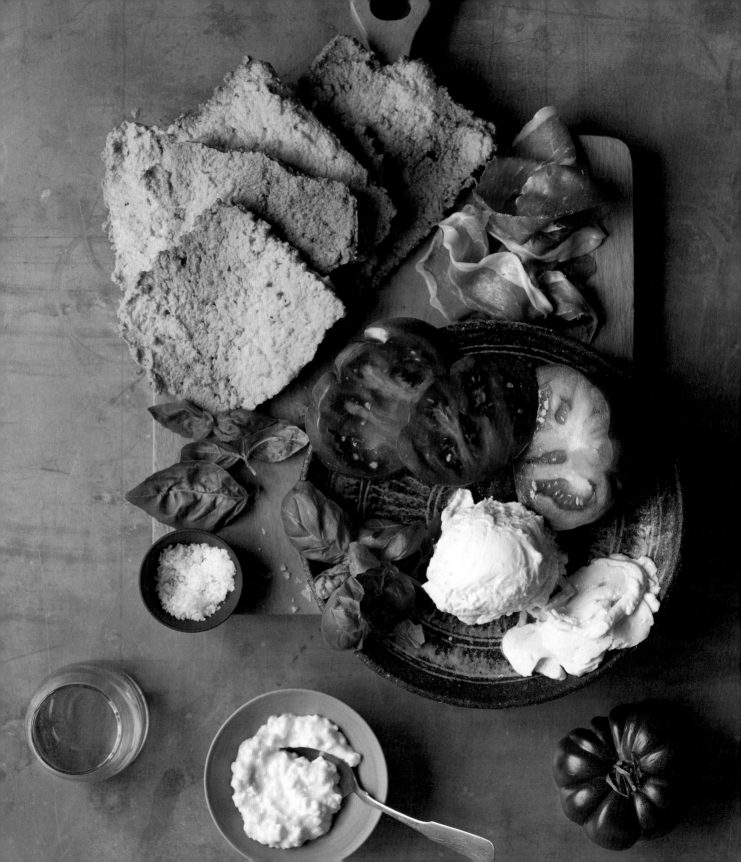

BRUSCHETTA
DUET

SERVES
4

If you're living a low-carb lifestyle, it doesn't mean you have to give up all the recipes you love, like bruschetta with two tasty toppings! The base of this one is flatbread, which is used for the Avocado Toast (page 142) and in a pinch can be a base for pizza, as well.

Flatbread dough

1 large egg

1 tablespoon extra-virgin olive oil

¼ cup cold water

1½ cups almond flour

½ cup grated Parmesan cheese

½ teaspoon baking powder

½ teaspoon stevia

¾ teaspoon dried oregano

¼ teaspoon crushed red pepper flakes

1 To make the flatbread: Place the egg, olive oil, and water in a large bowl, and whisk well. Set aside. Place the almond flour, Parmesan, baking powder, stevia, oregano, and crushed red pepper flakes in a large bowl, and stir well with a wooden spoon. Add the wet ingredients, stirring to form a thick, sticky dough.

2 Coat 2 sheets of parchment paper with olive oil spray. Roll out the dough into a large rectangle about ⅛ inch thick between the sheets of sprayed parchment paper. Slide onto a baking sheet and put in the freezer. Freeze for 15 minutes to make the dough easier to handle.

3 Preheat the oven to 375°F. Discard the top parchment sheet. Score the dough into 8 equal rectangles. Leaving the dough on the parchment paper–lined baking sheet, bake 20 to 25 minutes, until crisp around the edges. Cool completely on the baking sheet. Cut into pieces along the score marks. (Makes 4 servings of 2 flatbreads each.)

RECIPE CONTINUES

CRUST	
TIME	**PER SERVING**
Active: 15 minutes	*Net Carbs:* 7.3g
	Total Carbs: 12.5g
	Fiber: 5.2g
Total: 50 minutes	*Protein:* 22.1g
	Fat: 39.1g
	Calories: 466
	FV = 1.3

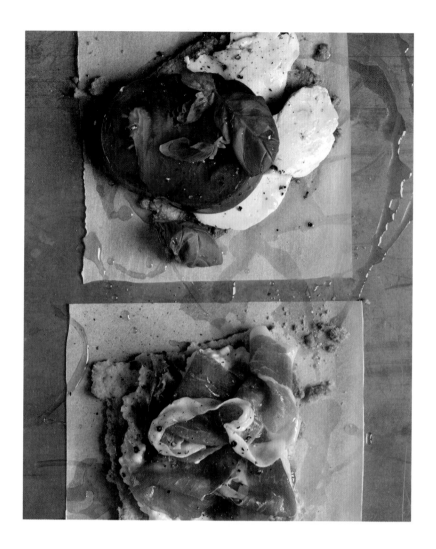

TOMATO-MOZZARELLA TOPPING

2 small tomatoes, sliced lengthwise

½ cup cubed fresh mozzarella

2 tablespoons chopped fresh basil

1 tablespoon olive oil

Place the tomatoes, mozzarella, basil, and olive oil in a medium bowl. Toss well, and divide among 4 flatbread pieces.

CHEESE AND PROSCIUTTO TOPPING

1 cup cottage cheese

1 tablespoon olive oil

1 thin slice of prosciutto, or
2 tablespoons crumbled cooked bacon or diced cooked pancetta

Place the cottage cheese and olive oil in a medium bowl and stir well. Divide among 8 flatbread pieces and top each with a piece of the slice of prosciutto.

TOMATO-MOZZARELLA TOPPING	
TIME	**PER SERVING**
Active: 15 minutes	*Net Carbs:* 7.3g
	Total Carbs: 12.5g
Total: 50 minutes	*Fiber:* 5.2g
	Protein: 22.1g
	Fat: 39.1g
	Calories: 466
	FV = 1.2

CHEESE AND PROSCIUTTO TOPPING	
TIME	**PER SERVING**
Active: 15 minutes	*Net Carbs:* 8.1g
	Total Carbs: 13.2g
Total: 50 minutes	*Fiber:* 5.1g
	Protein: 23.3g
	Fat: 36.1g
	Calories: 449
	FV = 0

ARTICHOKE DIP-STUFFED
MUSHROOMS

4.3g
NET CARBS

SERVES 4

275
CALORIES

Two appetizers in one, artichoke dip and stuffed mushrooms, no chips required! These richly stuffed, totally delicious mushrooms are ideal for parties and game night and can even be served as a meal when paired with any of the salads from Chapter 9.

TIME	PER SERVING
Active: 15 minutes	*Total Carbs:* 6.7g
	Fiber: 2.4g
	Protein: 8.3g
Total: 40 minutes	*Fat:* 24.8g
	FV = 3.8

10 ounces white cremini or button mushrooms

Olive oil spray

2 garlic cloves, minced

¼ cup chopped parsley

1 (9-ounce) box frozen artichokes, defrosted

½ cup mayonnaise

½ cup grated Parmesan cheese

1 Preheat the oven to 400°F. Remove the stems from the mushrooms, and chop finely. Coat a large skillet with olive oil spray and place over medium heat. Add the mushroom stems, garlic, and parsley to the skillet, and cook 3 to 4 minutes, until soft.

2 Place the defrosted artichokes in the bowl of a food processor, and pulse until finely chopped. Transfer the chopped artichokes to a clean kitchen towel, and squeeze out the water. Add the artichokes to a bowl, along with the cooked mushroom mixture, mayonnaise, and Parmesan. Mix well.

3 Fill the mushrooms with the artichoke mixture. Bake 15 to 20 minutes until the tops are golden and the mushrooms are soft. Serve immediately.

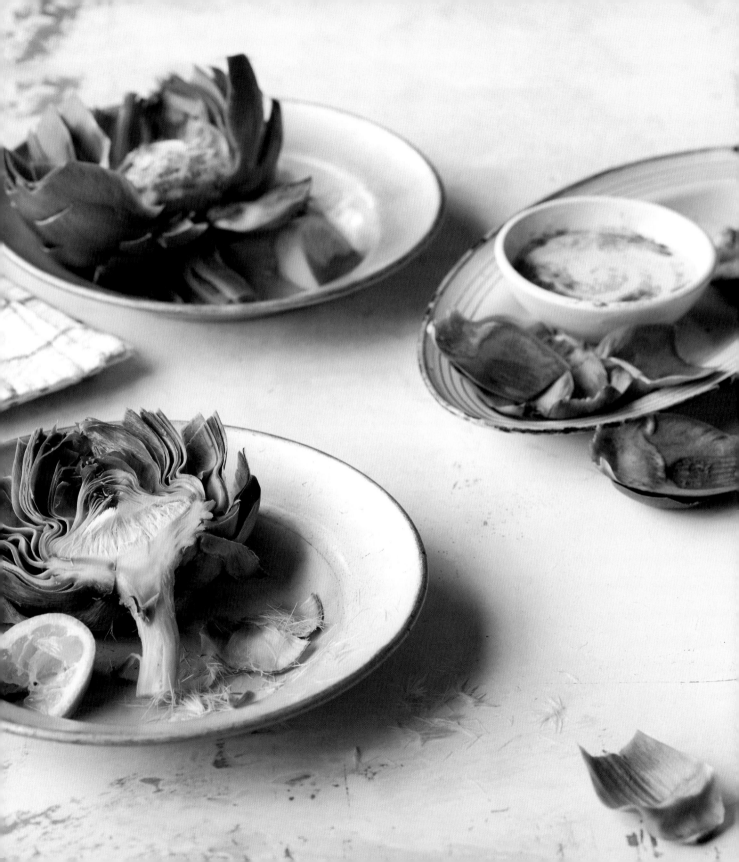

STEAMED
ARTICHOKE

with Homemade Lemon Mayonnaise

7.2g
NET CARBS

SERVES
4

323
CALORIES

Artichokes, which are part of the thistle family, are also superhealing for your liver.[1] Artichokes are also a prebiotic food, which means they are high in a certain kind of insoluble fiber that feeds the good bacteria in your gut and enhances digestion. If you want a healthier movie snack or finger food, this recipe is ideal, as you can pluck the artichoke leaves as you would popcorn and dip away!

TIME	PER SERVING
Active: 10 minutes	*Total Carbs:* **14.4g**
	Fiber: **7.2g**
Total: 30 minutes	*Protein:* **5.9g**
	Fat: **28.8g**
	FV = 6.6

4 medium artichokes

1 large egg

½ cup grape seed or safflower oil

Zest of 1 lemon, finely grated

1 tablespoon lemon juice

1 teaspoon Dijon mustard

½ teaspoon salt

¼ teaspoon freshly ground black pepper

¼ teaspoon sweet paprika

1 Cut the tops of the artichokes off and discard. Using a pair of scissors, clip the tops of any artichoke leaves that have thorns. Peel the outside of the stalk using a potato peeler or paring knife, and trim the bottom of the stem, retaining as much length as possible.

TIP

An immersion blender is a must-have in my kitchen because it allows me to make small portions of mayonnaise and hollandaise. Don't try to make these sauces in a food processor or standing blender, as they are too large and the recipes won't work.

2 Fit a large stockpot with a steamer basket, and fill with water to the edge of the basket. Bring to a boil on high heat. Add the artichokes and steam 15 to 20 minutes, until the stems are tender when pierced with a knife.

3 While the artichokes are steaming, make the mayonnaise: Place the egg in the bottom of an immersion blender cup or large measuring cup. Add the oil, lemon zest, lemon juice, mustard, salt, pepper, and paprika. Allow the egg to sink to the bottom. Add the nozzle of an immersion blender, pressing it to the bottom of the cup, and blend until a thick white cloud forms. Continue to blend until all the oil is incorporated. Divide the artichokes among four plates, and serve immediately with the mayonnaise.

BRIE-STUFFED
GRILLED JALAPEÑOS

3g
NET CARBS

SERVES 4

130
CALORIES

Jalapeño poppers are famous bar food loaded with carb-rich breading that can spike your blood sugar and leave you craving more fried and breaded food. These grilled poppers are lighter and still filled with satisfying, gooey cheese.

TIME	PER SERVING
Active: 10 minutes	*Total Carbs:* 5.9g
	Fiber: 2.9g
	Protein: 6.8g
Total: 20 minutes	*Fat:* 10.1g
	FV = 2.9

8 large jalapeños

3 ounces Brie cheese, sliced into 8 pieces

Olive oil spray

¼ teaspoon salt

¼ teaspoon freshly ground black pepper

½ cup olive tapenade from a jar (see Tip)

1 Cut off the tops of the jalapeños. Use the small end of a melon or small paring knife to remove the seeds. Place a piece of Brie into each jalapeño.

2 Set the oven to broil. Coat a grill or baking sheet with the olive oil spray. Coat the jalapeños with the olive oil spray. Grill the peppers or place them under the broiler on the middle rack for 5 to 6 minutes, until the peppers start to blister and the cheese melts. Serve immediately with the tapenade.

 TIP

If you can't find olive tapenade *(an olive-based dip), try serving these with a few tablespoons of the Ranch Dipping Sauce from the Fried Green Tomatoes recipe (page 153).*

TURMERIC ORANGE
SCALLOPS

9.4g
NET CARBS

SERVES 4

283
CALORIES

This gorgeous dish is ideal for your next dinner party or date night. Bright yellow turmeric gives a golden cast to the scallops and a flavorful health boost to your meal, since it is one of the most anti-inflammatory spices around. Pair it with black pepper, since the active compound in pepper, piperine, makes turmeric 100 percent more potent.[2] Cauliflower mash is a creamy, rich accompaniment to this special dish.

Cauliflower Mash

1 small head cauliflower, cut into florets (about 5 cups)

1 cup canned coconut milk

½ teaspoon garlic powder

¼ teaspoon freshly ground black pepper

Scallops

1 pound sea scallops

½ teaspoon ground turmeric

½ teaspoon hot or sweet paprika

½ teaspoon salt

¼ teaspoon freshly ground black pepper

1 tablespoon unsalted butter

Zest of 1 orange, finely grated

1 Prepare the cauliflower mash: Place the cauliflower florets in a large stockpot and add 2 inches of water. Bring to a boil over high heat. Steam for 4 to 5 minutes, until fork tender. Drain and transfer to a food processor along with the coconut milk, garlic powder, and pepper. Process until smooth. Set aside.

2 Place the scallops on a plate, and sprinkle both sides with the turmeric, paprika, salt, and pepper. Warm the butter in a large skillet over medium-high heat. Add the scallops and cook 2 to 3 minutes per side, until the scallops are well browned and no longer translucent when sliced with a knife. Serve immediately with the mash.

TIME	PER SERVING
Active: 15 minutes	*Total Carbs:* 13.1g
	Fiber: 3.7g
Total: 30 minutes	*Protein:* 20.7g
	Fat: 16.1g
	FV = 3.8

TURNIP
FRIES

9.8g NET CARBS   **SERVES 4**   **169** CALORIES

If you crave starchy fries, there's no reason to hit the drive-through when you can head to your oven for a tasty, fulfilling low-carb version: turnip fries! Turnips are the perfect vegetable to "fry" in the oven; the result is a delicious treat that is crispy on the outside and tender on the inside.

1½ pounds turnips

2 tablespoons olive oil

4 garlic cloves, minced

½ cup grated Parmesan cheese

½ teaspoon garlic salt

1 teaspoon sweet paprika (see Tip)

1 teaspoon onion powder

1 Preheat the oven to 425°F. Line a baking sheet with a piece of parchment paper.

2 Peel the turnips, and cut them into French fry–sized sticks, about ⅓ inch by 4 inches. Place in a large bowl, and toss with the olive oil and garlic to coat. Place the Parmesan, garlic salt, paprika, and onion powder on a sheet of wax paper and toss the fries in the mixture. Spread the fries out onto the prepared baking sheet. Bake until the outsides are crispy and the insides are tender, 20 to 25 minutes. Serve immediately.

TIP

For flavor variations, *you can replace the paprika with an equal amount of ground chipotle, herbes de Provence, or lemon pepper.*

TIME

Active:
20 minutes

Total:
40 minutes

PER SERVING

Total Carbs: 13.2g
Fiber: 3.4g
Protein: 6.7g
Fat: 10.6g
FV = 8.8

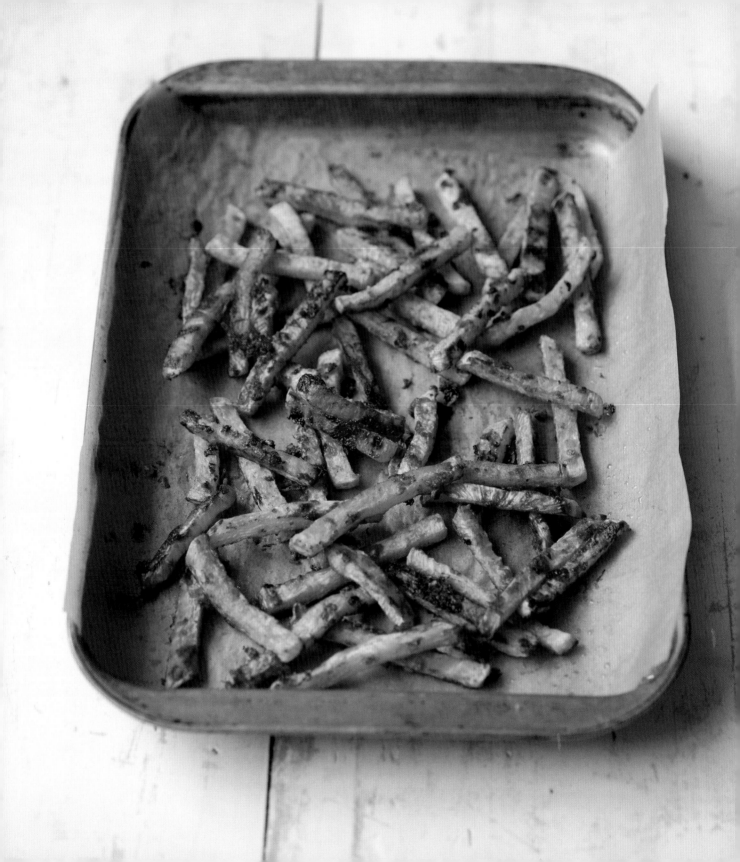

11

15-MINUTE MEALS

SIMPLE AND SATISFYING

MEALS FOR WEEKDAYS

Breakfast, Lunch, and Dinner

◆

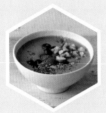 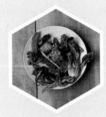 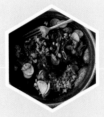

These 15-minute miracles will take your weeknight meals
from everyday to extraordinary. Less active cooking time and more flavor?
Yes, please! From supercharged smoothie bowls to
nutrient-filled, satisfying noodle dishes to skillet sensations inspired
by traditional favorites around the world, these recipes
have you covered.

RECIPES

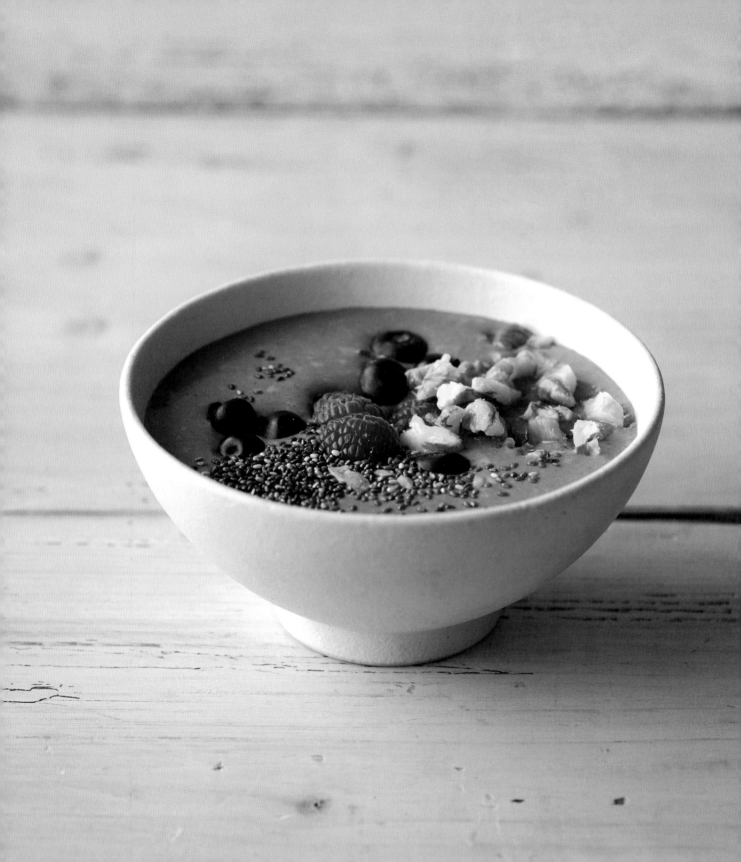

AVOCADO KALE BERRY

SMOOTHIE BOWL

12.5g
NET CARBS

SERVES 2

356
CALORIES

The vibrant colors of this spoonable smoothie bowl make it Instagram-worthy, but there's so much more to it—it is a blended plant-based meal that will supercharge your energy! Plus, blending breaks up plant fibers for easy digestion while you pack in nutrients for your thyroid, liver, and gut health. Smoothie bowls can also double as a light meal, a real treat when you're looking to cool down during scorching days.

TIME	PER SERVING
Active: 10 minutes	*Total Carbs:* **24.2g**
	Fiber: **11.8g**
Total: 10 minutes	*Protein:* **32.2g**
	Fat: **15.6g**
	FV = **3.5**

⅓ cup plain protein powder (see Tip, page 132)

1 cup plain full-fat Greek yogurt

¼ cup water

½ ripe Hass avocado

1 cup kale leaves

2 tablespoons chopped fresh mint

1 teaspoon stevia

½ cup fresh or frozen berries such as blackberries, strawberries, or raspberries

2 tablespoons almonds or walnut halves

2 tablespoons chia seeds

Place the protein powder, yogurt, water, avocado, kale, mint, and stevia in a blender. Blend until smooth, then divide between two bowls. Sprinkle the berries, almonds or walnut halves, and chia seeds over the smoothie. Serve immediately.

ALMOND BUTTER
SMOOTHIE BOWL

12.5g
NET CARBS

SERVES
2

417
CALORIES

Nuts, seeds, and greens are an energizing trio. High in hunger-busting, antioxidant-rich healthy fats, they also feature a wide spectrum of nutrients from which you can get most of your essential vitamins and some much-needed minerals (such as magnesium) in which many people are deficient.

TIME	PER SERVING
Active: 10 minutes	*Total Carbs:* 20g
	Fiber: 7.5g
Total: 10 minutes	*Protein:* 36.9g
	Fat: 22.5g
	FV = 4.8

- ⅓ cup plain protein powder
- 1 cup plain full-fat Greek yogurt
- ¼ cup water
- 8 ounces spinach or kale
- ¼ cup almond or peanut butter
- ½ cup fresh or frozen strawberries
- 2 tablespoons chopped almonds
- 2 tablespoons ground flaxseed

Place the protein powder, yogurt, water, spinach or kale, and almond or peanut butter in a blender. Blend until smooth, then divide between two bowls. Sprinkle the strawberries, almonds, and flaxseed in straight lines over the smoothie bowl. Serve immediately.

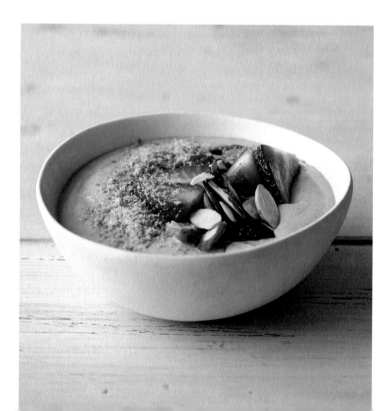

CARROT SPICE

SMOOTHIE BOWL

16.1g
NET CARBS

SERVES
2

434
CALORIES

Carrot and spice and everything nice, this deliciously sweet smoothie bowl could double as dessert! If you can't nosh on this bowl right away, pack it in an airtight container and store in the fridge for up to 5 hours or even overnight. As the flax sits in the mixture, it takes on a graham cracker–like flavor that cookie fans will cheer for.

TIME	PER SERVING
Active: 10 minutes	*Total Carbs:* 22g *Fiber:* 5.9g
Total: 10 minutes	*Protein:* 32.6g *Fat:* 25.8g *FV* = 2.5

- ⅓ cup plain protein powder
- 1 cup plain full-fat Greek yogurt
- ¼ cup water
- 1 carrot, peeled and chopped
- ¼ cup almond or peanut butter
- ½ teaspoon ground cinnamon
- ¼ teaspoon freshly grated nutmeg
- ¼ teaspoon ground turmeric
- ½ cup fresh or frozen sliced strawberries
- 2 tablespoons ground flaxseed
- 2 tablespoons unsweetened shredded or flaked coconut

Place the protein powder, yogurt, water, carrot, almond or peanut butter, cinnamon, nutmeg, and turmeric in a blender. Blend until smooth, then divide between two bowls. Sprinkle the strawberries, flaxseed, and coconut in straight lines over the smoothie bowl. Serve immediately.

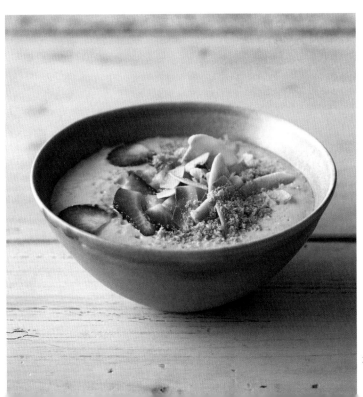

THAI PEANUT

BUDDHA BOWL

10.8g
NET CARBS

SERVES
4

427
CALORIES

Buddha bowls are filling, colorful meals bursting from a large bowl packed with nutritious veggies. Drizzle this bowl with a delectable peanut sauce, which adds crave-worthy flavor to otherwise plain proteins and vegetables.

TIME	PER SERVING
Active: **15 minutes**	*Total Carbs:* **18.1g**
	Fiber: **7.3g**
Total: **30 minutes**	*Protein:* **21.8g**
	Fat: **30.7g**
	FV = 6.3

Olive oil spray

2 skinless, boneless chicken breasts (12 ounces total)

½ cup peanut butter

3 tablespoons coconut milk

1 tablespoon fish sauce

2 teaspoons hot chili sauce

2 garlic cloves, minced

1 tablespoon minced fresh ginger

1 tablespoon sesame oil

3 tablespoons hot water

4 cups baby spinach

1 ripe Hass avocado, thinly sliced

1 medium zucchini, cut into noodle shapes

2 carrots, cut into noodle shapes

2 radishes, thinly sliced

8 sprigs cilantro

1 Preheat the oven to 400°F. Coat a small skillet with olive oil spray. Add the chicken and cook 3 to 4 minutes, turning once or twice to brown the chicken. Slide into the oven, and bake 6 to 8 minutes, until the chicken is cooked through and no longer pink in the center when sliced with a knife. Set aside to rest for 5 minutes, then shred.

2 Place the peanut butter, coconut milk, fish sauce, chili sauce, garlic, ginger, sesame oil, and hot water in a large bowl. Whisk well until smooth. Divide the spinach and avocado among four bowls. Top with the chicken, zucchini, carrots, radishes, and cilantro. Drizzle with the dressing, and serve immediately.

TIP

If you don't have a spiralizer, which is a convenient kitchen tool that allows you to slice vegetables such as zucchini, squash, carrots, and cucumbers into thin noodle shapes, you can achieve the same effect by using a vegetable peeler to shave thin ribbons (it's a little more time intensive and you won't get quite the same results as the "noodles" you get from a spiralizer, but your dish will taste just as delicious). You can also use a mandoline vegetable slicer and then use a knife to cut the strips into even thinner noodlelike strips.

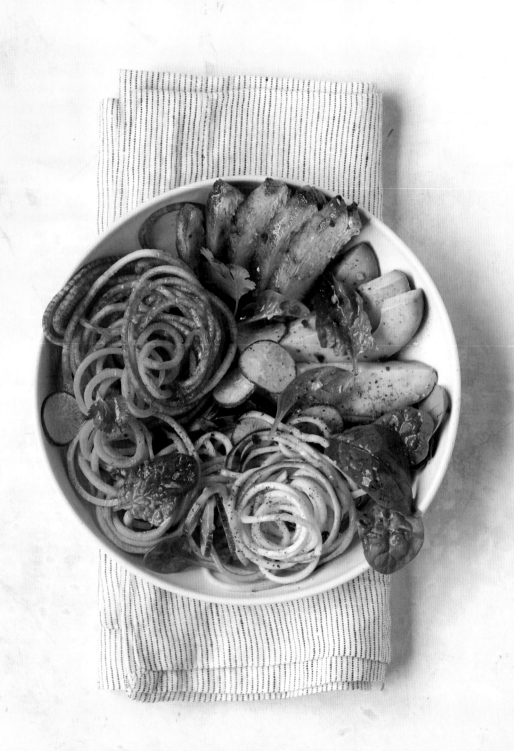

KUNG PAO
CHICKEN
with Cauliflower Rice

4.9g
NET CARBS

SERVES 4

366
CALORIES

Kung Pao Chicken gets its "pow" from Szechuan chilies and hot peppercorns that come from a province of central China. Szechuan chilies can be difficult to find, so this version uses hot chili paste, which you can find in the international aisle of your grocery store. The chopped peanuts and crisp radishes give this dish the classic "crunch" that turns it into a truly authentic Kung Pao Chicken experience.

TIME	PER SERVING
Active: 15 minutes	*Total Carbs:* 7.7g
	Fiber: 2.7g
Total: 30 minutes	*Protein:* 35.5g
	Fat: 22.2g
	FV = 2.9

½ head small cauliflower, cut into florets (about 2½ cups)

4 tablespoons sesame oil, divided

2 tablespoons Basic Bone Broth (page 161) or unsalted chicken broth

2 tablespoons tamari or soy sauce

1 to 2 tablespoons hot chili paste

1 tablespoon chopped garlic

1 teaspoon distilled white vinegar

2 teaspoons stevia

3 skinless, boneless chicken breasts, thinly sliced (18 ounces)

2 tablespoons Atkins Flour Mix (page 126)

4 radishes, thinly sliced

¼ cup chopped peanuts

2 scallions, thinly sliced

1 Place the cauliflower florets in a food processor and chop roughly. You will need to do this in two batches. Warm half the oil in a large skillet over medium heat, and cook the cauliflower 4 to 5 minutes, stirring occasionally, until it starts to brown and becomes tender. Transfer to a bowl and cover to keep warm.

2 In a medium bowl, whisk the broth, tamari or soy sauce, chili paste, garlic, vinegar, and stevia together. Toss the chicken in the Atkins Flour Mix. Heat the remaining oil in a large skillet, and add the coated chicken; cook 5 to 6 minutes, turning often, until crisp and cooked through. Transfer to a plate. Add the sauce to the skillet, and cook 1 minute more, stirring often. Pour the sauce over the chicken and garnish with the radishes. Sprinkle with the peanuts and scallions, and serve immediately with the cauliflower rice.

LEMON PEPPER
SHRIMP
with Snow Peas

4.8g
NET CARBS

SERVES 4

263
CALORIES

Bright lemon and pungent pepper flavor this fast meal that is just as delicious served hot or at room temperature (consider it for your next brunch buffet). For larger appetites or as part of a more elaborate meal, pair with a crepe (page 127) or a serving of Manchego Mini Muffins (page 211).

TIME	PER SERVING
Active: 15 minutes	*Total Carbs:* 6.6g *Fiber:* 1.9g *Protein:* 36.6g
Total: 30 minutes	*Fat:* 9.4g *FV* = 2.9

1½ pounds (about 40) medium shrimp

Zest of 1 lemon, finely grated

1 teaspoon freshly ground black pepper

1 tablespoon olive oil

1 tablespoon unsalted butter

½ pound snow peas

4 ounces green watercress, baby spinach, or baby kale

Combine the shrimp, lemon zest, and pepper in a large bowl, and toss well. Heat a large skillet over medium-high heat. Add the olive oil, butter, shrimp, and snow peas, and cook 5 to 6 minutes, tossing well, until the shrimp are cooked through. Turn off the heat, add the greens, and cover to wilt them, about 1 minute. Toss well, and serve immediately.

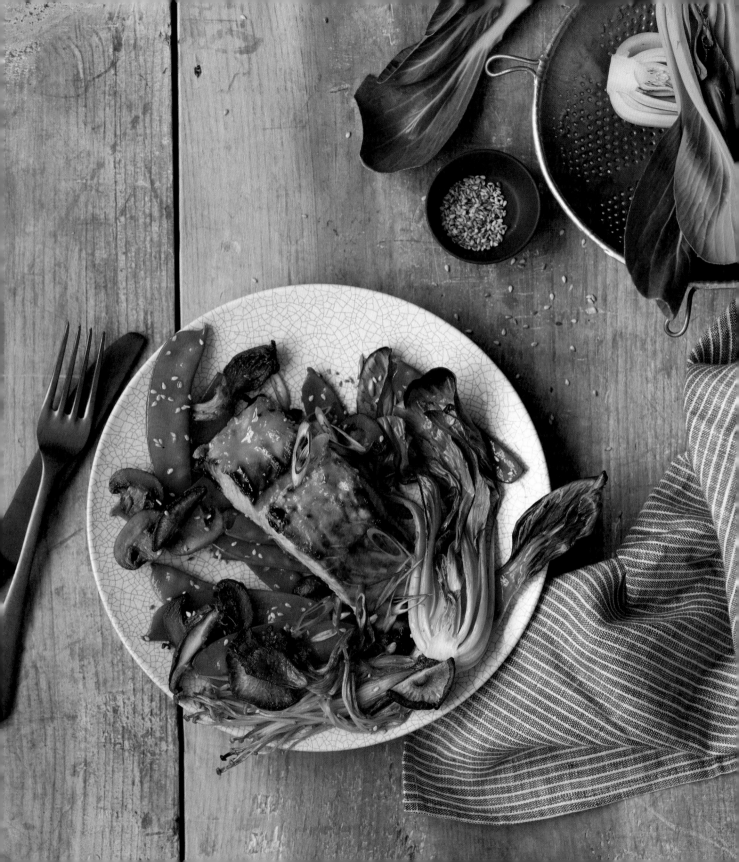

BROILER
MISO SALMON

9.1g
NET CARBS

SERVES
4

313
CALORIES

Miso is a fermented soybean paste that is bursting with savory and salty flavor, and that can be purchased in a health food store. You can keep leftover miso for up to 6 months in a refrigerated airtight container. The topping for this salmon also makes a tasty salad dressing (see Tip).

TIME	PER SERVING
Active: 5 minutes	*Total Carbs:* **10.6g**
	Fiber: **1.5g**
Total: 15 minutes	*Protein:* **27.9g**
	Fat: **17.7g**
	FV = **1.8**

Olive oil spray

4 tablespoons white miso paste

4 tablespoons lemon juice

2 teaspoons water

4 (4-ounce) salmon filets, skin on

4 ounces mushrooms, such as baby bella or shiitake, thinly sliced

8 ounces bok choy

4 ounces snow peas, trimmed

3 tablespoons sesame oil

½ teaspoon toasted sesame seeds

1 Cover a baking sheet with aluminum foil. Coat with a light layer of olive oil spray.

2 Set the oven to broil. Place the miso paste, lemon juice, and water in a medium bowl and whisk well. Place the salmon in the bowl and spoon the mixture over the top. Adjust the oven rack to the middle. Place the salmon filets on the prepared baking sheet, skin side down. Brush the remaining miso over the salmon. In a small bowl, toss the mushrooms, bok choy, and snow peas in the sesame oil, then transfer them to the baking sheet alongside the salmon.

3 Broil the salmon for 8 to 10 minutes, until it flakes when pressed with a fork. Check after 5 minutes so the miso does not burn. If the miso browns too quickly, cover the salmon loosely with a sheet of aluminum foil and return to the oven. After the salmon flakes, divide the vegetables among four plates. Top each with the salmon, sprinkle with the sesame seeds, and serve immediately.

TIP

Mix the miso paste and lemon juice mixture with 1 tablespoon olive oil and 1 tablespoon water **for a salad dressing with a zing!** *It will make ⅔ cup, about four servings.*

If you wish, substitute 8 ounces baby spinach for the bok choy and snow peas. Divide the spinach among four plates and top with the salmon and mushrooms.

MONGOLIAN
BEEF WRAPS

4.6g
NET CARBS

SERVES
4

327
CALORIES

Mongolian beef is an American/Asian restaurant creation that is usually packed with brown sugar and served over white rice, priming you for a sugar slump. This Atkins-approved makeover slashes the sugar (we swap the white rice for the pleasing crunch of a butter lettuce wrap) and lets the healing aromatic flavorings of ginger, garlic, and red chili flakes shine through.

TIME	PER SERVING
Active: 15 minutes	*Total Carbs:* 7.9g
	Fiber: 3.3g
Total: 30 minutes	*Protein:* 30g
	Fat: 20.9g
	FV = 3.5

1 pound flank steak, sliced against the grain

2 tablespoons Atkins Flour Mix (page 126)

½ teaspoon garlic salt

3 tablespoons sesame oil, divided

1 bunch asparagus, trimmed and thinly sliced on the bias

2 garlic cloves, minced

1 tablespoon minced fresh ginger

½ teaspoon crushed red pepper flakes

2 tablespoons tamari or soy sauce

¼ cup water

1 head butter lettuce, broken into leaves, for serving

4 scallions, thinly sliced

1 Place the steak on a plate, and sprinkle it with the Atkins Flour Mix and garlic salt. Toss well to coat. Warm 2 tablespoons of the oil over medium heat and add the beef, cooking 2 to 3 minutes, until the beef starts to brown. Transfer to a clean plate.

2 Warm the remaining sesame oil in the same skillet. Add the asparagus, garlic, ginger, and chili flakes; cook 4 to 5 minutes, stirring often, until the garlic becomes fragrant. Return the beef to the skillet, and reduce the heat to low. Add the tamari or soy sauce and water, tossing well until a thick sauce forms. Spoon the mixture into the lettuce leaves, sprinkle with the scallions, and serve immediately.

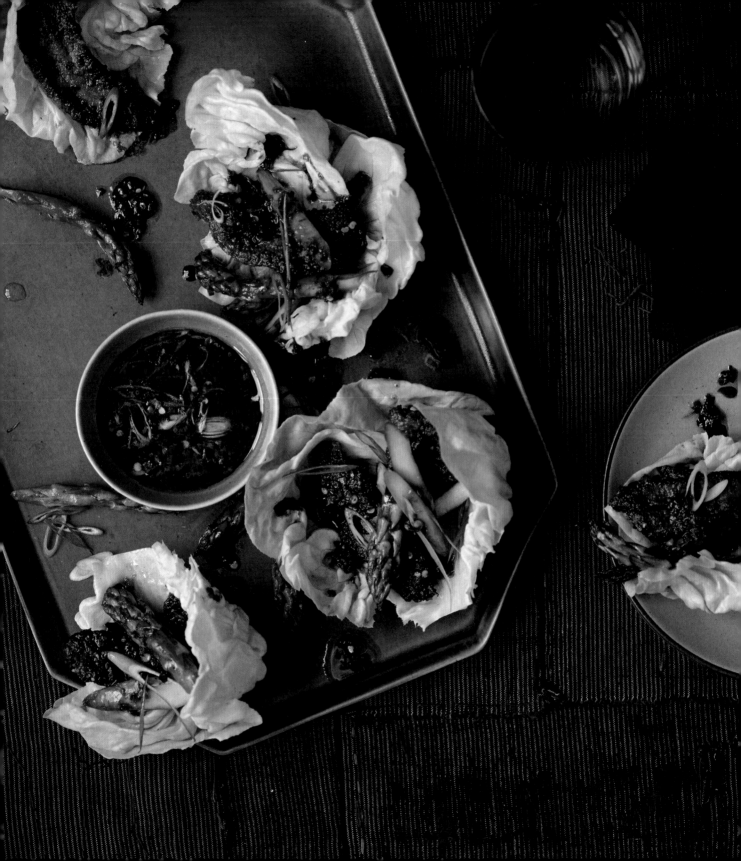

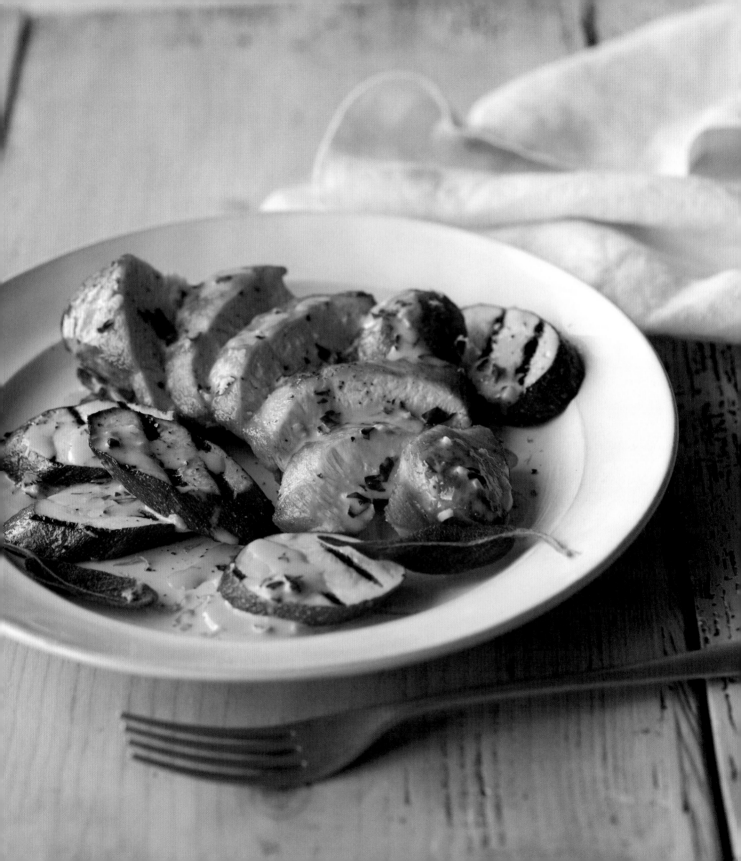

FRIED
SAGE
CHICKEN
AND ZUCCHINI

4.5g
NET CARBS

SERVES 4

328
CALORIES

Sage has long been prized in folk medicine for its ability to cleanse and protect against illness, and now we know why! Medical studies have revealed that sage is rich in potent antibacterial and antioxidant compounds.[1] Its flavor can be a bit overwhelming when it is raw, but cooking it in rich fats mellows it and makes it a perfect pairing for bright flavors such as lemon.

TIME	PER SERVING
Active: 15 minutes	*Total Carbs:* 5.9g
	Fiber: 1.4g
Total: 30 minutes	*Protein:* 28.5g
	Fat: 21.3g
	FV = 2.7

1 tablespoon unsalted butter

1 tablespoon olive oil

4 sage leaves, whole

¼ cup chopped fresh flat-leaf parsley

2 garlic cloves, minced

Zest of 1 lemon, finely grated

2 fresh sage leaves, thinly sliced

2 pounds skinless, boneless chicken breast, cubed

2 zucchini, thinly sliced

½ cup grated Parmesan cheese

½ cup unsalted chicken broth

¼ cup heavy cream

2 tablespoons lemon juice

1 Place the butter and olive oil in a large skillet over medium heat. When the mixture foams, add the whole sage leaves and fry until golden, 1 to 2 minutes. Remove the leaves from the skillet and set aside on paper towels. Add the parsley, garlic, and lemon zest; cook about 1 minute, until fragrant. Add the sliced sage leaves and chicken; cook 4 to 5 minutes more, until the chicken starts to brown. Add the zucchini, and cook 4 to 5 minutes, tossing well, until the zucchini is tender and the chicken is cooked through.

2 Reduce the heat to low, add the Parmesan, broth, and heavy cream, and cook 1 minute more, scraping any brown bits from the bottom of the pan. Add the lemon juice and mix. Garnish with the fried sage leaves, and serve immediately.

CHOP SUEY

4.7g
NET CARBS

SERVES 4

353
CALORIES

Chop Suey is a classic American dish that has its roots in Asian flavors such as soy and sesame but has no historical background. We update this recipe by mixing mild-tasting (and heart-healthy) oils such as sesame or coconut oil with butter, yielding a rich, slightly sweet base for the veggie-centric dish, which provides more flavor.

TIME	PER SERVING
Active: 15 minutes	*Total Carbs:* 7.2g
	Fiber: 2.6g
Total: 30 minutes	*Protein:* 27.1g
	Fat: 24.5g
	FV = 3.5

- 3 large pork chops on the bone (1½ pounds)
- ¼ teaspoon garlic salt
- ¼ teaspoon freshly ground black pepper
- 2 tablespoons Atkins Flour Mix (page 126)
- 3 tablespoons sesame or coconut oil
- 1 tablespoon unsalted butter
- 2 cups thinly sliced bok choy
- 5 ounces button or cremini mushrooms, thinly sliced
- 2 celery stalks, thinly sliced
- 1 green bell pepper, thinly sliced
- 4 scallions, thinly sliced
- ½ cup Basic Bone Broth (page 161) or unsalted chicken broth
- 2 tablespoons soy sauce or tamari

1   Thinly slice the meat off the pork chops, and discard the bone. Sprinkle the pork with the garlic salt, pepper, and Atkins Flour Mix.

2   In a large skillet, warm the oil and butter over medium heat. Add the pork slices and brown them, 2 to 3 minutes, stirring occasionally. Add the bok choy, mushrooms, celery, bell pepper, and scallions; cook 4 to 5 minutes, stirring often, until the vegetables are soft. Stir in the broth and soy sauce, scraping any brown bits from the bottom of the skillet. Serve immediately.

TIP

For a heartier dish, *pair with ½ cup cauliflower rice (page 118) per person for 2 added grams of Net Carbs.*

SUPERFAST
STROGANOFF

8.6g
NET CARBS

SERVES 4

425
CALORIES

Rich-tasting beef stroganoff has a gravy made by mixing sour cream with browned beef. It's a perfect cold-weather, creamy, iron-rich recipe that's fast to make and satisfying to eat. It's good enough to "stick to your ribs"—but not to worry, it won't! Depending on your carb intake, you can serve this stroganoff on top of 1 cup cooked zucchini noodles or with a veggie side that is lower in carbs, such as sautéed spinach.

TIME	PER SERVING
Active: 10 minutes	*Total Carbs:* 10.4g
	Fiber: 1.8g
Total: 20 minutes	*Protein:* 33.6g
	Fat: 29g
	FV = 5

2 tablespoons unsalted butter, divided

8 ounces button or cremini mushrooms, thinly sliced

1 onion, thinly sliced

2 garlic cloves, finely chopped

1 pound flank steak, sliced ½ inch thick

1 teaspoon garlic salt

1 cup Basic Bone Broth (page 161)

1 teaspoon Worcestershire sauce

¼ cup Atkins Flour Mix (page 126)

1 cup full-fat sour cream

1 Warm one tablespoon of butter in a large skillet over medium heat, and add the mushrooms, onion, and garlic; cook 4 to 5 minutes, stirring often, until the mushrooms start to brown. Transfer to a plate. Sprinkle the steak with the garlic salt. Add the remaining butter to the skillet over medium heat, then the steak, and cook 2 to 3 minutes, stirring occasionally, to brown the beef. Transfer to the plate with the mushroom mixture.

2 Stir in the broth and Worcestershire sauce, scraping up any brown bits from the bottom of the pan. Whisk in the Atkins Flour Mix, and simmer 1 minute, until the sauce begins to thicken. Return the steak and mushroom mixture to the skillet, and toss well. Turn the heat off. Stir in the sour cream, and serve immediately.

PARMESAN
SCALLOPS

14.3g NET CARBS

SERVES 4

299 CALORIES

This speedy seafood dish is ideal when you're in the mood for Italian fare. Fresh broccoli florets add a pleasing crunch as well as a boost of fiber, while the medley of scallops, bubbling Parmesan cheese, bright flavors of fresh herbs, and tangy marinara sauce completes the dish.

TIME	PER SERVING
Active: 15 minutes	*Total Carbs:* **17.4g**
	Fiber: **4.1g**
Total: 30 minutes	*Protein:* **29.2g**
	Fat: **13.3g**
	FV = 9.8

2 tablespoons olive oil

1 head broccoli, cut into small florets (about 4 cups)

¼ teaspoon garlic salt

¼ teaspoon freshly ground black pepper

2 cups low-sugar marinara sauce from a jar

½ cup water

1 pound fresh sea scallops (see Tip)

¼ cup chopped fresh flat-leaf parsley

½ cup grated Parmesan cheese

1 Warm the olive oil in a large skillet over medium heat. Add the broccoli, garlic salt, and black pepper; cook 7 to 8 minutes, until the broccoli starts to brown and soften. Set the oven to broil. Decrease the heat to low under the skillet, carefully add the marinara sauce and water, and stir well. Smooth the top of the broccoli sauce mixture, and place the scallops on top.

2 Sprinkle with the parsley and Parmesan, and place under the broiler. Broil 4 to 5 minutes, until the tops become golden and the scallops are cooked through and no longer translucent when sliced with a paring knife. Serve immediately.

TIP

Look for sea scallops that are "dry," *not treated with phosphates, a preserving method that makes them stringy when they are cooked.*

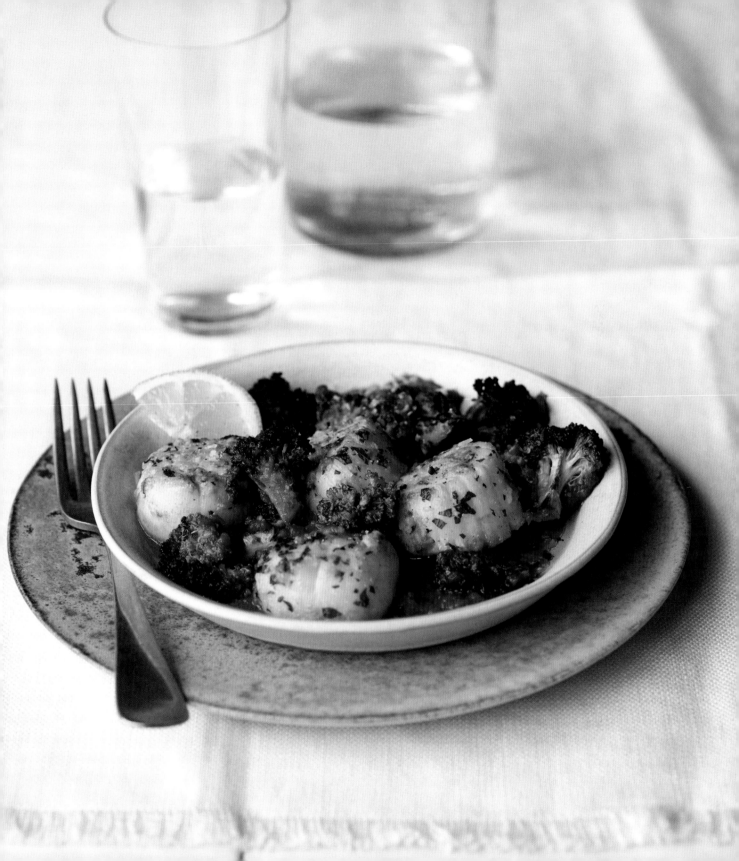

12

ONE-POT MEALS

EASY FAMILY FARE

for Tasty No-Fuss Meals

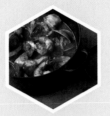 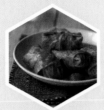 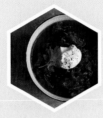

You'll love these budget-friendly one-pot meals,
which are super easy to cook and simple to clean up after. They are
flawless family meals and excellent crowd-pleasers.
Looking for something you can prepare in advance? Try the Italian
Stuffed Cabbage (page 251) or Year-Round Barbecued
Brisket (page 268), both of which are a breeze with the help of a slow
cooker. With their rich, hearty flavors and creamy sauces, you'll even
discover a few recipes perfect for a decadent date night!

RECIPES

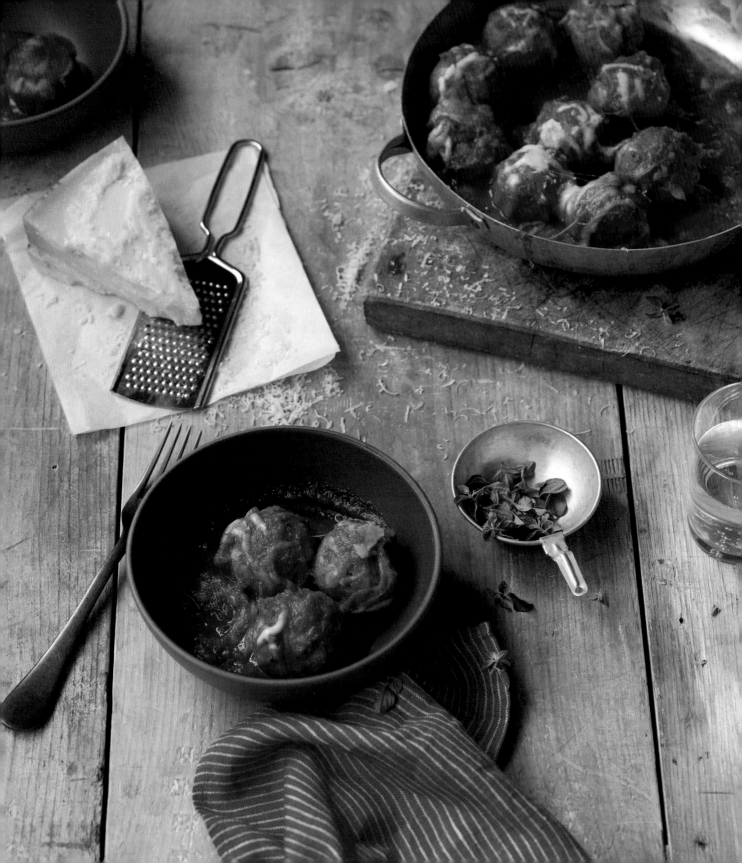

CHICKEN PARMESAN
MEATBALLS

5.1g
NET CARBS

SERVES 4

359
CALORIES

Craving the flavor of chicken Parm, but don't want to deal with the hassle and carbs of breading? These meatballs are bound to become your go-to for Italian Sunday-night meals. Grinding the chicken meat in your food processor is vital to the texture of this dish, since preground chicken meat is loaded with water and additives, making the meatball mixture too wet. Do it yourself for the flavor and the savings!

TIME	PER SERVING
Active: 15 minutes	*Total Carbs:* 6.7g *Fiber:* 1.6g
Total: 30 minutes	*Protein:* 37.7g *Fat:* 21.3g *FV = 1.8*

- 3 skinless, boneless chicken breasts (18 ounces total), cubed
- ½ cup **Atkins Flour Mix (page 126)**
- ½ cup full-fat cream cheese, room temperature
- 1 large egg
- 2 garlic cloves, minced
- 1 teaspoon dried oregano
- ½ teaspoon salt
- Olive oil spray
- 1 cup low-sugar marinara sauce from a jar
- ½ cup **Basic Bone Broth (page 161)** or unsalted chicken broth
- 2 slices (1 ounce) mozzarella cheese
- ¼ cup grated Parmesan cheese

1 Place the chicken in the food processor, pulsing to chop, for 6 to 7 minutes. Combine the chicken, Atkins Flour Mix, cream cheese, egg, garlic, oregano, and salt in a large bowl. Mix well with your hands until well incorporated. Roll into 2-inch balls (about 12).

2. Coat a large skillet with olive oil spray, and place over medium heat. Add the meatballs and cook 5 to 6 minutes, turning occasionally, until they are well browned. Reduce the heat to low, and add the marinara sauce and broth. Cover and cook 4 to 5 minutes more, until the meatballs are cooked through. Top with the sliced mozzarella and Parmesan. Cover and let rest 1 minute to melt the cheese. Serve immediately.

TIP

If you have the time, *put the cubed chicken on a baking sheet and freeze for about one hour, or until it is firmer but not solid, to help the chopping.*

ROAST BEEF

with Greek Yogurt Horseradish Sauce

1.2g
NET CARBS

SERVES
14

223
CALORIES

Need to feed a crowd with minimal work? This traditional roast beef feast gets a spicy kick from the creamy horseradish sauce. Serve with a delectable side such as Cauliflower Mac & Cheese (page 267) without the sausage, Cheesy Scallion Cheddar Cauliflower Mash (page 151), or sautéed spinach. Double the sauce and serve with cocktail shrimp as a festive, low-carb surf 'n' turf appetizer to kick off an evening.

TIME	PER SERVING
Active: 15 minutes	*Total Carbs:* 1.5g
	Fiber: 0.3g
Total: 1 hour 30 minutes	*Protein:* 37.7g
	Fat: 6.3g
	FV = 0

1 teaspoon garlic salt

1 teaspoon sweet paprika

1 teaspoon freshly ground black pepper

1 (5-pound) top or bottom round beef roast

Preheat the oven to 375°F. Place the garlic salt, paprika, and pepper in a small bowl, and mix well with a spoon. Sprinkle the roast with the spices, and transfer to a 2-quart baking dish. Transfer the roast to the oven, and cook for 1 hour to 1 hour, 30 minutes, until the outside of the roast is golden brown but the meat is still pinkish/red when sliced with a knife. Set aside for 5 minutes to allow the juices to redistribute. Slice the roast beef, and serve immediately with the Horseradish Sauce.

HORSERADISH SAUCE

2 tablespoons grated fresh horseradish

1 cup full-fat Greek yogurt

1 tablespoon lemon juice

1 cucumber, peeled, seeded, and grated

Place the horseradish, yogurt, lemon juice, and cucumber in a medium bowl. Stir well to combine, and refrigerate.

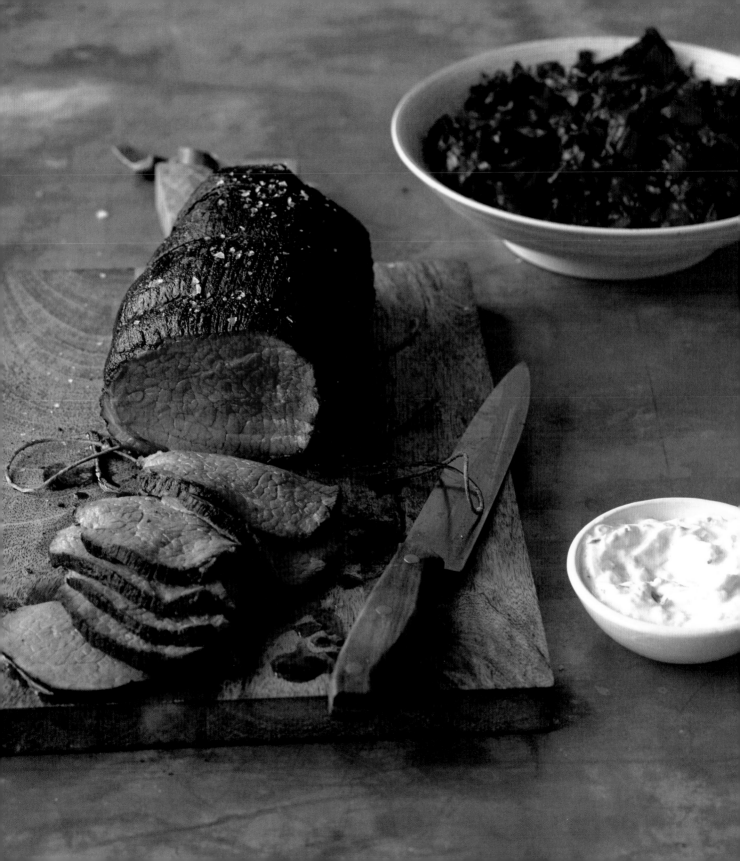

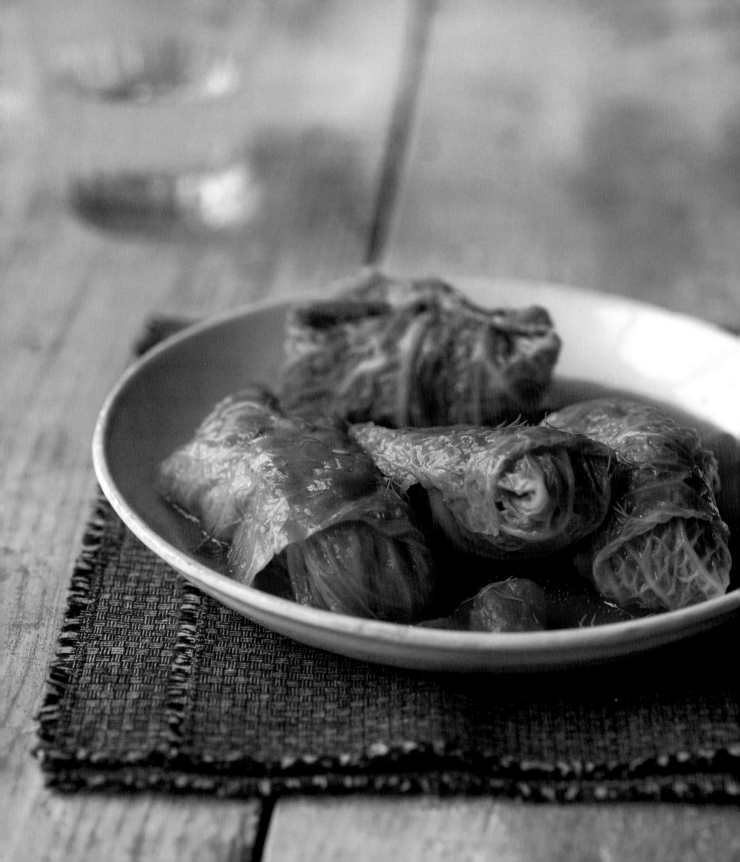

ITALIAN
STUFFED CABBAGE

5.3g NET CARBS

 SERVES **6**

291 CALORIES

Stuffed cabbage is a traditional Polish and Hungarian dish that's naturally healthy. Nutrient-dense cabbage is rich in vitamins C and K and fiber, and its softened leaves make the perfect casing for well-seasoned ground meat. This version uses Italian flavors, including basil and Parmesan, for a twist on an Eastern European classic.

TIME	PER SERVING
Active: 15 minutes	*Total Carbs:* 7g *Fiber:* 1.7g *Protein:* 29.7g
Total: 3 hours, 30 minutes	*Fat:* 15.3g *FV* = 4.6

- ½ cup grated Parmesan cheese
- 1 tablespoon ground flaxseed
- 1 large egg
- ½ teaspoon garlic salt
- ¼ teaspoon freshly ground black pepper
- 1 (3-pound) Napa cabbage
- 1 (14.5-ounce) can diced tomatoes
- 1 cup Basic Bone Broth (page 161) or beef broth
- 2 tablespoons tomato paste
- 1½ pounds ground beef or ground pork
- ¼ cup chopped basil leaves
- 1 teaspoon Italian seasoning or ½ teaspoon dried oregano
- ½ teaspoon ground turmeric
- Fresh dill for garnish, if desired

1 Stir together the Parmesan, flaxseed, egg, garlic salt, and pepper in a large bowl. Let rest for 30 minutes to allow the flaxseed to soften.

2 Meanwhile, bring a large stockpot filled halfway with water to a boil over high heat. Trim the tough root end of the cabbage so that you can easily remove 24 of the outer leaves; reserve the remaining cabbage for another use, such as Hot-and-Sour Soup (page 179). When the water boils, turn off the heat and add half of the leaves, pressing to submerge them in the hot water. Cover the stockpot, and let soak for 4 to 5 minutes, until the leaves begin to soften. Remove the cabbage leaves with tongs, and drain them in a colander.

RECIPE CONTINUES

3 Bring the water to a boil again, and cook the remaining cabbage leaves until they slowly start to soften but aren't fully cooked. Drain them in a colander. Alternatively, working in batches, wrap the leaves in a damp paper towel and microwave for 1 minute, until softened. Set aside to cool.

4 Put the diced tomatoes, broth, and tomato paste into a slow cooker, and mix together.

5 Add the ground beef or pork, basil, Italian seasoning or oregano, and turmeric to the flaxseed mixture, and mix together with your fingers. Place a cabbage leaf on a cutting board and trim the tough bottom. Place 3 tablespoons of the meat mixture close to the bottom edge of the leaf, and roll up. Tuck in the edges, and place the cabbage roll seam side down over the tomato mixture in the slow cooker. Repeat with the remaining leaves and filling.

6 Cover the slow cooker, and cook on the low setting for 3 to 3½ hours, until the filling is cooked through and no longer pink in the middle. To check for doneness, slice a cabbage roll open with a paring knife. Transfer four stuffed cabbage leaves to each of 6 soup plates and serve immediately. Garnish with fresh dill, if desired.

MUSHROOM
SPINACH
EGG SKILLET

7.8g NET CARBS

SERVES 4

237 CALORIES

Of all the quick weeknight meals, this simple skillet is the most beautiful. Serve it alongside one of our salad recipes for dinner or a relaxed weekend brunch along with some Cauliflower Hash Browns (page 118).

TIME	PER SERVING
Active: **15 minutes**	*Total Carbs:* **11.7g**
Total: **30 minutes**	*Fiber:* **3.9g**
	Protein: **16.2g**
	Fat: **15g**
	FV = **6.5**

Olive oil spray

1 pound baby spinach or spinach leaves, chopped

1 pound button or cremini mushrooms, thinly sliced

½ small yellow onion, finely chopped

3 small garlic cloves, minced

½ teaspoon salt

¼ teaspoon freshly ground black pepper

¼ teaspoon freshly grated nutmeg

⅓ cup heavy cream

4 large eggs

¼ cup grated Parmesan cheese

1 Coat a large skillet with olive oil spray, and place over high heat. Add the spinach in batches and stir to wilt, cooking each batch 1 to 2 minutes and transferring the wilted spinach to a bowl as you work. Coat the skillet with the olive oil spray again. Add the mushrooms, onion, garlic, salt, pepper, and nutmeg. Cook 4 to 5 minutes, stirring often, until the mushrooms and onions soften. Return the spinach to the skillet, and stir well. Turn the heat to low, and stir in the cream. Using a wooden spoon, make four wells in the vegetable mixture to hold the eggs.

2 Crack the eggs into the wells, and cover. Cook on low for 3 to 4 minutes. Sprinkle with the Parmesan and cover, cooking 1 minute more, until the Parmesan is melted and the whites are cooked through. Spoon out an egg and the vegetable mixture it is nestled in, and serve in a soup plate. Repeat with the remaining eggs.

GARLIC ROSEMARY
PORK LOIN

with Creamed Spinach

4.7g
NET CARBS

SERVES 4

429
CALORIES

Garlic and rosemary, two flavor staples of many cuisines, are also high in health-promoting antiviral and antibacterial compounds. Pork loin is a naturally low-fat cut of meat that benefits from the gentle roasting in this recipe. If your loin comes with a large fat cap (the fat on the top of the roast), you can trim it back before cooking.

TIME	PER SERVING
Active: 15 minutes	*Total Carbs:* **7.9g**
	Fiber: **3.2g**
Total: 1 hour	*Protein:* **37g**
	Fat: **28.1g**
	FV = 2.5

1 pound boneless pork loin

Olive oil spray

1 tablespoon Dijon mustard

3 garlic cloves, minced

2 tablespoons thinly sliced fresh rosemary

1 Preheat the oven to 350°F. Place the pork loin, fatty side down, in a small skillet over medium heat. Cook 4 to 5 minutes to brown the top and render some of the fat.

2 Coat a 7-by-11-inch baking dish with olive oil spray. Place the pork loin into the dish. Place the mustard, garlic, and rosemary in a small bowl and stir well. Spoon the mixture over the pork.

3 Bake for 45 minutes to 1 hour, until the loin is cooked through but still slightly pink in the center. About 15 minutes before the loin is done, prepare the Creamed Spinach. When the pork is cooked, let rest 5 minutes before slicing. Slice and serve immediately with the creamed spinach.

CREAMED SPINACH

16 ounces baby spinach or spinach leaves, chopped

2 tablespoons unsalted butter

2 tablespoons Atkins Flour Mix (page 126)

½ cup heavy cream

½ cup Basic Bone Broth (page 161) or unsalted chicken broth

¼ teaspoon freshly grated nutmeg

Zest of one lemon

½ cup grated Parmesan cheese

Heat a large skillet over high heat. Add the spinach in batches and stir to wilt, cooking each batch 1 to 2 minutes and transferring the wilted spinach to a bowl as you work. Melt the butter in the same skillet over medium heat. When the butter is melted, sprinkle in the Atkins Flour Mix and cook 1 to 2 minutes, stirring often, until the flour coats the pan. Whisk in the cream, broth, nutmeg, and lemon zest; cook 1 minute more, until the mixture forms a thick sauce. Stir in the reserved spinach and the Parmesan, stirring well until smooth and creamy.

TIP

Creamed Spinach is a rich side dish that is a traditional steakhouse favorite. It pairs well with grilled steak, salmon, poultry, or Year-Round Barbecued Brisket (page 268). Here are some other suggestions for starters and hearty sides to round out these meals.

- *Instead of bread, start with the Steamed Artichoke (page 219) or a crudité platter, which is a plate of sliced vegetables. Experiment with colorful vegetables that are in season, in addition to carrots, celery, bell peppers, and cherry tomatoes. Try sliced beets, grilled radicchio, or purple Brussels sprouts. You can also add marinated artichoke hearts, mushrooms, and olives, found at most grovery store salad or olive bars. Dip your veggies in hummus or any of the homemade salad dressings in Chapter 9.*

- *Skip the mashed potatoes in favor of Cheesy Scallion Cheddar Cauliflower Mash (page 151) or steamed broccoli or asparagus drizzled with rich hollandaise sauce.*

- *If you're still craving potatoes, cut up half a potato and toss it with olive oil and vegetables lower in carbs, such as pieces of sweet potato, cauliflower, broccoli, and mushrooms. Season with salt and pepper and roast in the oven.*

CHICKEN AND DUMPLINGS

7.7g NET CARBS

SERVES 4

346 CALORIES

Homey, creamy chicken topped with tender dumplings that steam directly inside the pot is the ultimate comfort food combination. If you've never had drop dumplings before, imagine cakelike clouds of goodness that you can use to sop up a delicious sauce.

TIME	PER SERVING
Active: 15 minutes	*Total Carbs:* 11.3g
	Fiber: 3.6g
Total: 30 minutes	*Protein:* 37.8g
	Fat: 17.6g
	FV = 2.2

Chicken

2 tablespoons unsalted butter

2 skinless, boneless chicken breasts, cubed (about 12 ounces)

½ teaspoon garlic salt

½ teaspoon paprika

¼ teaspoon freshly ground black pepper

5 ounces cremini or button mushrooms, thinly sliced

2 celery stalks, thinly sliced

4 garlic cloves, minced

¾ cup Basic Bone Broth (page 161) or unsalted chicken broth

2 tablespoons full-fat cream cheese

¼ cup chopped fresh flat-leaf parsley

Dumplings

1 cup Atkins Flour Mix (page 126)

2 teaspoons baking powder

½ teaspoon salt

¼ cup whole milk

2 teaspoons olive oil

1 Prepare the chicken: Warm the butter in a large stockpot over medium heat. Add the chicken, and sprinkle with the garlic salt, paprika, and pepper; cook 4 to 5 minutes, stirring occasionally, until the chicken starts to brown. Add the mushrooms, celery, and garlic; cook 4 to 5 minutes more, until the vegetables are tender. Add the broth, scraping up any brown bits from inside the stockpot. Turn the heat to low, and stir in the cream cheese and parsley.

2 Prepare the dumplings: Place the Atkins Flour Mix, baking powder, and salt in a small bowl. Mix well. Stir in the milk and oil, until a thick, wet dough forms. Spoon the dough on top of the chicken mixture in heaping spoonfuls, leaving an inch in between as they will expand. Cover and simmer 4 to 5 additional minutes to steam the dumplings. Serve immediately with the chicken.

GREEN BEAN
CHICKEN
SKILLET

4.6g
NET CARBS

SERVES 4

384
CALORIES

Inspired by the standard holiday green bean casserole, this skillet meal is a faster and more protein-rich version that uses fresh green beans in place of canned. Swap the typical dehydrated onion topping—which can be a haven for hidden carbs and preservatives—for the pleasing, heart-healthy crunch of nuts and unsweetened coconut. To save time on prep, shop for presliced green beans and nuts that are labeled as "pieces," meaning there is no need to chop them.

TIME	PER SERVING
Active: 15 minutes	*Total Carbs:* 9g
	Fiber: 4.4g
Total: 30 minutes	*Protein:* 28.1g
	Fat: 27.5g
	FV = 2

- 4 skinless, boneless chicken breasts, diced (1½ pounds)
- 2 tablespoons Atkins Flour Mix (page 126)
- ½ teaspoon garlic salt
- ½ teaspoon sweet paprika
- ¼ teaspoon freshly ground black pepper
- 2 tablespoons coconut or olive oil, divided
- 8 ounces green beans, trimmed, cut in half
- ¾ cup unsalted chicken broth or **Basic Bone Broth** (page 161)
- 2 tablespoons full-fat cream cheese
- ½ cup unsweetened shredded coconut
- ¼ cup chopped pecans, macadamia nuts, or walnuts

1 Place the chicken on a plate, and sprinkle with the Atkins Flour Mix, garlic salt, paprika, and pepper, tossing with tongs to coat evenly. Heat 1 tablespoon of the oil in a large skillet over medium heat. Add the chicken, and cook 3 to 4 minutes, until the chicken starts to brown. Transfer to a plate. Add the remaining oil and the green beans to the skillet, and cook 6 to 8 minutes, until the green beans begin to soften.

2 Set the oven to broil. Return the chicken to the skillet, add the broth, and bring to a simmer; cook 1 minute more, stirring well. Decrease the heat to low, and stir in the cream cheese until it melts. Turn the heat off. Sprinkle the coconut and nuts over the chicken mixture, and place under the broiler on the middle rack for 30 to 40 seconds, until the tops are golden brown. Serve immediately.

BOLOGNESE
SKILLET
LASAGNA

8.7g
NET CARBS

SERVES
4

403
CALORIES

Lasagna, filled with a rich meat ragù, is delicious but a lot of work to assemble and cook. This "cheat" version, which is made in one skillet, uses the crepe recipe (page 127) as the lasagna sheet and takes half the time. If you want to make this novel recipe for date night, just cut the ingredients in half, use a small skillet, and serve the skillet tableside for just the two of you.

TIME	PER SERVING
Active: 25 minutes	*Total Carbs:* 10.7g
	Fiber: 2.7g
Total: 45 minutes	*Protein:* 45.8g
	Fat: 26.1g
	FV = 4.9

⅓ crepe recipe (page 127)

1 pound lean ground beef

½ teaspoon salt

¼ teaspoon freshly ground black pepper

Olive oil spray

4 garlic cloves, minced

2 tablespoons tomato paste

1 (14-ounce) can diced tomatoes

½ cup dry white wine, Basic Bone Broth (page 161), beef broth, or chicken broth

6 fresh basil leaves

½ cup chopped fresh flat-leaf parsley

1 cup thinly sliced fresh mozzarella

½ cup grated Parmesan cheese

1 Prepare the 4 crepes, and set aside. Sprinkle the beef with the salt and pepper. Coat a large skillet with olive oil spray and place over medium heat. Add the beef and garlic; cook 5 to 6 minutes, stirring occasionally, until the beef is well browned. Add the tomato paste, and cook 1 to 2 minutes more, until fragrant.

2 Add the tomatoes, wine, basil, and parsley. Increase the heat to high, and bring to a rapid simmer. Reduce the heat to low, and cook covered 25 to 30 minutes, stirring occasionally, until the sauce thickens. Top the sauce with the four crepes, layering them slightly over each other to completely cover the surface of the meat. Cover with the mozzarella slices, and sprinkle with the Parmesan. Coat the inside of the pan lid with olive oil spray to prevent it from sticking, and cover the lasagna. Simmer 10 to 15 minutes more, until the cheese is melted and bubbly. Serve immediately.

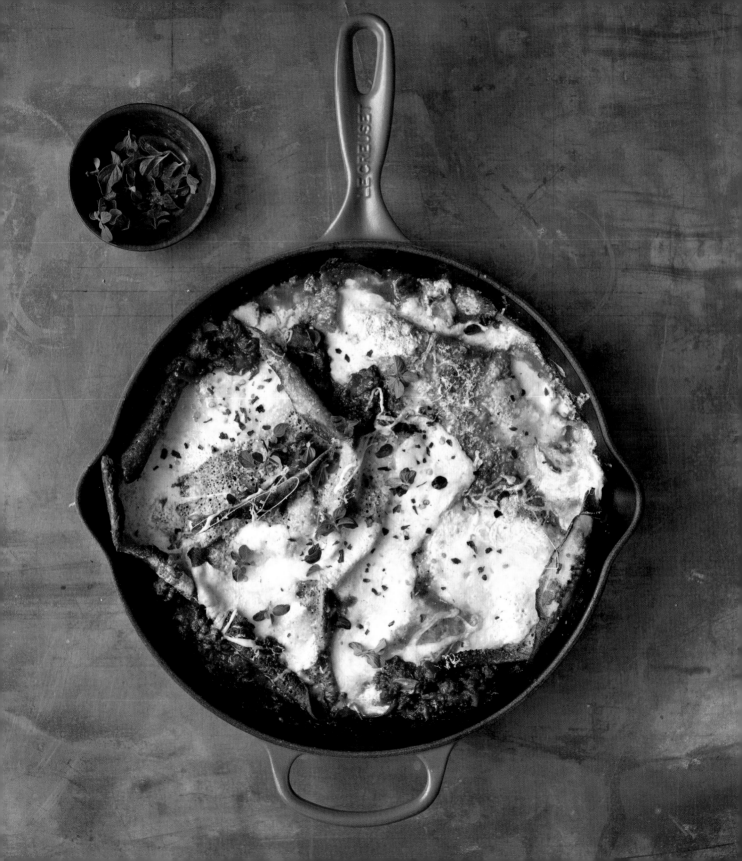

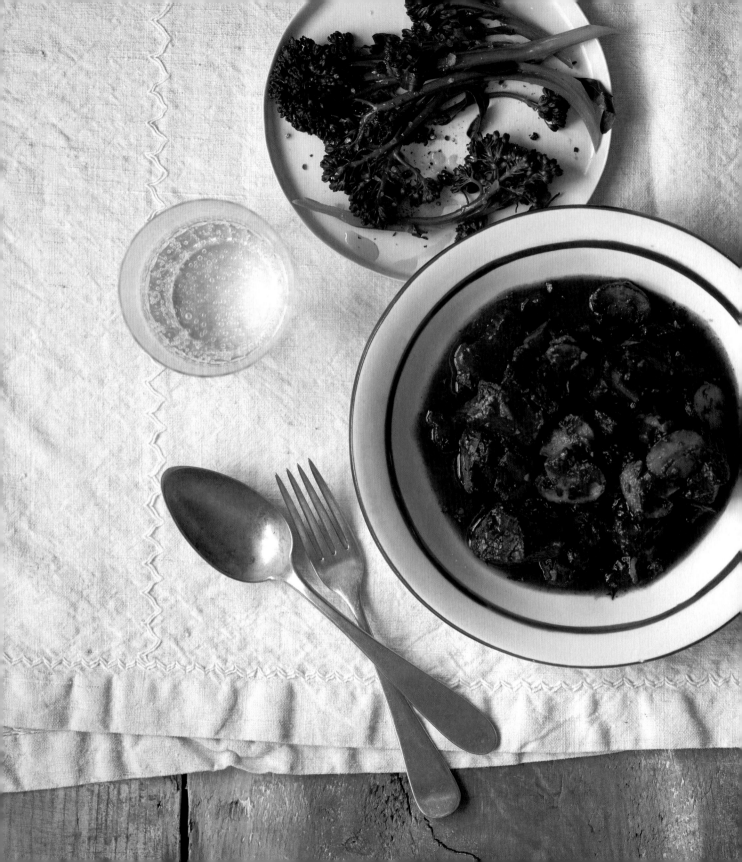

BEEF
BOURGUIGNON

7.2g
NET CARBS

SERVES
4

461
CALORIES

This delectable French stew gets its flavors from bacon, herbs, and red wine. The combination of aromatic ingredients will make your home smell like a French bistro. Serve this stew over 1 cup of steamed broccoli (for 4 grams of Net Carbs) or a simple mixed green side salad tossed in olive oil and a teaspoon of red wine vinegar (for 2 grams of Net Carbs). You don't have to be Julia Child to master this mouthwatering, home-cooked recipe.

TIME	PER SERVING
Active: 30 minutes	*Total Carbs:* 8.9g
	Fiber: 1.7g
Total: 3 hours	*Protein:* 28.2g
	Fat: 30.3g
	FV = 3.7

1 pound beef stew meat

1 tablespoon Atkins Flour Mix (page 126)

½ teaspoon salt

¼ teaspoon freshly ground black pepper

2 tablespoons unsalted butter

2 tablespoons olive oil

¼ pound bacon, chopped

10 ounces mushrooms, such as button or cremini, trimmed and sliced

½ onion, chopped

4 garlic cloves, minced

2 tablespoons tomato paste

1 teaspoon fresh thyme leaves

1 cup red wine, Basic Bone Broth (page 161), or beef broth

2 cups Basic Bone Broth (page 161) or beef broth

Chopped fresh flat-leaf parsley for garnish (optional)

1   Place the beef on a plate, and sprinkle with the Atkins Flour Mix, salt, and pepper. Toss to coat evenly. Set aside. Warm the butter and olive oil in a large stockpot over medium-high heat. Add the beef and cook 4 to 5 minutes, turning occasionally, until the coating browns. Transfer the beef to a plate.

2   Add the bacon and cook 4 to 5 minutes, stirring often, scraping up any brown bits that stick to the inside of the pot. Add the mushrooms, onion, and garlic; cook 4 to 5 minutes, stirring often, until the mushrooms soften and the onion is brown. Reduce the heat to low, and add the tomato paste and thyme, cooking 1 minute more, until the tomato paste is fragrant. Add the red wine and broth, and increase the heat to high. Return the beef to the stockpot, and bring to a boil, then immediately reduce to a simmer and cover. Cook 2½ to 3 hours, until the beef is tender and the sauce thickens. Serve immediately. Garnish with chopped parsley, if desired.

SHELLFISH
CIOPPINO

13.2g
NET CARBS

SERVES 4

372
CALORIES

Cioppino, a San Francisco tradition created by Italian immigrants who settled in California in the 1800s, is a delectable seafood stew bursting with the flavors of the sea in a savory broth that is great for celebrations or date night. This dish is easy to make even if you're not used to cooking fish, and the minerals and B vitamins in the variety of seafood give your brain and energy levels a natural boost.

TIME	PER SERVING
Active: 15 minutes	*Total Carbs:* 15.8g
	Fiber: 2.6g
Total: 30 minutes	*Protein:* 41.8g
	Fat: 12g
	FV = 7.7

2 tablespoons olive oil

1 medium fennel bulb, thinly sliced, fronds reserved and chopped

2 shallots, chopped

2 large garlic cloves, finely chopped

½ teaspoon salt

¼ teaspoon freshly ground black pepper

1 teaspoon crushed red pepper flakes, divided

2 tablespoons tomato paste

1 (14-ounce) can diced tomatoes in juice

¾ cup dry white wine or unsalted chicken broth

2 cups unsalted chicken broth

1 bay leaf

½ pound Manila clams, scrubbed

½ pound mussels, scrubbed, debearded

½ pound uncooked large shrimp (about 20), peeled and deveined

¾ pound assorted firm-fleshed fish fillets such as halibut

1 lemon, quartered

1 Heat the oil in a large stockpot over medium heat. Add the fennel, shallots, garlic, salt, pepper, and half the red pepper flakes; cook 8 to 10 minutes, stirring occasionally, until the vegetables start to brown. Stir in the tomato paste. Add the diced tomatoes with their juice, wine, broth, and bay leaf. Cover and bring to a simmer. Reduce the heat to medium-low. Simmer for 10 minutes to allow the flavors to meld.

RECIPE CONTINUES

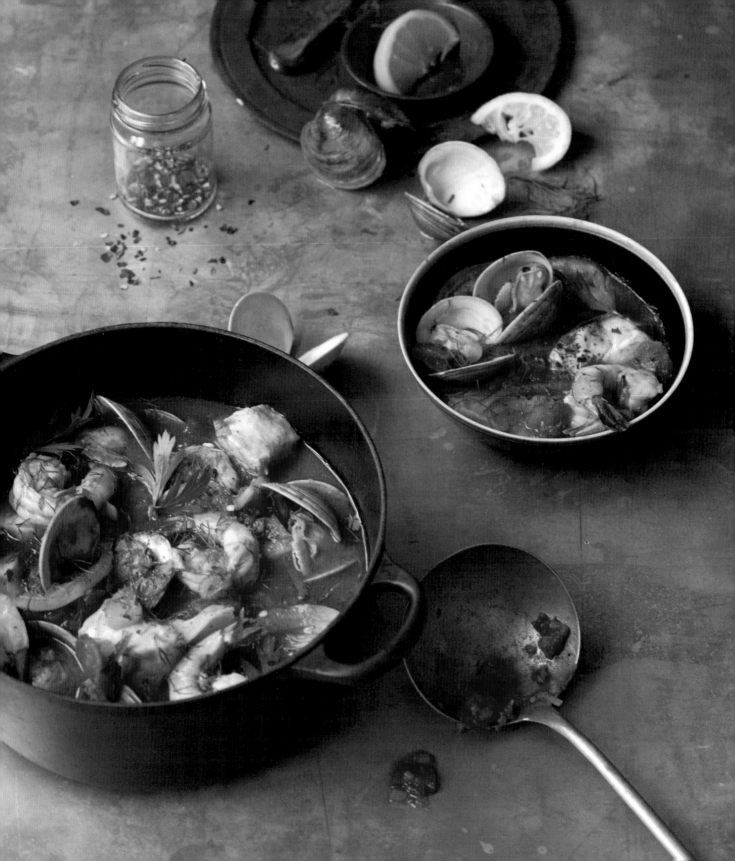

TIPS

For date night, *cut the recipe in half and serve with Wilted Brussels Sprout Salad with Warm Pancetta Dressing (page 190) or Pear and Manchego Mesclun Salad with Caramelized Onions (page 195).*

Though crusty sourdough bread is traditionally used to sop up the savory broth in this dish, depending on how many carbs you are consuming, a slice of **Low-Carb Flax Meal Bread** *(page 202) works equally well.*

2 Add the clams and mussels to the cooking liquid; cover and cook until the clams and mussels begin to open, about 4 to 5 minutes. Add the shrimp and fish. Simmer 4 to 5 minutes longer, stirring gently, until the fish and shrimp are just cooked through and the clams are completely open (discard any clams and mussels that do not open). Remove the bay leaf, ladle the stew into bowls, and garnish with the remaining red pepper flakes, reserved fennel fronds, and the lemon.

ROASTED FENNEL AND
COD

with Moroccan Olives

6.4g
NET CARBS

SERVES **4**

335
CALORIES

Refreshing, slightly sweet, aromatic fennel makes a light base for flaky, well-seasoned cod in this simple roasted fish recipe. Any olives will work for this recipe, but to make it even more flavorful, look for firm, salty black Moroccan olives cured in oil. Or use large, tart Italian Cerignola olives, which are sold in gourmet Italian markets, removing the pits before you bake.

TIME	PER SERVING
Active: 15 minutes	*Total Carbs:* **11.2g**
	Fiber: **4.8g**
Total: 45 minutes	*Protein:* **32.4g**
	Fat: **18.4g**
	FV = **5.3**

- **2 fennel bulbs, trimmed and thinly sliced**
- **1 lemon**
- **1 tablespoon olive oil**
- **½ teaspoon garlic salt**
- **1½ pounds cod fillets**
- **½ cup black Moroccan olives, pitted**
- **¼ cup chopped dill or cilantro**
- **½ teaspoon hot paprika or ¼ teaspoon crushed red pepper flakes**
- **¼ teaspoon salt**
- **¼ teaspoon freshly ground black pepper**
- **4 tablespoons unsalted butter**

1 Preheat the oven to 400°F. Place the fennel in a 7-by-11-inch baking dish. Zest the lemon over the fennel, and add the olive oil and garlic salt. Toss well. Transfer to the oven, and bake for 10 to 15 minutes, until the edges of the fennel start to brown.

2 Cut the zested lemon into quarters. Place the fish on top of the fennel, as well as the lemon wedges, and sprinkle with the olives, dill or cilantro, paprika or chili flakes, salt, and pepper. Place a tablespoon of butter onto each piece of fish. Bake 20 to 25 minutes, until the fish flakes when pressed with a fork. Squeeze lemon juice from the lemon wedges over the fish, and serve immediately.

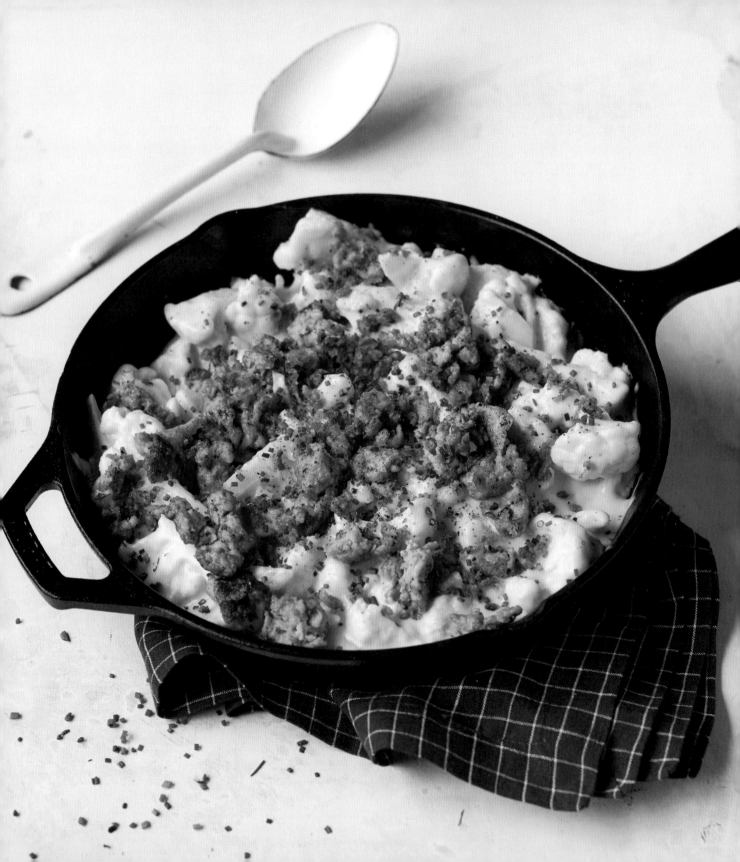

CAULIFLOWER
MAC & CHEESE

SERVES
8

In this cheesy comfort food classic, tender cauliflower florets are a "super" low-carb swap for pasta. Cauliflower, a member of the cruciferous family, is considered a superfood because it's rich in certain compounds that may ward off heart disease, plus it's a good source of fiber, vitamins, and minerals. You'll be hooked when you pair it with a medley of bubbling cheeses and savory chunks of chicken sausage, which turn it into a full, protein-rich meal.

1 small head cauliflower, cut into florets (about 5 cups)

Olive oil spray

12 ounces chicken sausage, chopped (optional)

2 tablespoons unsalted butter

4 garlic cloves, minced

3 tablespoons Atkins Flour Mix (page 126)

½ cup whole milk

½ cup Basic Bone Broth (page 161) or unsalted chicken broth

1 cup shredded cheddar cheese

1 cup grated Parmesan cheese

4 ounces full-fat cream cheese, room temperature

½ teaspoon freshly grated nutmeg, divided

2 tablespoons chopped fresh chives

1 Place the cauliflower florets into a large stockpot, and add 2 inches of water. Bring to a boil over high heat. Cook 4 to 5 minutes, until fork tender. Drain and set aside.

2 Coat a large skillet with olive oil spray, and place over high heat. Add the sausage, if using, and cook 8 to 10 minutes, stirring often, until browned and cooked through. Transfer to a plate. Reduce the heat to low, add the butter and garlic, and cook 1 to 2 minutes, until the garlic is fragrant. Add the Atkins Flour Mix, and cook 1 to 2 minutes, whisking continuously until a thick paste forms. Add the milk, broth, cheddar cheese, Parmesan, cream cheese, and half the nutmeg.

3 Reduce the heat to low, and cook 1 to 2 minutes, stirring well, until the cheese is melted and the mixture is smooth. Stir in the cauliflower and toss well to coat in the sauce. Sprinkle with the sausage, if using, garnish with the remaining nutmeg and the chives, and serve.

WITH SAUSAGE	
TIME	**PER SERVING**
Active: 15 minutes	*Net Carbs:* **5.7g**
	Total Carbs: **7.6g**
Total: 30 minutes	*Fiber:* **1.9g**
	Protein: **21.8g**
	Fat: **21.8g**
	Calories: **311**
	FV = 2.2

WITHOUT SAUSAGE	
TIME	**PER SERVING**
Active: 15 minutes	*Net Carbs:* **5.1g**
	Total Carbs: **6.9g**
Total: 30 minutes	*Fiber:* **1.9g**
	Protein: **14.3g**
	Fat: **17.6g**
	Calories: **238**
	FV = 2.2

YEAR-ROUND
BARBECUED
BRISKET

2.6g
NET CARBS

SERVES
14

270
CALORIES

Brisket is a picnic and outdoor barbecue treat that you can easily make any time of year when you use a slow cooker. It's the perfect hands-off dish that takes minimal prep time—just throw the ingredients into your slow cooker, set the timer, and forget about it until the pleasing aroma of barbecue fills your house. So go ahead, have a picnic indoors anytime you get the hankering by pairing this with Cauliflower Mac & Cheese (page 267) without the sausage or Creamed Spinach (page 255).

TIME	PER SERVING
Active: 15 minutes	*Total Carbs:* 3.6g
	Fiber: 1g
Total: 10 hours	*Protein:* 35.1g
	Fat: 12.3g
	FV = 1.7

1 (6-ounce) can tomato paste

⅓ cup apple cider vinegar

1 tablespoon chili powder

2 teaspoons onion powder

2 teaspoons garlic salt

1 teaspoon freshly ground black pepper

1 teaspoon smoked paprika

1 teaspoon cayenne pepper

2 tablespoons stevia

2 tablespoons Atkins Flour Mix (page 126)

1 (5-pound) beef brisket

1 Place the tomato paste, vinegar, chili powder, onion powder, garlic salt, black pepper, paprika, cayenne pepper, stevia, and Atkins Flour Mix in the slow cooker. Whisk to combine. Spoon out ¼ cup of the sauce to top the brisket.

2 Add the brisket, and top with the sauce. Set the slow cooker to low, and cook 9 to 10 hours, until the meat is very tender. Shred and serve immediately.

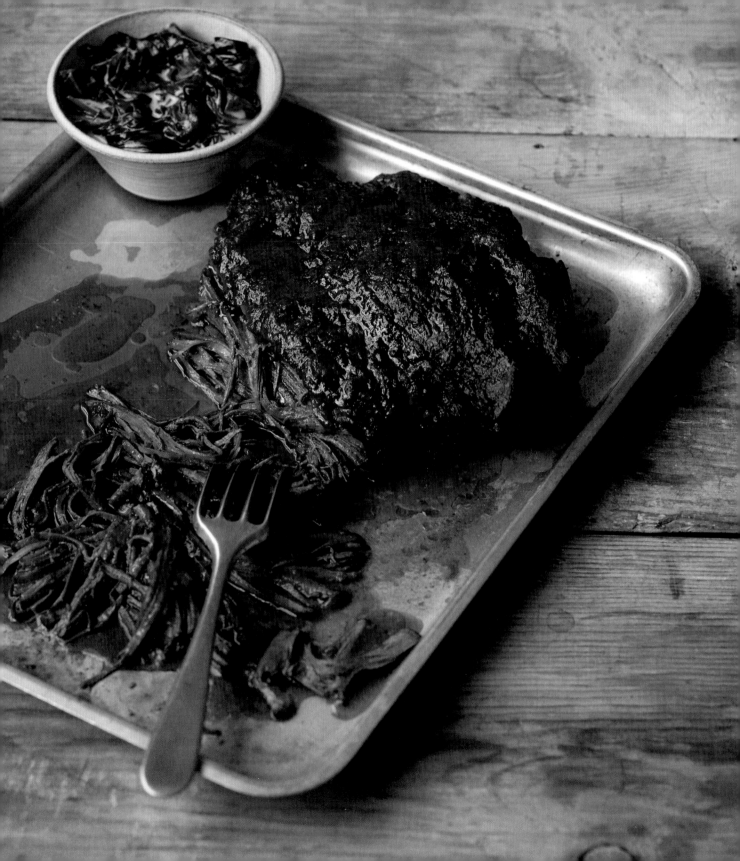

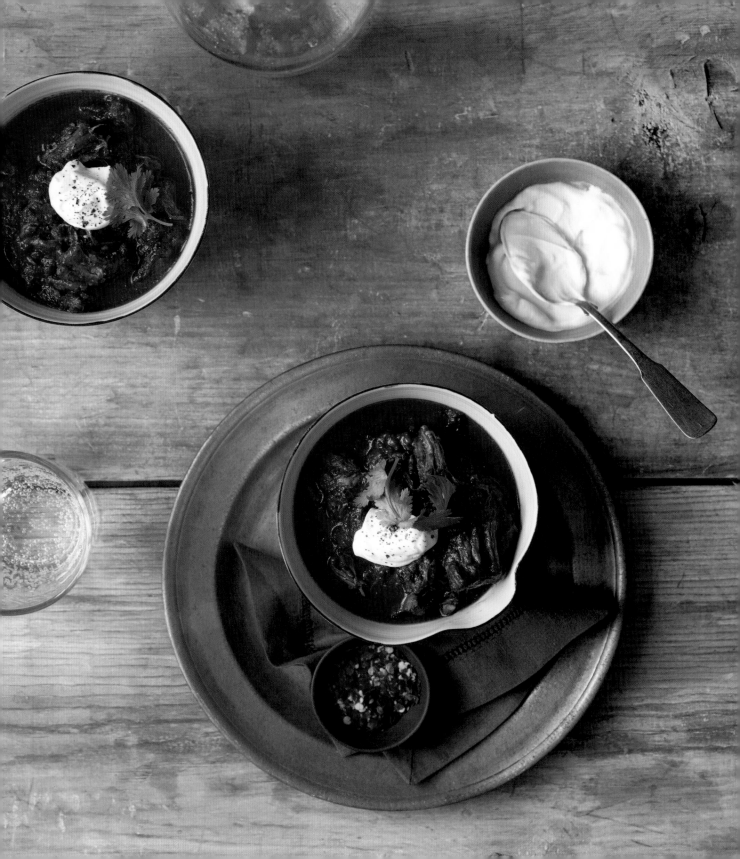

SMOKY
HABANERO
CHILI

4.8g
NET CARBS

SERVES 8

296
CALORIES

Smoky sea salt and chilies lend fiery southwestern flavors to this delicious chili that easily feeds a group. Pair this meat-centric dish with a leafy green salad, Sautéed Spinach with Caramelized Shallots (page 154), or steamed broccoli to make it more nutritionally balanced.

TIME	PER SERVING
Active: 15 minutes	*Total Carbs:* 6.1g
	Fiber: 1.3g
Total: 3 hours, 15 minutes	*Protein:* 23.1g
	Fat: 19.5g
	FV = 2.7

2 pounds beef stew meat

1 teaspoon smoked sea salt or steak seasoning

1 teaspoon freshly ground black pepper

2 tablespoons grape seed or safflower oil

1 red onion, minced

4 garlic cloves, minced

1 habanero chili, seeded and minced

2 tablespoons mild chili powder

1 teaspoon crushed red pepper flakes

¼ teaspoon dried oregano

2 tablespoons tomato paste

4 cups Basic Bone Broth (page 161) or unsalted chicken broth

½ cup full-fat sour cream

½ cup chopped fresh cilantro leaves and stems

1 Season the beef with the salt or steak seasoning and pepper. Warm the oil in a large stockpot over high heat. Add the beef, and cook 3 to 4 minutes, turning occasionally, until it browns. Add the onion, garlic, habanero, chili powder, red pepper flakes, oregano, and tomato paste, and cook 2 to 3 minutes more, until fragrant.

2 Add the broth, and bring to a simmer. Cover and reduce the heat to low, and cook 2½ to 3 hours, until the beef begins to fall apart. Shred the beef with a fork, and serve immediately with the sour cream and cilantro.

13
JUST DESSERTS

THE GRAND FINALE IS JUST AS SWEET,

Minus the Carbs and Sugar

◆

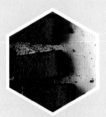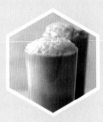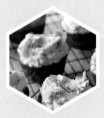

Desserts are definitely not a thing of the past if you're living a low-carb, low-sugar lifestyle. Guilty pleasures? Nothing could be further from the truth! Get ready to indulge in these sweet, sometimes no-bake, often chocolate-y, deliciously sinful but guilt-free delicacies.

RECIPES

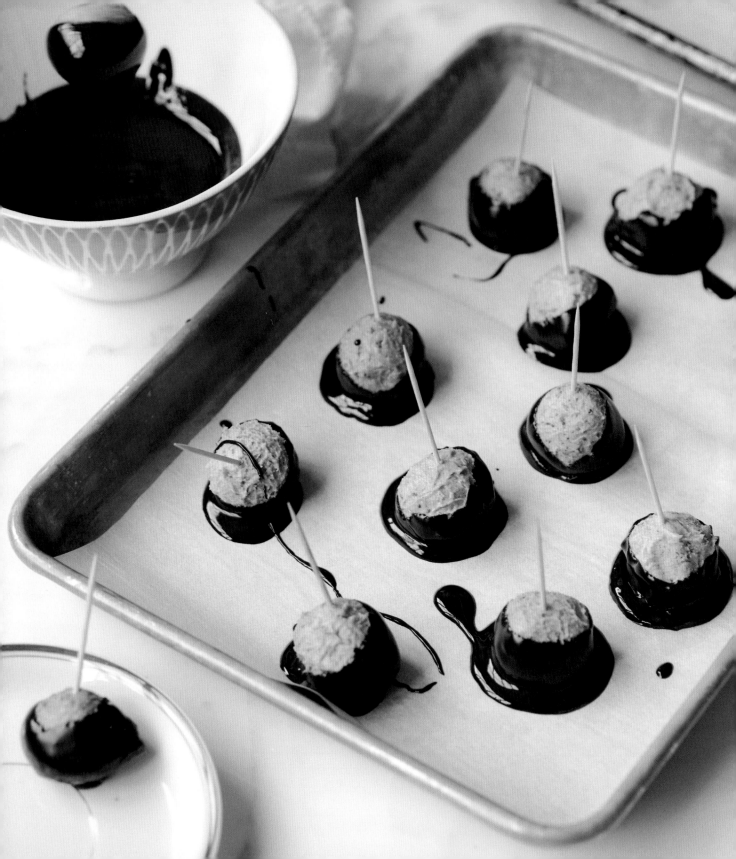

BUCKEYE
TRUFFLES

2.3g
NET CARBS

MAKES
24

141
CALORIES

Buckeye trees, which are indigenous to Ohio and Pennsylvania, are the inspiration for the buckeye candy that resembles the nuts from these trees. This "truffled" version has a softer filling that is dunked in 100 percent antioxidant-rich chocolate.

TIME	PER SERVING
Active: 10 minutes	*Total Carbs:* 3.8g
	Fiber: 1.5g
Total: 45 minutes	*Protein:* 4.7g
	Fat: 12.6g

Truffles

1 cup no-sugar-added peanut butter

½ cup unsalted butter, softened

¼ cup stevia

⅓ cup plain protein powder

2 tablespoons ground flaxseed

1 teaspoon vanilla extract

Chocolate Coating

4 ounces unsweetened baking chocolate, chopped

2 tablespoons unsalted butter

1 **Make the truffles:** Place the peanut butter, butter, stevia, protein powder, flaxseed, and vanilla extract in a stand mixer, and blend until smooth.

2 Line a tray that will fit into your freezer with wax paper. Using a soup spoon to scoop the peanut mixture, make 24 (1-inch) mounds. Transfer them to the prepared tray, and freeze for 30 minutes.

With wet fingers, roll into balls. Return to the freezer on a separate plate while you prepare the chocolate coating. Reserve the tray with the wax paper for the dipped truffles.

3 Melt the chocolate and butter in a microwavable bowl for 30 seconds to 1 minute. Stir until smooth. Since the entire batch won't fit on one plate, dip half the batch while you keep the other half in the freezer (which also prevents the other half from melting while you dip the first half).

4 Insert a toothpick or fork in the center of each peanut butter ball, and dunk in the melted chocolate.

5 Return the dipped truffles to the wax paper–lined baking sheet. Repeat with the remaining truffles. Keep refrigerated until ready to serve. You can also freeze these in an airtight container for up to 6 months.

CHOCOLATE
EGG CREAM

6.4g **208**
NET CARBS   SERVES 2   CALORIES

Don't be fooled by the name "egg cream." This classic soda shop drink received that nickname from the frothy top, which is made with a combination of seltzer and milk and is as light as whipped egg whites. It's the ideal low-carb swap when you crave chocolate milk or a chocolate milk shake.

TIME	PER SERVING
Active: 5 minutes	*Total Carbs:* 7.4g
	Fiber: 1g
Total: 5 minutes	*Protein:* 2.4g
	Fat: 19.3g

½ cup canned coconut milk

¼ cup heavy cream

¼ cup sugar-free chocolate syrup

1½ cups unflavored seltzer water

Divide the coconut milk, heavy cream, and chocolate between two glasses. Stir each glass well. Top off each with ¾ cup of the seltzer, and serve immediately.

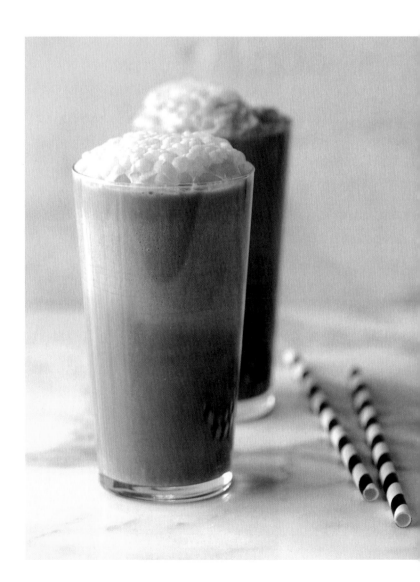

MEXICAN
WEDDING
COOKIES

2.4g **NET CARBS**

 MAKES 22

124 **CALORIES**

Almost every culture has its version of a crumbly nut-and-butter-based cookie, such as Russian tea cake, butter balls, and Italian wedding cookies. This version is made with fiber-rich almond flour spiked with healing spices—ground cardamom and cinnamon—that add another layer of wonderful flavor with each bite.

TIME	PER COOKIE
Active: 10 minutes	*Total Carbs:* **4.2g**
	Fiber: **1.8g**
Total: 30 minutes	*Protein:* **4.4g**
	Fat: **11.1g**

2 cups almond flour

1 cup finely chopped walnuts

¼ cup Atkins Flour Mix (page 126)

1 teaspoon baking powder

1 teaspoon ground cardamom

¼ teaspoon salt

¼ cup unsalted butter, softened

1 large egg

1 teaspoon vanilla extract

½ cup stevia, divided

1 tablespoon ground cinnamon

1 Preheat the oven to 325°F, and line two baking sheets with parchment paper.

2 In a medium bowl, whisk together the almond flour, walnuts, Atkins Flour Mix, baking powder, cardamom, and salt.

3 In a large bowl, beat the butter until light and fluffy, about 2 minutes. Beat in the egg, vanilla extract, and half the stevia and beat in the almond flour mixture until the dough comes together. Form the dough into ¾-inch balls, and place on the baking sheets about 1 inch apart.

4 Bake for 16 to 18 minutes, until just lightly golden brown. In a medium bowl, add the remaining stevia and cinnamon, and mix well. While the cookies are still warm, roll them around in the cinnamon mixture to coat. Transfer to a plate to cool completely. Serve or store in an airtight container on the countertop for up to 4 days.

LIME
COCONUT RUM
CUPCAKES

3.8g
NET CARBS

MAKES
12

287
CALORIES

Island flavors of lime, coconut, and rum give an otherwise plain vanilla cupcake some serious gourmet flair. These are ideal for an adult birthday, paired with artisanal low-carb rum drinks, or for a kids' birthday bash, using vanilla extract and water in place of the rum. Zest the lime for the icing first, then juice the lime for the cupcakes.

TIME	PER SERVING
Active: 10 minutes	*Total Carbs:* **5.3g** *Fiber:* **1.6g**
Total: 24 minutes	*Protein:* **11.2** *Fat:* **25.1g**

Cupcakes

½ cup unsalted butter, melted

⅓ cup stevia

Juice of 1 lime, reserve 2 teaspoons for icing

2 tablespoons dark rum or coconut rum or 1 teaspoon vanilla extract mixed with 1 tablespoon water

1 teaspoon vanilla extract

4 large eggs

1 cup Atkins Flour Mix (page 126)

⅓ cup unsweetened shredded coconut

1¼ teaspoons baking powder

¼ teaspoon salt

Icing

4 ounces full-fat cream cheese, room temperature

2 tablespoons stevia

Zest of 1 lime, plus reserved 2 teaspoons lime juice

1 teaspoon vanilla extract

½ cup unsalted butter, room temperature

½ cup unsweetened shredded coconut

1 **Make the cupcakes:** Heat the oven to 350°F. Line a 12-cup muffin tin with cupcake liners. Place the butter, stevia, lime juice, rum, and vanilla in a large bowl, and beat with an electric mixer until smooth and creamy. Beat in the eggs. In a separate bowl place the Atkins Flour Mix, coconut, baking powder, and salt, and stir well.

2 Using a stand or hand mixer, slowly add the flour and coconut mixture to the wet ingredients. Beat until smooth, about 1 minute. Pour into the prepared muffin tin. Bake for 14 to 16 minutes, until the cake springs back when lightly touched in the middle. Cool in the pan on a wire rack for 5 minutes.

3 **Make the icing:** Place the cream cheese in a medium mixing bowl along with the stevia, lime zest, reserved lime juice, and vanilla extract. Whip well until smooth, 30 seconds to 1 minute. Add the butter and mix until smooth. Ice the cooled cupcakes, and sprinkle with the coconut. Serve immediately, or store in an airtight container at room temperature for up to 4 days.

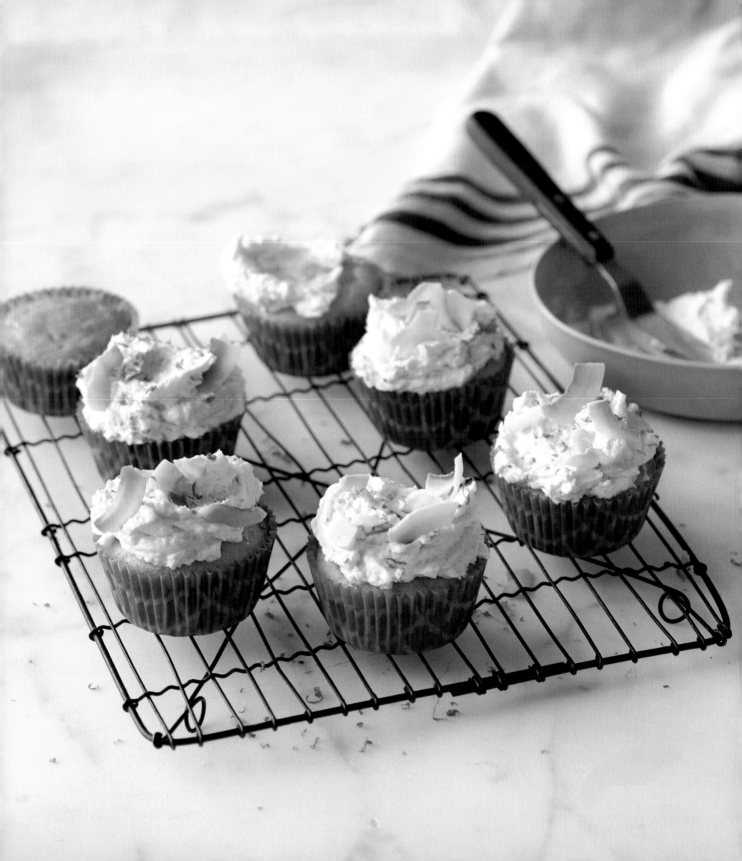

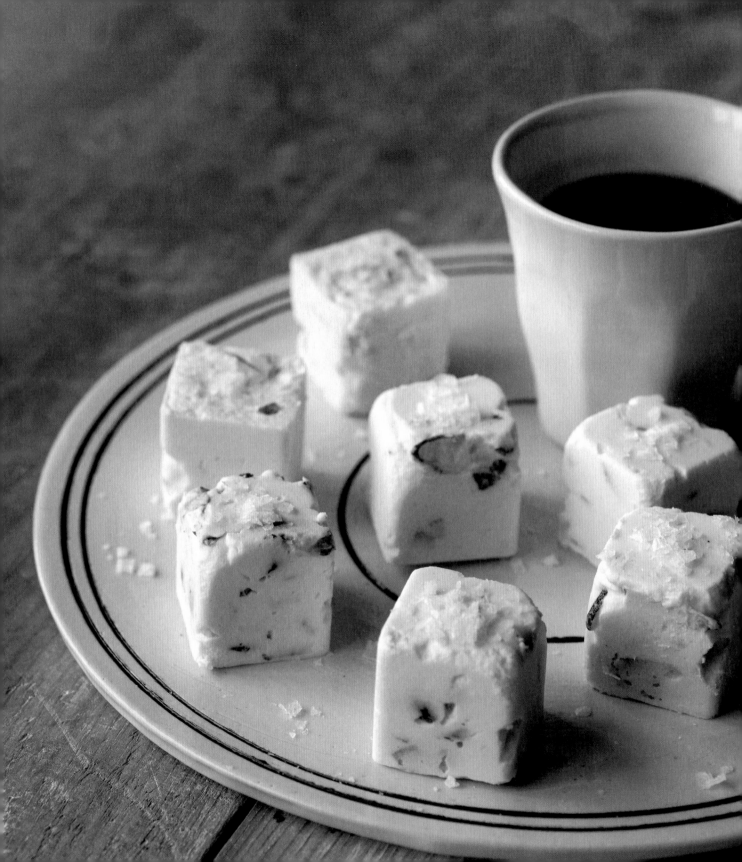

SALTED CARAMEL CHEESECAKE BITES

0.9g
NET CARBS

MAKES 18

81
CALORIES

Caramel fans will freak over these cheesecake bites that pack a creamy punch, with the perfect taste combo of sweet and salty. If you have xanthan gum on hand, it will improve the texture, but you can also leave it out.

½ cup heavy cream

⅓ cup plain protein powder

2 tablespoons stevia

6 ounces full-fat cream cheese, room temperature

⅓ cup chopped almonds or macadamia nuts

1 tablespoon sugar-free caramel syrup

1 teaspoon vanilla extract

⅛ teaspoon xanthan gum (optional)

¼ teaspoon sea salt or Maldon sea salt flakes

1 Place the heavy cream in a large mixing bowl with the protein powder and stevia. Whisk until smooth. Add the cream cheese, almonds or macadamia nuts, caramel syrup, and vanilla extract, and blend until smooth. If the cream cheese clumps slightly, mix with a rubber spatula, breaking up the bits of cream cheese against the side of the bowl. Sprinkle the mixture with the xanthan gum, if desired, and mix again for about 30 seconds. The mixture will thicken slightly.

2 Cover a tray that will fit into your freezer with a sheet of wax paper. Using a soup spoon to scoop the mixture onto the tray, make 18 mounds. Alternatively, you can use two silicone candy molds or coat an empty ice cube tray with olive oil spray, and press spoonfuls of the cheesecake mixture into 18 of the molds. Sprinkle with the sea salt. Freeze at least one hour before serving. Store in the freezer for up to 1 month.

TIP

Switch up flavors *by using sugar-free hazelnut syrup in place of the caramel and hazelnuts or walnuts instead of the almonds or macadamia nuts.*

TIME	PER SERVING
Active: 10 minutes	*Total Carbs:* 1.1g
	Fiber: 0.3g
Total: 1 hour, 10 minutes	*Protein:* 2.6g
	Fat: 7.6g

DOUBLE CHOCOLATE BROWNIES

2.1g
NET CARBS

MAKES
18

108
CALORIES

Chocolate-y cakes, cookies, and brownies are sweets that may seem more "forbidden" when living a low-carb, low-sugar lifestyle. However, real chocolate, which you'll find in two forms here—bar and powdered—can actually double as a healing food when it's unsweetened. Recent studies show that chocolate is a powerful brain booster, with detoxifying compounds that may boost memory and help sweeten your cognition as you age.[1]

TIME	PER SERVING
Active: 15 minutes	*Total Carbs:* 3.3g *Fiber:* 1.3g
Total: 45 minutes	*Protein:* 2.8g *Fat:* 10.7g

Olive oil spray

4 ounces unsweetened chocolate, chopped

½ cup unsalted butter

¼ cup canned coconut milk

½ cup stevia

¼ cup almond flour

3 tablespoons unsweetened cocoa powder, divided

1 teaspoon baking powder

4 large eggs, whisked

1 Preheat the oven to 325°F. Coat an 8-by-8-inch pan with olive oil spray. Place the chocolate, butter, and coconut milk in a bowl and microwave on high power for approximately 2 minutes, until the chocolate is melted. Whisk well, and cool for 5 minutes while you prepare the dry ingredients.

2 Place the stevia, almond flour, 2 tablespoons of the cocoa powder, and baking powder in a large bowl, and mix well. Whisk in the eggs and the cooled chocolate. Transfer to the prepared pan, and smooth the top with a spatula. Bake for 20 to 25 minutes, until the edges are firm but the center is still soft. Cool completely in the pan, then cut into 18 pieces (three rows of six brownies). Sprinkle with the remaining cocoa powder. Store in an airtight container in the fridge for up to 5 days.

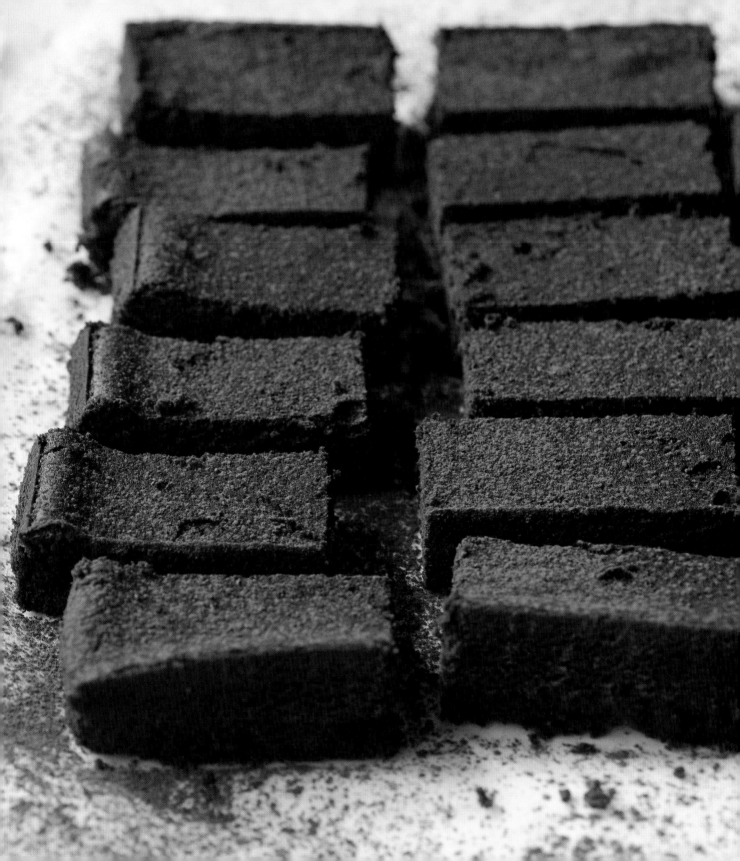

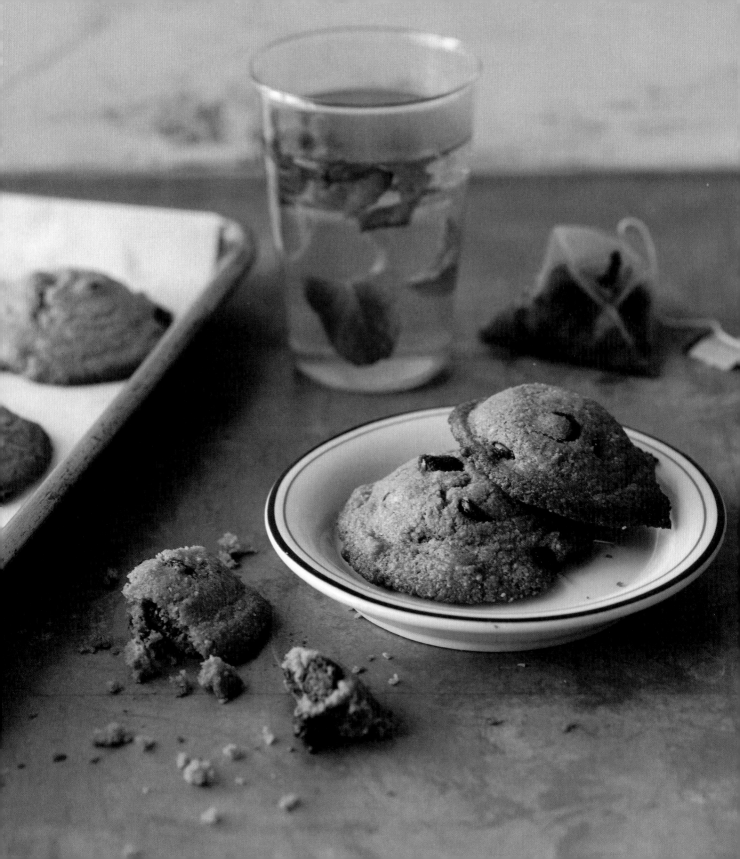

CHOCOLATE CHIP COOKIES

1.4g NET CARBS

MAKES 24

111 CALORIES

An American institution, chocolate chip cookies can still be part of your low-carb lifestyle when made with nutritious almond flour and unsweetened chocolate.

TIME	PER SERVING
Active: 10 minutes	*Total Carbs:* 2.5g
	Fiber: 1.1g
Total: 25 minutes	*Protein:* 2.4g
	Fat: 10.1g

Olive oil spray

½ cup coconut oil, at room temperature

2 large eggs

1 teaspoon vanilla extract

½ teaspoon almond extract (optional)

1½ cups almond flour

¼ cup stevia

½ teaspoon baking soda

1 teaspoon ground cinnamon

¼ teaspoon salt

½ cup sugar-free chocolate chips

TIP

For a flavor twist *and gooey, softer cookies, add 1 teaspoon sugar-free vanilla or caramel syrup to the batter, and bake 1 to 2 additional minutes.*

1 Preheat the oven to 375°F. Coat a large baking sheet with olive oil spray. Place the coconut oil, eggs, vanilla extract, and almond extract (if using) in a large mixing bowl, and beat with an electric mixer until smooth and creamy, 30 seconds to 1 minute.

2 In a medium bowl, whisk together the almond flour, stevia, baking soda, cinnamon, and salt. Beat the almond flour mixture into the wet ingredients until the dough comes together.

3 Drop the cookie dough onto the prepared baking sheet by teaspoonfuls, Gently flatten the cookies by pressing with a fork or spatula. Press a few chocolate chips onto the top of each cookie. Bake 10 to 12 minutes, until lightly browned. Remove the cookies from the baking sheet and place on a wire rack to cool completely, then serve. Store in an airtight container on the countertop for up to 4 days.

APPLE
CRUMBLE

7.3g
NET CARBS

SERVES
6

227
CALORIES

This is the perfect summertime dessert that will bring back childhood memories, while satisfying your sweet tooth. This hybrid pie/crumble has bottom and top crusts to satisfy apple pie fans, and sandwiches a delectable filling that includes zucchini to help reduce the carbs of the typical apple dessert. Mild zucchini mimics the apple flavor as they cook together and pick up the fragrance of spices.

TIME	PER SERVING
Active: 15 minutes	*Total Carbs:* 11g
	Fiber: 3.7g
Total: 40 minutes	*Protein:* 6.2g
	Fat: 19.7g

Topping

Olive oil spray

1 medium zucchini, peeled and diced

1 apple, cored and diced

3 tablespoons stevia

1 tablespoon ground cinnamon

1 tablespoon Atkins Flour Mix (page 126)

1 tablespoon coconut oil

⅓ cup water

1 teaspoon vanilla extract

Crust

1 cup almond flour

2 tablespoons stevia

2 teaspoons Atkins Flour Mix (page 126)

¼ teaspoon salt

¼ cup unsalted butter, chilled and cut into chunks

1 Preheat the oven to 350°F. Coat an 8-by-8-inch pan with olive oil spray. Place the zucchini, apple, stevia, cinnamon, and Atkins Flour Mix in a medium bowl. Mix well.

2 Heat the coconut oil in a large skillet over medium heat. Cook the zucchini-apple mixture, tossing well, 1 to 2 minutes. Reduce the heat to low, add the water, and cover. Simmer 6 to 8 minutes, until the apple and zucchini are tender and a thick sauce forms. Set aside.

3 Combine the crust ingredients in a food processor, and pulse until a crumbly dough forms. Press half the crust mixture into the prepared pan. Bake 10 to 15 minutes, until the crust is golden. Spoon the zucchini-apple mixture over the crust, and sprinkle the remaining crust mixture on top. Return to the oven, and bake 8 to 10 minutes more, until the top starts to brown. Serve immediately or cool to room temperature, and store in the refrigerator in an airtight container for up to 3 days.

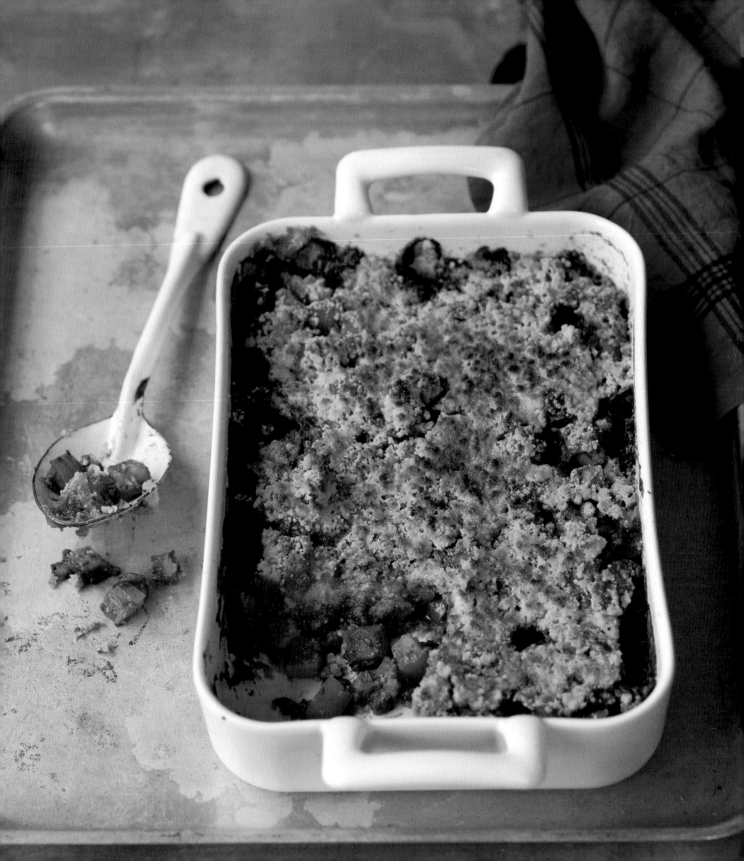

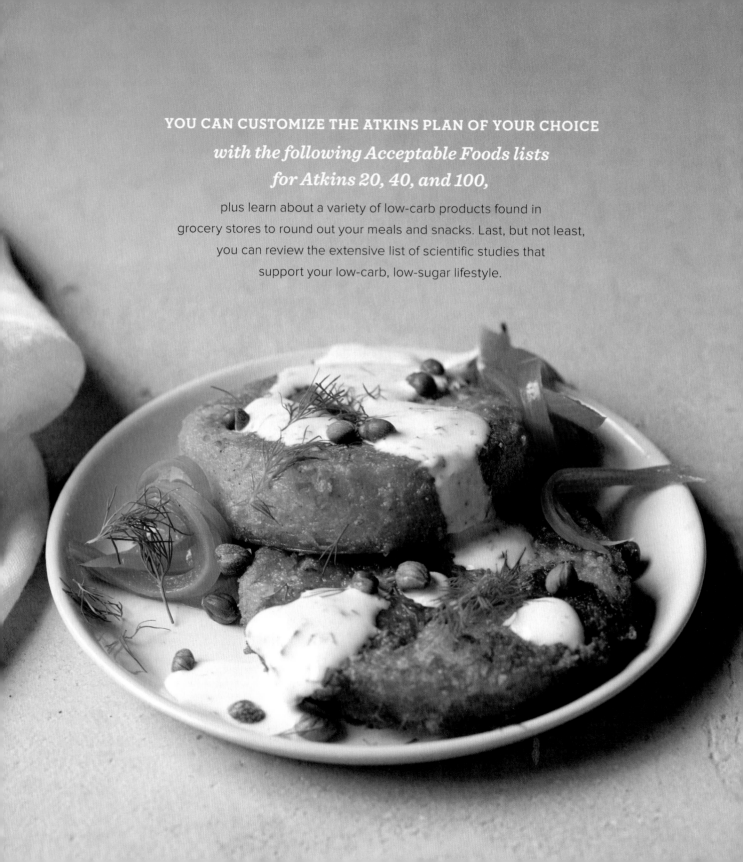

YOU CAN CUSTOMIZE THE ATKINS PLAN OF YOUR CHOICE
*with the following Acceptable Foods lists
for Atkins 20, 40, and 100,*
plus learn about a variety of low-carb products found in
grocery stores to round out your meals and snacks. Last, but not least,
you can review the extensive list of scientific studies that
support your low-carb, low-sugar lifestyle.

This is an extensive list, but it may not include all
possible Acceptable Foods.

FISH AND SHELLFISH

- Most fish and shellfish contain no carbs. All are acceptable with the following exceptions:
- Avoid pickled herring prepared with sugar, artificial crab (surimi), sold as "sea legs," and other processed shellfish products.
- Oysters and mussels contain carbs, so limit to about 4 ounces day.
- Do not bread seafood.

POULTRY

- All pure poultry products are acceptable.
- Do not use any products with breading or fillers.

MEAT

- All pure meat products are acceptable.
- Avoid any processed meats with fillers (some salami, pepperoni, hog dogs, meatballs) or breaded or cured with sugar (bacon, ham).

EGGS

- Eggs in any style are acceptable.

SOY AND VEGETARIAN PRODUCTS

- Quorn products contain milk and eggs, making them unsuitable for vegans.
- Soy cheeses that contain casein, a milk product, are also unsuitable for vegans.
- Many veggie burgers have carb counts higher than 2 grams of Net Carbs and ingredients that may not be acceptable in Level 1.

PRODUCT	SERVING SIZE	NET CARBS* (Grams)
Almond milk, unsweetened	1 cup	1.0
Quorn burger	1	4.0
Quorn roast	4 ounces	4.0
Quorn unbreaded cutlet	1	3.0
Seitan	1 piece	2.0
Shirataki soy noodles	½ cup cooked	1.0
Soy "cheese"	1 slice	1.0
Soy "cheese"	1 ounce	2.0
Soy milk, plain, unsweetened	8 ounces	1.2
Tempeh	½ cup	3.3
Tofu, firm	4 ounces	2.5
Tofu, silken, soft	4 ounces	3.1
Tofu "bacon"	2 strips	2.0
Tofu "Canadian bacon"	3 slices	1.5
Tofu "hot dogs" *(depending on brand)*	1	2.0–5.0
Tofu bulk "sausage"	2 ounces	2.0
Tofu link "sausage"	2 links	4.0
Vegan "cheese," no casein	1 slice	5.0
Vegan "cheese," no casein	1 ounce	6.0
Veggie burger	1 burger	2.0
Veggie crumbles	⅓ cup	2.0
Veggie "meatballs"	4–5 balls	4.0

* Check individual products for exact carb counts.

CHEESE

- All cheese except ricotta and cottage cheese (they can be added in Level 2).
- Up to 4 ounces a day. A tablespoon or two of any grated cheese contains a negligible amount of carbs.
- Avoid cheese spreads that contain other ingredients—strawberry cream cheese, for example—"diet" cheese, "cheese products," and whey cheeses, none of which is 100 percent cheese.
- Soy or rice "cheese" is acceptable, but check the carb count.

FOUNDATION VEGETABLES

These include both salad vegetables and others that are usually cooked.

Salad Vegetables

- Measure the following salad vegetables raw (except for artichoke hearts).
- Tomatoes, onions, and bell peppers are higher in carbs than other salad vegetables, so use them in smaller portions.
- Included are fruits generally thought of as vegetables, such as avocados and olives.

VEGETABLE	SERVING SIZE	NET CARBS (Grams)
Alfalfa sprouts	½ cup	0.2
Artichoke hearts, canned	1	1.0
Artichoke hearts, marinated	4 pieces	2.0
Arugula	1 cup	0.4
Avocado, Hass	½ fruit	1.8
Beans, green, snap, string, wax	½ cup, raw	2.1
Bok choy (pak choi)	1 cup, raw	0.4
Boston/Bibb lettuce	1 cup, raw	0.8
Broccoli florets	½ cup	0.8
Cabbage, green, red, Savoy	½ cup, shredded	1.1
Cauliflower florets	½ cup	1.4
Celery	1 stalk	0.8
Celery root (celeriac)	½ cup, grated	3.5
Chicory greens	½ cup	0.1
Chinese cabbage	½ cup, shredded	0.0
Chives	1 tbsp	0.1
Cucumber	½ cup	1.0
Daikon radish	½ cup	1.0
Endive	½ cup	0.4
Escarole	½ cup	0.1
Fennel	½ cup	1.8
Greens, mixed	1 cup	0.4
Iceberg lettuce	1 cup	0.2
Jicama	½ cup	2.5
Loose-leaf lettuce	1 cup	1.0
Mesclun	1 cup	0.5
Mung bean sprouts	½ cup	2.1
Mushrooms, button, fresh	½ cup	1.2
Olives, black	5	0.7
Olives, green	5	0.0
Onion	2 tablespoons, chopped	0.5
Parsley (and all fresh herbs)	1 tablespoon	0.1
Pepper, green bell	½ cup	2.1
Pepper, red bell	½ cup	2.9
Radicchio	½ cup	0.7
Radishes	6	0.5
Rhubarb, unsweetened	½ cup	1.7
Romaine lettuce	1 cup	0.4
Scallion/green onion	¼ cup	1.2
Spinach	1 cup	0.2
Tomato	1 small (3–4 ounces)	2.5
Tomato	1 medium	3.3
Tomato, cherry	5	2.2
Watercress	½ cup	0.0

Cooked Vegetables

- Some also appear on the salad vegetable list, but cooking compacts them, which explains the differences in carb counts.
- Some, such as celery root, kohlrabi, leeks, mushrooms, onions, and pumpkin, are higher in carbs than most, which accounts for the smaller portions.
- Vegetables *not* on this list should not be consumed in Level 1.

VEGETABLE	SERVING SIZE	NET CARBS (Grams)
Artichoke	½ medium	3.5
Asparagus	6 spears	2.4
Bamboo shoots, canned, sliced	½ cup canned	1.2
Beans, green, wax, string, snap	½ cup	2.9
Beet greens	½ cup	3.7
Bok choy (pak choi)	½ cup	0.2
Broccoflower	½ cup	2.3
Broccoli	½ cup	1.7
Broccoli rabe	½ cup	2.0
Brussels sprouts	¼ cup	1.8
Cabbage, green	½ cup	1.6
Cabbage, red	½ cup	2.0
Cabbage, Savoy	½ cup	1.9
Cardoon	½ cup	2.7
Cauliflower	½ cup	0.9
Celery	½ cup	1.2
Chard, Swiss	½ cup	1.8
Chayote	½ cup	1.8
Collard greens	½ cup	2.0
Dandelion greens	½ cup	1.8
Eggplant	½ cup	2.0
Escarole	½ cup	0.1
Fennel	½ cup	1.5
Hearts of palm	1	0.7
Kale	½ cup	2.4
Kohlrabi	¼ cup	2.3
Leeks	½ cup	3.4
Mushrooms, button	¼ cup	2.3
Mushrooms, shiitake	¼ cup	4.4
Mustard greens	½ cup	0.1
Nopales (cactus pads)	½ cup	1.0
Okra	½ cup	2.4
Onion	¼ cup	4.3
Peppers, green bell, chopped	¼ cup	1.9
Peppers, red bell, chopped	¼ cup	1.9
Pumpkin	¼ cup	2.4
Rhubarb, unsweetened	½ cup	1.7
Sauerkraut	½ cup, drained	1.2
Scallions	½ cup	2.4
Shallots	2 tablespoons	3.1
Snow peas/snap peas in the pod	½ cup	3.4
Sorrel	½ cup	0.2
Spaghetti squash	¼ cup	2.0
Spinach	½ cup	2.2
Summer squash	½ cup	2.6

VEGETABLE	SERVING SIZE	NET CARBS (Grams)
Tomatillo	½ cup	2.6
Tomato	¼ cup	4.3
Turnips, white, mashed	½ cup	3.3
Water chestnuts, canned	¼ cup	3.5
Zucchini	½ cup	1.5

SALAD DRESSINGS

- Any salad dressing with no more than 2 grams of Net Carbs per 2-tablespoon serving is acceptable.
- Do *not* use sugar, honey, maple syrup, or other caloric sweeteners in salad dressings.

FATS AND OILS

- Butter, canola oil, coconut oil, flaxseed oil, grape seed oil, olive oil, high-oleic safflower oil, sesame oil, and walnut oil are acceptable.
- Oils labeled "cold pressed" or "expeller pressed" are preferable.
- Mayonnaise should be made with olive, canola, or high-oleic safflower oil.
- Use extra-virgin olive oil for dressing salads and vegetables and sautéing.
- Use olive, canola, or high-oleic safflower oil for other cooking.
- Use walnut, sesame, or other specialty oils to season a dish after removing it from the heat.
- Avoid products labeled "lite" or "low fat" and all margarines and shortening products, which contain small amounts of trans fats.
- Avoid corn, soy, sunflower seed, and other vegetable oils.

NONCALORIC SWEETENERS

- The following are acceptable in moderation: Splenda (sucralose), Truvia or SweetLeaf (stevia), Sweet'N Low (saccharin), xylitol.

BEVERAGES

The following are acceptable:

- Broth/bouillon
- Club soda
- Cream, heavy or light, or half-and-half (1 to 1.5 ounces a day)
- Caffeinated or decaffeinated coffee and tea
- Diet soda sweetened with noncaloric sweeteners
- Lemon juice or lime juice; limit to 2 to 3 tablespoons a day.
- Plain or essence-flavored seltzer (must say "no calories")
- Herb tea (without added barley or fruit sugars)
- Unsweetened, unflavored soy or almond milk

CONDIMENTS, HERBS, AND SPICES

- All herbs, spices, and seasonings are acceptable.
- Avoid herb or spice mixtures that contain added sugar.
- Avoid condiments made with added sugar or flour, cornstarch, and other carb-filled thickeners.

CONDIMENT, HERB, OR SPICE	SERVING SIZE	NET CARBS (Grams)
Ancho chili pepper	1	5.1
Anchovy paste	1 tablespoon	0.0
Black bean sauce	1 teaspoon	3.0
Capers	1 tablespoon	0.1
Chipotle en adobe	2	2.0
Clam juice	1 cup	0.0
Enchilada sauce	¼ cup	2.0
Fish sauce	1 teaspoon	0.2
Garlic	1 large clove	0.9
Ginger	1 tablespoon grated root	0.8
Horseradish sauce	1 teaspoon	0.4
Jalapeño pepper	½ cup sliced	1.4
Miso paste	1 tablespoon	2.6
Mustard, Dijon	1 teaspoon	0.5
Mustard, yellow	1 teaspoon	0.0
Olives, black	5	0.7
Olives, green	5	2.5
Pasilla pepper	1	1.7
Pesto sauce	1 tablespoon	0.6
Pickapeppa sauce	1 teaspoon	1.0
Pickle, dill or kosher	½	1.0
Pimento/roasted red pepper	1 ounce	2.0
Salsa, green (no added sugar)	1 tablespoon	0.6
Salsa, red (no added sugar)	1 tablespoon	1.0
Serrano chili pepper	½ cup	1.6
Soy sauce	1 tablespoon	0.9
Tabasco or other hot sauce	1 teaspoon	0.0
Taco sauce	1 tablespoon	1.0
Tahini (sesame paste)	2 tablespoons	1.0
Vinegar, balsamic	1 tablespoon	2.3
Vinegar, cider	1 tablespoon	0.9
Vinegar, red wine	1 tablespoon	1.5
Vinegar, rice (unsweetened)	1 tablespoon	0.0
Vinegar, sherry	1 tablespoon	0.9
Vinegar, white wine	1 tablespoon	1.5
Wasabi paste	1 teaspoon	0.0

In addition to the Acceptable Foods for Level 1,
the following foods are acceptable in Level 2.

NUTS AND SEEDS

- Most nuts and seeds and butters made from them are acceptable.
- Consume no more than 2 ounces (about ¼ cup) a day.
- Nut meals and flours broaden your cooking options.
- Avoid honey-roasted and smoked products.
- Chestnuts are very starchy and high in carbs, making them unsuitable for this level.
- Avoid products such as Nutella that include sugar or other sweeteners.

The following listing provides portions equivalent to 1 ounce.

NUT OR SEED	SERVING SIZE	NET CARBS (Grams)
Almonds	24	2.3
Almond butter	1 tablespoon	2.5
Almond meal/flour	¼ cup	3.0
Brazil nuts	5	2.0
Cashew butter	1 tablespoon	4.1
Cashew nuts	9	4.4
Coconut, shredded, unsweetened	¼ cup	1.3
Macadamias	6	2.0
Macadamia butter	1 tablespoon	2.5
Hazelnuts	12	0.5
Peanuts	22	1.5
Peanut butter, natural	1 tablespoon	2.4
Peanut butter, smooth	1 tablespoon	2.2
Pecans	10 halves	1.5
Pine nuts (piñons)	2 tablespoons	1.7
Pistachios	25	2.5
Pumpkin seeds, hulled	2 tablespoons	2.0
Sesame seeds	2 tablespoons	1.6
Soy "nuts"	2 tablespoons	2.7
Soy "nut" butter	1 tablespoon	3.0
Sunflower seeds, hulled	2 tablespoons	1.1
Sunflower seed butter	1 tablespoon	0.5
Tahini (sesame paste)	1 tablespoon	0.8
Walnuts	7 halves	1.5

BERRIES AND OTHER FRUITS

- All berries are acceptable, as are melon (but not watermelon) and cherries.
- All fruits should be regarded as garnishes, not major components of a dish.
- Also acceptable are small (1-tablespoon) portions of preserves made without added sugar. Each tablespoon should provide no more than 2 grams of Net Carbs.

FRUIT	SERVING SIZE	NET CARBS (Grams)
Blackberries, fresh	¼ cup	2.7
Blackberries, frozen	¼ cup	4.1
Blueberries, fresh	¼ cup	4.1
Blueberries, frozen	¼ cup	3.7
Boysenberries, fresh	¼ cup	2.7
Boysenberries, frozen	¼ cup	2.8
Cherries, sour, fresh	¼ cup	2.8
Cherries, sweet, fresh	¼ cup	4.2
Cranberries, raw	¼ cup	2.0
Currants, fresh	¼ cup	2.5
Gooseberries, raw	½ cup	4.4
Loganberries, raw	¼ cup	2.7
Melon, cantaloupe balls	¼ cup	3.7
Melon, Crenshaw balls	¼ cup	2.3
Melon, honeydew balls	¼ cup	3.6
Raspberries, fresh	¼ cup	1.5
Raspberries, frozen	¼ cup	1.8
Strawberries, fresh, sliced	¼ cup	1.8
Strawberries, frozen	¼ cup	2.6
Strawberry, fresh	1 large	1.0

FRESH CHEESE AND OTHER DAIRY PRODUCTS

- You can now reintroduce the remaining fresh cheeses.
- Use only plain, unsweetened, whole milk yogurt or Greek yogurt.
- Avoid processed yogurt made with fruit or other flavorings or with any added sugar.
- Avoid low-fat and no-fat cottage cheese and yogurt products.

CHEESE OR DAIRY PRODUCT	SERVING SIZE	NET CARBS (Grams)
Cottage cheese	½ cup	4.1
Cottage cheese, creamed	½ cup	2.8
Milk, whole, evaporated	2 tablespoons	3.0
Ricotta, whole milk	½ cup	3.8
Yogurt, low carb	4 ounces	3.0
Yogurt, plain, unsweetened, whole	4 ounces	5.5
Yogurt, Greek, plain, unsweetened whole	4 ounces	3.5

LEGUMES

- Use small portions and regard legumes as a garnish.
- Avoid baked beans, which are full of sugar, and other products such as beans in tomato sauce with sugar or starches and bean dips.
- Black soybeans are far lower in carbs than black (or turtle) beans with no trade-off in taste.

LEGUME	SERVING SIZE	NET CARBS (Grams)
Black-eyed peas	¼ cup	6.2
Black/turtle beans	¼ cup	6.5
Cannellini beans	¼ cup	8.5
Chickpeas/garbanzo beans	¼ cup	6.5
Cranberry/Roman beans	¼ cup	6.3
Fava beans	¼ cup	6.0
Great Northern beans	¼ cup	6.3
Hummus	2 tablespoons	4.6
Kidney beans	¼ cup	5.8
Lentils	¼ cup	6.0
Lima beans, baby	¼ cup	7.1
Lima beans, large	¼ cup	6.5
Navy beans	¼ cup	9.1
Peas, split	¼ cup	6.3
Pigeon peas	¼ cup	7.0
Pink beans	¼ cup	9.6
Pinto beans	¼ cup	7.3
Refried beans, canned	¼ cup	6.5
Soybeans, black	½ cup	1.0
Soybeans, green edamame	¼ cup	3.1

Note: *Serving sizes for dried legumes are after cooking. Serving sizes for fresh legumes are for shelled beans.*

VEGETABLE AND FRUIT JUICES

- Most fruit juices are completely off limits.
- In Level 2, you can double the amount of lemon and lime juice.
- You can now also introduce small portions of tomato juice or tomato juice cocktail.

JUICES	SERVING SIZE	NET CARBS (Grams)
Lemon juice	¼ cup	5.2
Lime juice	¼ cup	5.6
Tomato juice	4 ounces	4.2
Tomato juice cocktail	4 ounces	4.5

LOW-CARB PRODUCTS SUITABLE FOR LEVEL 2

- In each case, we've provided the *maximum* acceptable carb count for a single serving. If the carb count of a specific product exceeds the amount listed here, pass it up.

LOW-CARB PRODUCT	SERVING SIZE	NET CARBS (Grams)
Low-carb bagels	1	5.0
Atkins All-Purpose Bake Mix	¾ cup	5.0
Low-carb bread	1 slice	6.0
Low-carb chocolate/candy	1.2 ounces	3.0
Low-carb dairy drink	8 ounces	4.0
Low-carb pancake mix	2 pancakes	6.0
Low-carb pita	One 6-inch	4.0
Low-carb roll	1	4.0
Low-carb soy chips	1 ounce	5.0
Low-carb tortillas	One 7-inch	4.0
No-added-sugar ice cream	½ cup	4.0

In addition to the foods you can eat in Levels 1 and 2,
the following foods are acceptable in Levels 3 and 4.

FRUITS OTHER THAN BERRIES

- All fruit is high in sugar and should be treated as a garnish.
- Avoid canned fruit, even packed in juice concentrate or "lite" syrup.
- Continue to avoid fruit juice, other than lemon and lime juice.
- Avoid dried fruit.

The following carb counts are for fresh fruit:

FRUIT	SERVING SIZE	NET CARBS (Grams)
Apple	½ medium	8.7
Apricot	3 medium	9.2
Banana	1 small	21.2
Carambola (star fruit)	½ cup sliced	2.8
Cherimoya	½ cup	24.3
Figs, fresh	1 small	6.4
Grapes, green	½ cup	13.7
Grapes, purple Concord	½ cup	7.4
Grapes, red	½ cup	13.4
Grapefruit, red	½	7.9
Grapefruit, white	½	8.6
Guava	½ cup	5.3
Kiwi	1	8.7
Kumquat	4	7.5
Loquat	10	14.2
Lychee	½ cup	14.5
Mango	½ cup	12.5
Orange	1 medium	12.9
Orange sections	½ cup	8.4
Nectarine	1 medium	13.8
Papaya	½ small	6.1
Passion fruit	¼ cup	7.7
Peach	1 small	7.2
Pear, Bartlett	1 medium	21.1
Pear, Bosc	1 small	17.7
Persimmon	½	12.6
Pineapple	½ cup	8.7
Plantain	½ cup	21
Plum	1 small	3.3
Pomegranate	¼	6.4
Quince	1	12.3
Tangerine	1	6.2
Watermelon	½ cup balls	5.1

STARCHY VEGETABLES

All vegetables are measured after cooking, except for Jerusalem artichoke.

VEGETABLES	SERVING SIZE	NET CARBS (Grams)
Beets	½ cup	6.8
Burdock	½ cup	12.1
Calabaza (Spanish pumpkin), mashed	½ cup	5.9
Carrot	1 medium	5.6
Cassava (yuca), mashed	½ cup	25.1
Corn	½ cup	12.6
Corn on the cob	1 ear	17.2
Jerusalem artichoke	½ cup	11.9
Parsnips, cooked	½ cup	10.5
Potato, baked	½	10.5
Rutabaga	½ cup	5.9
Squash, acorn, baked	½ cup	7.8
Squash, acorn, steamed	½ cup	7.6
Squash, butternut, baked	½ cup	7.9
Sweet potato, baked	½	12.1
Taro	½ cup	19.5
Yam, sliced	½ cup	16.1
Yautia (arracache), sliced	½ cup	29.9

WHOLE GRAINS

- Note that these are *whole* grains, not simply grains.
- Avoid refined grains, such as white flour, "enriched flour," and white rice.
- Baked goods should be made with 100 percent whole grains.
- All measurements are for cooked grains, except for cornmeal, oat bran, rolled oatmeal, and steel cut oatmeal.

WHOLE GRAIN	SERVING SIZE	NET CARBS (Grams)
Barley, hulled	½ cup	13.0
Barley, pearled	½ cup	19.0
Bulgur wheat	½ cup	12.8
Cornmeal	2 tablespoons	10.6
Couscous, whole wheat	½ cup	17.1
Cracked wheat	½ cup	15.0
Hominy	½ cup	9.7
Kasha (buckwheat groats)	½ cup	14.0
Millet	½ cup	19.5
Oat bran	2 tablespoons	6.0
Oatmeal, rolled	⅓ cup	19.0
Oatmeal, steel cut	¼ cup	19.0
Quinoa	¼ cup	27.0
Rice, brown	½ cup	20.5
Rice, wild	½ cup	16.0
Wheat berries	½ cup	14.0

DAIRY PRODUCTS

- You can also add small portions of whole milk (4 ounces contain almost 6 grams of Net Carbs) or buttermilk.
- Avoid skim, nonfat, and low-fat milk.

APPENDIX D
ATKINS 40 AND ATKINS 100 ACCEPTABLE FOODS

On Atkins 40 and Atkins 100, you can eat all the foods
shown previously for Atkins 20, Levels 1 through 4, in addition to the
following foods, which are listed with serving sizes that
correspond to either 5 or 10 grams of Net Carbs, so that you can easily
keep track. An asterisk indicates a rounded Net Carbs value.

NUTS AND SEEDS AND THEIR BUTTERS

NUTS OR SEEDS	SERVING SIZE	NET CARBS (Grams)
Almonds	½ cup	5*
Almond butter	¼ cup	5*
Brazil nuts	¾ cup	5*
Cashews	2 tablespoons	5*
Cashew butter	1 tablespoon	5*
Coconut, unsweetened	1 cup	5*
Hazelnuts	½ cup	5*
Macadamia nuts	½ cup	5*
Peanuts	3 tablespoons	5*
Peanut butter	3 tablespoons	5*
Pecans	1 cup	5*
Pine nuts	½ cup	5*
Pistachios	3 tablespoons	5*
Pumpkin seeds	½ cup	5*
Sesame seeds	¼ cup	5*
Soy nuts	3 tablespoons	5*
Sunflower seeds	½ cup	5*
Walnuts	¾ cup	5*

CHEESE AND OTHER DAIRY PRODUCTS

CHEESE & OTHER DAIRY	SERVING SIZE	NET CARBS (Grams)
Almond milk (unsweetened, plain)	1 cup	1
Blue cheese	2 tablespoons	.4
Brie	1 ounce	.1
Buttermilk	½ cup	5*
Cheddar	1 ounce	.4
Coconut milk (unsweetened, plain)	1 cup	1
Colby cheese	1 ounce	.7
Cottage cheese	½ cup	5*
Cream, heavy (liquid)	¾ cup	5*
Cream, sour	¾ cup	5*
Cream cheese (full fat, plain)	5 tablespoons	5*
Feta	1 ounce	1.2
Goat cheese (chèvre)	1 ounce	.3
Gouda	1 ounce	.6
Half-and-half	1 cup	5*
Havarti	1 ounce	0
Jarlsberg	1 ounce	1.2
Laughing Cow	1 wedge	1
Milk, whole	½ cup	5*
Mozzarella (whole milk)	1 ounce	.6
Parmesan, chunk	1 ounce	.9
Parmesan, grated	1 tablespoon	.2
Ricotta (whole milk)	¼ cup	2
Romano (chunk)	1 ounce	1
Soy milk (unsweetened, plain)	1 cup	2
String cheese (whole milk)	1 ounce	1
Swiss cheese	1 ounce	1.5
Yogurt, Greek, plain, unsweetened whole milk	½ cup	5*

LEGUMES

LEGUME	SERVING SIZE	NET CARBS (Grams)
Black beans	3 tablespoons/½ cup	5/10*
Black-eyed peas	3 tablespoons/½ cup	5/10*
Cannellini	3 tablespoons/½ cup	5/10*
Chickpeas	2 tablespoons/¼ cup	5/10*
Edamame	10 tablespoons/¼ cup	5/10*
Great Northern beans	2 tablespoons/¼ cup	5/10*
Hummus, plain	5 tablespoons/⅔ cup	5/10*
Kidney beans	3 tablespoons/½ cup	5/10*
Lima beans	3 tablespoons/½ cup	5/10*
Peas, split	3 tablespoons/½ cup	5/10*
Pinto beans	3 tablespoons/½ cup	5/10*
Soybeans, white	5 tablespoons/⅔ cup	5/10*

FRUIT

FRUIT	SERVING SIZE	NET CARBS (Grams)
Apple	⅓/⅔	5/10*
Apricot	½/⅓	5/10*
Blackberries	¾ cup/1½ cups	5/10*
Banana (small)	¼/½	5/10*
Blueberries	¼ cup/½ cup	5/10*
Boysenberries	¾ cup/1½ cups	5/10*
Cantaloupe	½ cup/1 cup	5/10*
Clementine	⅔ cup/1⅓ cups	5/10*
Cranberries	⅔ cup/1⅓ cups	5/10*
Cherries	3 tablespoons/6 tablespoons	5/10*
Coconut	1 cup/2 cups	5/10*
Dates	½	5/10*
Figs	¾/1½	5/10*
Gooseberries	⅓ cup/⅔ cup	5/10*
Grapefruit	¼ /½	5/10*
Grapes	3 tablespoons/6 tablespoons	5/10*
Guava	⅓ cup/⅔ cup	5/10*
Honeydew melon	⅓ cup/⅔ cup	5/10*
Kiwi	⅔/1⅓	5/10*
Lemon juice	5 tablespoons/10 tablespoons	5/10*
Lime juice	4½ tablespoons/9 tablespoons	5/10*
Mango	¼ cup/½ cup	5/10*
Orange	½/1	5/10*
Peach	½/1	5/10*
Pear	¼/½	5/10*
Pineapple	¼ cup/½ cup	5/10*
Plum	¾/1½	5/10*
Raisins	¾ tablespoon/1½ tablespoons	5/10*
Raspberries	¾ cup/1½ cups	5/10*
Rhubarb	1½ cups/3 cups	5/10*
Strawberries	½ cup/1 cup	5/10*
Watermelon	½ cup/1 cup	5/10*

STARCHY VEGETABLES

STARCHY VEGETABLE	SERVING SIZE	NET CARBS (Grams)
Acorn squash	¼ cup/½ cup	5/10*
Beets	¼ cup/½ cup	5/10*
Butternut squash	⅓ cup/⅔ cup	5/10*
Carrots, sliced	½ cup/1 cup	5/10*
Corn	¼ cup/½ cup	5/10*
Parsnips	¼ cup/½ cup	5/10*
Peas	¼ cup/½ cup	5/10*
Potato, baked, small	¼/½	5/10*
Rutabaga	½ cup/1 cup	5/10*
Sweet potato, baked, medium	¼/½	5/10*

WHOLE GRAINS

GRAIN	SERVING SIZE	NET CARBS (Grams)
Barley, cooked	2 tablespoons/¼ cup	5/10*
Brown rice, cooked	2 tablespoons/¼ cup	5/10*
Coconut flour	2½ tablespoons/⅓ cup	5/10*
Couscous, cooked	2½ tablespoons/⅓ cup	5/10*
Grits, cooked	2½ cups/⅓ cup	5/10*
Millet, cooked	2 tablespoons/¼ cup	5/10*
Oat bran, raw	2 to 4 tablespoons	5/10*
Oatmeal, steel cut, dry	2 tablespoons/¼ cup	5/10*
Polenta, dry	1 to 2 tablespoons	5/10*
Quinoa, cooked	2½ tablespoons/⅓ cup	5/10*
Wheat bran, raw	6 tablespoons/¾ cup	5/10*
Wheat germ	2 tablespoons/¼ cup	5/10*
Whole wheat bread	½ slice/1 slice	5/10*
Whole wheat pasta, cooked	2½ tablespoons/⅓ cup	5/10*

ALCOHOLIC BEVERAGES

BEVERAGE	SERVING SIZE	NET CARBS (Grams)
Beer, light	12 ounces	5.6
Beer, low carb	12 ounces	2.5
Bourbon	1 ounce	0
Champagne	1 ounce	2–3
Rum	1 ounce	0
Scotch	1 ounce	0
Vodka	1 ounce	0
Wine, red	3.5 ounces	2.6
Wine, white	3.5 ounces	2

You can find a variety of delicious low-carb products,
and the selections and quality continue to expand, which
makes snacking or mealtimes that much easier.

BREADS, TORTILLAS, NOODLES, AND PASTA

MAHLER'S
Low-carb bread made from soy and flax
www.mahlersbakery.com

GREAT LOW-CARB BREAD COMPANY
Low-carb bread, bagels, buns, muffins, pizza crust, and pasta
www.shop.greatlowcarb.com

TUMARO'S AND MISSION
Low-carb tortillas and wraps
www.tumaros.com
www.missionmenus.com

MIRACLE NOODLE
Almost zero-calorie and no-carb noodles and rice made from a yam-like tuber called Devil's Tongue
www.miraclenoodle.com

CALI'FLOUR FOODS
Pizza crust made from cauliflower
www.califlourfoods.com

SNACKS

HARVEST SNAPS
Lentil, green pea, and black bean snaps in various flavors
www.harvestsnaps.com

JULIAN BAKERY
Low-carb crackers in salt-and-pepper and organic Parmesan flavors
www.julianbakery.com

SUZIE'S
Thin puffed cakes made from flax and spelt
www.goodgroceries.com

SEAPOINT FARMS
Dry-roasted edamame
www.seapointfarms.com

WONDERFUL
Roasted and shelled pistachios
www.getcrackin.com

KITCHEN TABLE BAKERS
Oven-baked Parmesan crisps in a variety of savory flavors
www.kitchentablebakers.com

PROTES
Protein chips in spicy chili lime, tangy southern BBQ, toasted coconut, and zesty nacho flavors
www.eatprotes.com

JUST THE CHEESE
Crunchy baked cheese snacks in a variety of flavors
www.justthecheese.com

MEAT SNACKS

CHEF'S CUT REAL JERKY
Hand-cut jerky that's also gluten and nitrite free
www.chefscutrealjerky.com

DUKE'S JERKY
Grass-fed steak and brisket strips and smoked sausages with no added sugar
www.dukesmeats.com

4505 MEATS
Chicharrones (fried pork rinds) in classic chili and salt, jalapeno, and smokehouse barbecue flavors
www.4505meats.com

MEALS AND SNACKS

ATKINS NUTRITIONALS, INC.
Low-carb nutrition bars and shakes, treats, snacks, and frozen meals
www.atkins.com

YOGURT AND ICE CREAM

SIGGI'S AND CHOBANI
Whole milk and Greek yogurt
www.siggisdairy.com
www.chobani.com

HALO TOP
Low-calorie, low-sugar, low-carb, high-protein ice cream in a variety of delicious flavors
www.halotop.com

BEVERAGES

TORANI
Sugar-free flavored syrups
www.torani.com

MARQUIS
A no-sugar, no-carb organic energy drink that comes in super berry, mango ginger, and citrus lime flavors.
www.drinkmarquis.com

BAI
This is a low-calorie, low-sugar beverage that contains an antioxidant-rich superfruit called coffee fruit and is sweetened with stevia leaf.
www.drinkbai.com

COOKING AND BAKING SUPPLIES AND CONDIMENTS

PRIMAL KITCHEN
Sugar-free or low-sugar salad dressings, mayo, cooking oil, and protein bars and powder
www.primalkitchen.com

HEALTH GARDEN
Natural sugar substitutes such as xylitol, erythritol, stevia, coconut sugar, and monk sugar
www.healthgardenusa.com

APPENDIX F
SCIENTIFIC STUDIES SUPPORTING ATKINS 20, 40, AND 100

ATKINS 20

Austin, G. L., Dalton, C. B., Hu, Y., Morris, C. B., Hankins, J., Weinland, S. R., et al. (2009). A very-low-carbohydrate diet improves symptoms and quality of life in diarrhea-predominant irritable bowel syndrome. *Clinical Gastroenterology and Hepatology* 7(6). doi:10.1016/j.cgh.2009.02.023.

Bailes, J. R., Strow, M. T., Werthammer, J., McGinnis, R. A., and Elitsur, Y. (2003). Effect of low-carbohydrate, unlimited calorie diet on the treatment of childhood obesity: a prospective controlled study. *Metabolic Syndrome and Related Disorders* 1(3): 221–225. doi:10.1089/154041903322716697.

Ben-Avraham, S., Harman-Boehm, I., Schwarzfuchs, D., and Shai, I. (2009). Dietary strategies for patients with type 2 diabetes in the era of multi-approaches; review and results from the Dietary Intervention Randomized Controlled Trial (DIRECT). *Diabetes Research and Clinical Practice* 86. doi:10.1016/s0168-8227(09)70008-7.

Boden, G., Sargrad, K., Homko, C., Mozzoli, M., and Stein, T. P. (2005). Effect of a low-carbohydrate diet on appetite, blood glucose levels, and insulin resistance in obese patients with type 2 diabetes. *Annals of Internal Medicine* 142(6): 403. doi:10.7326/0003-4819-142-6-200503150-00006.

Brinkworth, G. D., Noakes, M., Buckley, J. D., Keogh, J. B., and Clifton, P. M. (2009). Long-term effects of a very-low-carbohydrate weight-loss diet compared with an isocaloric low-fat diet after 12 months. *American Journal of Clinical Nutrition* 90(1): 23–32. doi:10.3945/ajcn.2008.27326.

Coleman, M. D., and Nickols-Richardson, S. M. (2005). Urinary ketones reflect serum ketone concentration but do not relate to weight loss in overweight premenopausal women following a low-carbohydrate/high-protein diet. *Journal of the American Dietetic Association* 105(4), 608–611. doi:10.1016/j.jada.2005.01.004.

Davis, N. J., Tomuta, N., Schechter, C., Isasi, C. R., Segal-Isaacson, C. J., Stein, D., et al. (2009). Comparative study of the effects of a 1-year dietary intervention of a low-carbohydrate diet versus a low-fat diet on weight and glycemic control in type 2 diabetes. *Diabetes Care* 32(7): 1147–1152. doi:10.2337/dc08-2108.

DiLorenzo, C., Curra, A., Sirianni, G., Coppola, G., Bracaglia, M., Cardillo, A., et al. (2013). Diet transiently improves migraine in two twin sisters: possible role of ketogenesis? *Functional Neurology* 28(4): 305–308. doi:10.11138/FNeur/2013.28.4.305.

Fine, E. J., Segal-Isaacson, C., Feinman, R. D., Herszkopf, S., Romano, M. C., Tomuta, N., et al. (2012). Targeting insulin inhibition as a metabolic therapy in advanced cancer: a pilot safety and feasibility dietary trial in 10 patients. *Nutrition* 28(10): 1028–1035. doi:10.1016/j.nut.2012.05.001.

Foster, G. D. (2010). Weight and metabolic outsomes after 2 years on a low-carbohydrate versus low-fat diet. *Annals of Internal Medicine* 153(3): 147. doi:10.7326/0003-4819-153-3-201008030-00005.

Foster, G., Wyatt, H., Hill, J., McGuckin, B., Brill, C., Mohammed, B., et al. (2003). A randomized trial of a low-carbohydrate diet for obesity. *New England Journal of Medicine* 348(21): 2082–2090. https://www.ncbi.nlm.nih.gov/pubmed/12761365.

Friedman, A., Ogden, L., Foster, G., Klein, S., Stein, R., Miller, B., et al. (2012). Comparative effects of low-carbohydrate high-protein versus low-fat diets on the kidney. *Clinical Journal of the American Society of Nephrology* 7(7): 1103–1111. doi:10.2215/CJN.11741111.

Gann, D. (2004). A low-carbohydrate diet in overweight patients undergoing stable statin therapy raises high-density lipoprotein and lowers triglycerides substantially. *Clinical Cardiology* 27(10): 563–564. doi:10.1002/clc.4960271008.

Gardner, C. D., Kiazand, A., Alhassan, S., Kim, S., Stafford, R. S., Balise, R. R., et al. (2007). Comparison of the Atkins, Zone, Ornish, and LEARN diets for change in weight and related risk factors among overweight premenopausal women. *Journal of the American Medical Association* 297(9): 969. doi:10.1001/jama.297.9.969.

Hickey, J. T., Hickey, L., Yancy, W. S., Hepburn, J., and Westman, E. C. (2003). Clinical use of a carbohydrate-restricted diet to treat the dyslipidemia of the metabolic syndrome. *Metabolic Syndrome and Related Disorders* 1(3): 227–232. doi:10.1089/154041903322716705.

Hussain, T. A., Mathew, T. C., Dashti, A. A., Asfar, S., Al-Zaid, N., and Dashti, H. M. (2012). Effect of low-calorie versus low-carbohydrate ketogenic diet in type 2 diabetes. *Nutrition* 28(10): 1016–1021. doi:10.1016/j.nut.2012.01.016.

Krebs, N. F., Gao, D., Gralla, J., Collins, J. S., and Johnson, S. L. (2010). Efficacy and safety of a high-protein, low-carbohydrate diet for weight loss in severely obese adolescents. *Journal of Pediatrics* 157(2): 252–258. doi:10.1016/j.jpeds.2010.02.010.

Martin, C. K., Rosenbaum, D., Han, H., Geiselman, P. J., Wyatt, H. R., Hill, J. O., et al. (2011). Change in food cravings, food preferences, and appetite during a low-carbohydrate and low-fat diet. *Obesity* 19(10): 1963–1970. doi:10.1038/oby.2011.62.

Mavropoulos, J., Yancy, W., Hepburn, J., and Westman, E. (2005). The effects of a low-carbohydrate, ketogenic diet on the polycystic ovary syndrome: a pilot study. *Nutrition & Metabolism* 2(35). https://www.ncbi.nlm.nih.gov/pubmed/16359551.

McAuley, K. A., Hopkins, C. M., Smith, K. J., McLay, R. T., Williams, S. M., Taylor, R. W., and Mann, J. I. (2004). Comparison of high-fat and high-protein diets with a high-carbohydrate diet in insulin-resistant obese women. *Diabetologia* 48(1): 8–16. doi:10.1007/s00125-004-1603-4.

Morgan, L., Griffin, B., Millward, D., Delooy, A., Fox, K., Baic, S., et al. (2008). Comparison of the effects of four commercially available weight-loss programmes on lipid-based cardiovascular risk factors. *Public Health Nutrition* 12(6): 799. doi:10.1017/s1368980008003236.

Paoli, A., Grimaldi, K., D'Agostino, D., Cenci, L., Moro, T., Bianco, A., and Palma, A. (2012). Ketogenic diet does not affect strength performance in elite artistic gymnasts. *Journal of the International Society of Sports Nutrition* 9(1): 34. doi:10.1186/1550-2783-9-34.

Phinney, S., Bistrian, B., Wolfe, R., and Blackburn, G. (1983). The human metabolic response to chronic ketosis without caloric restriction: physical and biochemical adaptation. *Metabolism* 32(8): 757–768. doi:10.1016/0026-0495(83)90105-1.

Seshadri, P., Iqbal, N., and Stern, L. (2005). A randomized study comparing the effects of a low-carbohydrate diet and a conventional diet on lipoprotein subfractions and C-reactive protein levels in patients with severe obesity. *ACC Current Journal Review* 14(1): 19. doi:10.1016/j.accreview.2004.12.027.

Sharman, M., and Volek, J. (2004). Weight loss leads to reductions in inflammatory biomarkers after a very-low-carbohydrate diet and a low-fat diet in overweight men. *Clinical Science* 107(4): 365–369. doi:10.1042/cs20040111.

Tay, J., Brinkworth, G. D., Noakes, M., Keogh, J., and Clifton, P. M. (2008). Metabolic effects of weight loss on a very-low-carbohydrate diet compared with an isocaloric high-carbohydrate diet in abdominally obese subjects. *Journal of the American College of Cardiology* 51(1): 59–67. doi:10.1016/j.jacc.2007.08.050.

Thomson, C. A., Stopeck, A. T., Bea, J. W., Cussler, E., Nardi, E., Frey, G., and Thompson, P. A. (2010). Changes in body weight and metabolic indexes in overweight breast cancer survivors enrolled in a randomized trial of low-fat vs. reduced carbohydrate diets. *Nutrition and Cancer* 62(8): 1142–1152. doi:10.1080/01635581.2010.513803.

Vernon, M. C., Kueser, B., Transue, M., Yates, H. E., Yancy, W. S., and Westman, E. C. (2004). Clinical experience of a carbohydrate-restricted diet for the metabolic syndrome. *Metabolic Syndrome and Related Disorders* 2(3): 180–186. doi:10.1089/met.2004.2.180.

Vernon, M. C., Mavropoulos, J., Transue, M., Yancy, W. S., and Westman, E. C. (2003). Clinical experience of a carbohydrate-restricted diet: effect on diabetes mellitus. *Metabolic Syndrome and Related Disorders* 1(3): 233–237. doi:10.1089/154041903322716714.

Westman, E. C., Yancy, W. S., Mavropoulos, J. C., Marquart, M., and McDuffie, J. R. (2008). The effect of a low-carbohydrate, ketogenic diet versus a low-glycemic index diet on glycemic control in type 2 diabetes mellitus. *Nutrition & Metabolism* 5(1): 36. doi:10.1186/1743-7075-5-36.

Westman, E. C., Yancy, W. S., Edman, J. S., Tomlin, K. F., and Perkins, C. E. (2002). Effect of 6-month adherence to a very-low-carbohydrate diet program. *American Journal of Medicine* 113(1): 30–36. doi:10.1016/s0002-9343(02)01129-4.

Yancy, W. S., Westman, E. C., McDuffie, J. R., Grambow, S. C., Jeffreys, A. S., Bolton, J., et al. (2010). A randomized trial of a low-carbohydrate diet vs Orlistat plus a low-fat diet for weight loss. *Archives of Internal Medicine* 170(2), 136. doi:10.1001/archinternmed.2009.492.

Yancy, W. S., Almirall, D., Maciejewski, M. L., Kolotkin, R. L., McDuffie, J. R., and Westman, E. C. (2009). Effects of two weight-loss diets on health-related quality of life. *Quality of Life Research* 18(3): 281–289. doi:10.1007/s11136-009-9444-8.

Yancy, W., Foy, M., Chalecki, A., Vernon, M., and Westman, E. C. (2005). A low-carbohydrate, ketogenic diet to treat type 2 diabetes. *Nutrition & Metabolism* 2(34). https://www.ncbi.nlm.nih.gov/pubmed/16318637.

Yancy, W. S. (2004). A low-carbohydrate, ketogenic diet versus a low-fat diet to treat obesity and hyperlipidemia. *Annals of Internal Medicine* 140(10): 769. doi:10.7326/0003-4819-140-10-200405180-00006.

Yancy, W. S., Vernon, M. C., and Westman, E. C. (2003). A pilot trial of a low-carbohydrate, ketogenic diet in patients with type 2 diabetes. *Metabolic Syndrome and Related Disorders* 1(3):, 239–243. doi:10.1089/154041903322716723.

Yancy, W., Provenzale, D., and Westman, E. C. (2001). Improvement of gastroesophageal reflux disease after initiation of a low-carbohydrate diet: five brief case reports. *Alternative Therapies in Health and Medicine* 7(6): 116–119. https://www.ncbi.nlm.nih.gov/pubmed/11712463.

ATKINS 40

Ballard, K., et al. (2013). Dietary carbohydrate restriction improves insulin sensitivity, blood pressure, microvascular function, and cellular adhesion markers in individuals taking statins. *Nutrition Research* 33(11): 905–912. doi: 10.1016/j.nutres.2013.07.022.

Bazzano, L. A., et al. (2014). Effects of low-carbohydrate and low-fat diets: a randomized trial. *Annals of Internal Medicine* 161(5): 309–318. doi:10.7326/M14-0180.

Brehm, B. J., et al. (2003). A randomized trial comparing a very low carbohydrate diet and a calorie-restricted low-fat diet on body weight and cardiovascular risk factors in healthy women. *Journal of Clinical Endocrinology and Metabolism* 88(4): 1617–1623. doi:10.1210/jc.2002-021480.

Brehm, B. J., et al. (2005). The role of energy expenditure in the differential weight loss in obese women on low-fat and low-carbohydrate diets. *Journal of Clinical Endocrinology and Metabolism* 90(3): 1475–1482. doi:10.1210/jc.2004-1540.

Dashti, H. M., et al. (2004). Long-term effects of a ketogenic diet in obese patients. *Experimental & Clinical Cardiology* 9(3): 200–205. https://www.ncbi.nlm.nih.gov/pubmed/19641727.

Dashti, H. M., et al. (2003). Ketogenic diet modifies the risk factors of heart disease in obese patients. *Nutrition* 19(10): 901–902. https://www.ncbi.nlm.nih.gov/pubmed/14559328.

Ebbeling, C. B., et al. (2012). Effects of dietary composition on energy expenditure during weight-loss maintenance. *Journal of the American Medical Association* 307(24): 2627–2634. doi:10.1001/jama.2012.6607.

Forsythe, C. E., et al. (2008). Comparison of low-fat and low-carbohydrate diets on circulating fatty acid composition and markers of inflammation. *Lipids* 43(1): 65–77. doi:10.1007/s11745-007-3132-7.

Forsythe, C. E., et al. (2010). Limited effect of dietary saturated fat on plasma saturated fat in the context of a low carbohydrate diet. *Lipids* 45(10): 947–962. doi:10.1007/s11745-010-3467-3.

Iqbal, N., et al. (2010). Effects of a low-intensity intervention that prescribed a low-carbohydrate vs. a low-fat diet in obese, diabetic participants. *Obesity* (Silver Spring) 18(9): 1733–1738. doi:10.1038/oby.2009.460.

Nickols-Richardson, S. M., et al. (2005). Perceived hunger is lower and weight loss is greater in overweight premenopausal women consuming a low-carbohydrate/high-protein vs high-carbohydrate/low-fat diet. *Journal of the American Dietary Association* 105(9): 1433–1437. dx.doi.org/10.1016/j.jada.2005.06.025.

O'Brien, K. D., et al. (2005). Diet-induced weight loss is associated with decreases in plasma serum amyloid and C-reactive protein independent of dietary macronutrient composition in obese subjects. *Journal of Clinical Endocrinology & Metabolism* 90(4): 2244–2249. doi:10.1210/jc.2004-1011.

Paoli, A., et al. (2013). Long-term successful weight loss with a combination biphasic ketogenic Mediterranean diet and Mediterranean diet maintenance protocol. *Nutrients* 5(12): 5205–5217. doi:10.3390/nu5125205.

Ruth, M. R., et al. (2013). Consuming a hypocaloric high-fat, low-carbohydrate diet for 12 weeks lowers C-reactive protein, and raises serum adiponectin and high-density lipoprotein-cholesterol in obese subjects. *Metabolism* 62(12): 1779–1787. doi:10.1016/j.metabol.2013.07.006.

Saslow, L. R., et al. (2014). A randomized pilot trial of a moderate-carbohydrate diet compared to a very-low-carbohydrate diet in overweight or obese individuals with type 2 diabetes mellitus or prediabetes. *PLOS ONE*. dx.doi.org/10.1371/journal.pone.0091027.

Sharman, M. J., et al. (2002). A ketogenic diet favorably affects serum biomarkers for cardiovascular disease in normal-weight men. *Journal of Nutrition* 132(7): 1879–1885. jn.nutrition.org /content/132/7/1879.abstract.

Sharman, M. J., et al. (2004). Weight loss leads to reductions in inflammatory biomarkers after a very-low-carbohydrate diet and a low-fat diet in overweight men. *Clinical Science* 107(4): 365–369. doi:10.1042/CS20040111.

Siegel, R. M., et al. (2009). A 6-month, office-based, low-carbohydrate diet intervention in obese teens. *Clinical Pediatrics* 48(7): 745–749. doi:10.1177/0009922809332585.

Sondike, S. B., et al. (2003). Effects of a low-carbohydrate diet on weight loss and cardiovascular risk factor in overweight adolescents. *Journal of Pediatrics* 142(3): 253–258. doi:10.1067/mpd.2003.4.

Stern, L., et al. (2004). The effects of low-carbohydrate versus conventional weight loss diets in severely obese adults: one-year follow-up of a randomized trial. *Annals of Internal Medicine* 140(10): 778–785. www.ncbi.nlm.nih.gov/pubmed /15148064.

Tay, J., et al. (2014). A very-low-carbohydrate, low-saturated-fat diet for type 2 diabetes management: a randomized trial. *Diabetes Care*. doi:https://doi.org/10.2337/dc14-0845.

Velhorst, M. A., et al. (2010). Presence or absence of carbohydrates and the proportion of fat in a high-protein diet affects appetite suppression but not energy expenditure in normal-weight human subjects fed in energy balance. *British Journal of Nutrition* 104(9), 1395–1405. doi:10.1017/ S0007114510002060.

Volek, J. S., et al. (2000). Fasting lipoprotein and postprandial triacylglycerol responses to a low-carbohydrate diet supplemented with n-3 fatty acids. *Journal of the American College of Nutrition* 19(3): 383–391. https://www.ncbi.nlm.nih .gov/pubmed/10872901.

Volek, J. S., et al. (2002). Body composition and hormonal responses to a carbohydrate-restricted diet. *Metabolism* 51(7): 864–870. https://www.ncbi.nlm.nih.gov/pubmed/12077732.

Volek, J. S., et al. (2004). Comparison of a very-low-carbohydrate and low-fat diet on fasting lipids, LDL subclasses, insulin resistance, and postprandial lipemic responses in overweight women. *Journal of the American College of Nutrition* 23(2): 177–184. https://www.ncbi.nlm.nih .gov/pubmed/15047685.

Volek, J. S., et al. (2004). Comparison of energy-restricted very low-carbohydrate and low-fat diets on weight loss and body composition in overweight men and women. *Nutrition & Metabolism* 1(13). doi:10.1186/1743-7075-1-13.

Volek, J. S., et al. (2009). Effects of dietary carbohydrate restriction versus low-fat diet on flow-mediated dilation. *Metabolism* 58(12): 1769–1777. doi:10.1016/ j.metabol.2009.06.005.

Walsh, C. O., et al. (2013). Effects of diet composition on postprandial energy availability during weight-loss maintenance. *PLOS ONE* 8(3). doi:10.1371/journal. pone.0058172.

ATKINS 100

Accurso, A., Bernstein, R., Dahlqvist, A., Draznin, B., Feinman, R., Fine, E., et al. (2008). Dietary carbohydrate restriction in type 2 diabetes millitus and metabolic syndrome: time for a critical appraisal. *Nutrition & Metabolism* 5(9). doi:10.1186/1743-7075-5-9.

Ajala, O., English, P., and Pinkney, J. (2013). Systematic review and meta-analysis of different dietary approaches to the management of type 2 diabetes. *American Journal of Clinical Nutrition* 97(3): 505–516. doi:10.3945/ajcn.112.042457.

Aude, Y. W., Agatston, A. S., Lopez-Jimenez, F., Lieberman, E. H., Almon, M., Hansen, M., et al. (2004). The National Cholesterol Education Program diet vs a diet lower in carbohydrates and higher in protein and monunsaturated fat. *Archives of Internal Medicine* 164(19): 2141. doi:10.1001/ archinte.164.19.2141.

Bueno, N. B., Melo, I. S., Oliveira, S. L., and Ataide, T. D. (2013). Very-low-carbohydrate ketogenic diet vs low-fat diet for long-term weight loss: a meta-analysis of randomised controlled trials. *British Journal of Nutrition* 110(7): 1178–1187. doi:10.1017/ s000711451300548.

Chiu, S., Bergeron, N., Williams, P., Bray, G., Sutherland, B., and Krauss, R. (2015). Comparison of the DASH (Dietary Approaches to Stop Hypertension) diet and a higher-fat DASH diet on blood pressure and lipids and lipoproteins: a randomized controlled trial. *American Journal of Clinical Nutrition* 103(2): 341–347. doi:10.3945/ajcn.115.123281.

Daly, M. E., Paisey, R., Paisey, R., Millward, B. A., Eccles, C., Williams, K., et al. (2006). Short-term effects of severe dietary carbohydrate-restriction advice in Type 2 diabetes—a randomized controlled trial. *Diabetic Medicine* 23(1): 15–20. doi:10.1111/j.1464-5491.2005.01760.x.

DeSouza, R. J., Mente, A., Maroleanu, A., Cozma, A., Ha, V., Kishibe, T., et al. (2015). Intake of saturated and trans unsaturated fatty acids and risk of all cause mortality, cardiovascular disease, and type 2 diabetes: systematic review and meta-analysis of observational studies. *British Medical Journal*. doi:10.1136/bmj.h3978.

DiNicolantonio, J. (2014). The cardiometabolic consequences of replacing saturated fats with carbohydrates or ŒΩ-6 polyunsaturated fats: do the dietary guidelines have it wrong? *Open Heart (British Medical Journal)* 1(1). http://dx.doi.org/10.1136/openhrt-2013-000032.

Feinman, R. D., Pogozelski, W. K., Astrup, A., Bernstein, R. K., Fine, E. J., Westman, E. C., et al. (2015). Dietary carbohydrate restriction as the first approach in diabetes management: critical review and evidence base. *Nutrition* 31(1), 1–13. doi:10.1016/j.nut.2014.06.011.

Gannon, M. C., and Nuttall, F. Q. (2004). Effect of a high-protein, low-carbohydrate diet on blood glucose control in people with type 2 diabetes. *Diabetes* 53(9), 2375–2382. doi:10.2337/diabetes.53.9.2375.

Gutierrez, M., Akhavan, M., Jovanovic, L., and Peterson, C. M. (1998). Utility of a short-term 25% carbohydrate diet on improving glycemic control in type 2 diabetes mellitus. *Journal of the American College of Nutrition* 17(6): 595–600. doi:10.1080/07315724.1998.10718808.

Hays, J. H., Gorman, R. T., and Shakir, K. M. (2002). Results of use of metformin and replacement of starch with saturated fat in diets of patients with type 2 diabetes. *Endocrine Practice* 8(3), 177–183. doi:10.4158/ep.8.3.177.

Johnston, B. C., Kanters, S., Bandayrel, K., Wu, P., Naji, F., Siemieniuk, R. A., et al. (2014). Comparison of weight loss among named diet programs in overweight and obese adults. *Journal of the American Medical Association* 312(9): 923. doi:10.1001/jama.2014.10397.

Lin, P.-J., and Borer, K. T. (2016). Third exposure to a reduced carbohydrate meal lowers evening postprandial insulin and GIP responses and HOMA-IR estimate of insulin resistance. *PLOS ONE* 11(10): e0165378. https://doi.org/10.1371/journal.pone.0165378.

Maekawa, S., Kawahara, T., Nomura, R., Murase, T., Ann, Y., Oeholm, M., and Harada, M. (2014). Retrospective study on the efficacy of a low-carbohydrate diet for impaired glucose tolerance. *Diabetes, Metabolic Syndrome and Obesity: Targets and Therapy* 195. doi:10.2147/dmso.s62681.

Meckling, K. A., O'Sullivan, C., and Saari, D. (2004). Comparison of a low-fat diet to a low-carbohydrate diet on weight loss, body composition, and risk factors for diabetes and cardiovascular disease in free-living, overweight men and women. *Journal of Clinical Endocrinology & Metabolism* 89(6): 2717–2723. doi:10.1210/jc.2003-031606.

Moreno, B., Bellido, D., Sajoux, I., Goday, A., Saavedra, D., Crujeiras, A. B., and Casanueva, F. F. (2014). Comparison of a very-low-calorie-ketogenic diet with a standard low-calorie diet in the treatment of obesity. *Endocrine* 47(3): 793–805. doi:10.1007/s12020-014-0192-3.

Nielsen, J. V., and Joensson, E. A. (2008). Low-carbohydrate diet in type 2 diabetes: stable improvement of body weight and glycemic control during 44 months follow-up. *Nutrition & Metabolism* 5(1): 14. doi:10.1186/1743-7075-5-14.

Rosedale, R., Westman, E., and Konhilas, J. (2009). Clinical experience of a diet designed to reduce aging. *Journal of Applied Research* 9(4): 159–165. https://www.ncbi.nlm.nih.gov/pmc/articles/PMC2831640/.

Sackner-Bernstein, J., Kanter, D., and Kaul, S. (2015). Dietary intervention for overweight and obese adults: comparison of low-carbohydrate and low-fat diets. A meta-analysis. *PLOS ONE* 10(10). doi:10.1371/journal.pone.0139817.

Samaha, F. F., Iqbal, N., Seshadri, P., Chicano, K. L., Daily, D. A., McGrory, J., et al. (2003). A low-carbohydrate as compared with a low-fat diet in severe obesity. *New England Journal of Medicine* 348(21): 2074–2081. doi:10.1056/nejmoa022637.

Santos, F. L., Esteves, S. S., Pereira, A. D., Yancy Jr., W. S., and Nunes, J. P. (2012). Systematic review and meta-analysis of clinical trials of the effects of low carbohydrate diets on cardiovascular risk factors. *Obesity Reviews* 13(11): 1048–1066. doi:10.1111/j.1467-789x.2012.01021.x.

Sasakabe, T., Haimoto, H., et al. (2011). Effects of a moderate low-carbohydrate diet on preferential abdominal fat loss and cardiovascular risk factors in patients with type 2 diabetes. *Diabetes, Metabolic Syndrome and Obesity: Targets and Therapy* 167. doi:10.2147/dmso.s19635.

Shai, I., Spence, J. D., Schwarzfuchs, D., Henkin, Y., Parraga, G., Rudich, A., et al. (2010). Dietary intervention to reverse carotid atherosclerosis. *Circulation* 121(10): 1200–1208. doi:10.1161/circulationaha.109.879254.

Shai, I., Schwarzfuchs, D., Henkin, Y., Shahar, D., Witcow, S., Greenberg, I., et al. (2008). Weight loss with a low-carbohydrate, Mediterranean, or low-fat diet. *New England Journal of Medicine* 359(20): 2169–2172. doi:10.1056/nejmc081747.

Siri-Tarino, P. W., Sun, Q., Hu, F. B., and Krauss, R. M. (2010). Meta-analysis of prospective cohort studies evaluating the association of saturated fat with cardiovascular disease. *American Journal of Clinical Nutrition* 91(3): 535–546. doi:10.3945/ajcn.2009.27725.

Stewart, K. J., Dobrosielski, D. A., Sibler, H. A., Zakaria, S., Shapiro, E. P., and Ouyang, P. (2011). Losing 10 lbs with a low-CHO diet plus exercise does not impair vascular function. *Medicine & Science in Sports & Exercise* 43(suppl. 1): 154. doi:10.1249/01.mss.0000400404.56488.57.

Tirosh, A., Golan, R., Harman-Boehm, I., Henkin, Y., Schwarzfuchs, D., Rudich, A., et al. (2013). Renal function following three distinct weight loss dietary strategies during 2 years of a randomized controlled trial. *Diabetes Care* 36(8): 2225–2232. doi:10.2337/dc12-1846.

Volek, J. S., Volk, B. M., and Phinney, S. D. (2012). The twisted tale of saturated fat. *Lipid Technology* 24(5): 106–107. doi:10.1002/lite.201200189.

Volek, J. S., and Westman, E. C. (2002). Very-low-carbohydrate weight-loss diets revisited. *Cleveland Clinic Journal of Medicine* 69(11): 849, 853, 856–858 passim. doi:10.3949/ccjm.69.11.849.

Volk, B. M., Kunces, L. J., Freidenreich, D. J., Kupchak, B. R., Saenz, C., Artistizabal, J. C., et al. (2014). Effects of step-wise increases in dietary carbohydrate on circulating saturated fatty acids and palmitoleic acid in adults with metabolic syndrome. *PLOS ONE* 9(11). doi:10.1371/journal.pone.0113605.

Westman, E. C., Mavropoulos, J., Yancy, W. S., and Volek, J. S. (2003). A review of low-carbohydrate ketogenic diets. *Current Atherosclerosis Reports* 5(6), 476–483. doi:10.1007/s11883-003-0038-6.

Yamada, Y., Uchida, J., Izumi, H., Tsukamoto, Y., Inoue, G., Watanabe, Y., et al. (2014). A non-calorie-restricted low-carbohydrate diet is effective as an alternative therapy for patients with type 2 diabetes. *Internal Medicine* 53(1), 13–19. doi:10.2169/internalmedicine.53.0861.

ACKNOWLEDGMENTS

I'm proud to say that writing this book was a team effort. It began with the realization that we had this amazing opportunity to speak to a very important part of our population that is interested in making small changes and embracing a better way of eating by learning how to live a low-carb, low-sugar lifestyle. You are done with diets, but you are passionate about the quality and quantity of the food you eat and how it impacts your overall health and wellness.

I am thankful to the leadership and vision of Scott Parker, Chief Marketing Officer (CMO) at Atkins, and Jennifer Livingston, Director of Public Relations, who were enormously helpful with insightful comments and additions from the very beginning, when this book was simply just a glimmer in our eyes, and during the continual process of bringing it to life. Gretchen Ferraro, freelance writer, was the editorial director who collaborated with me, and without her contributions, this book would not have been possible. Nutritionist Vicki Cox, Director of Nutrition Communications at Atkins, pored over every word for accuracy and supplied scientific references and insight where needed. Jennifer Knollenberg created our delicious and useful meal plans, which incorporated the recipes in this book; it was no easy task to meet all our nutritional targets, but she did it. And I would like

to extend a special thanks to Joe Scalzo, Atkins' Chief Executive Officer, and Hanno Holm, Atkins' Chief Operations Officer, for their insights in supporting this book and assembling this talented team.

The key to this book is the mouthwatering low-carbohydrate and low-sugar recipes created by Jennifer Iserloh, which demonstrate once and for all that eating the Atkins way—eating right, not less—is wonderfully flexible and can be personalized to suit your individual needs. With Atkins, food should be an experience worth sharing and savoring with others, and these recipes are a testament to that.

Finally, this book would not have been possible without Joy Tutela, from the David Black Literary Agency, who went above and beyond in coordinating the moving pieces, and many thanks to the superb editorial efforts of Cara Bedick and David Falk at Touchstone/Simon & Schuster.

Last, but far from least, I am so thankful to Ellen Silverman for contributing her beautiful photography to this project, and to Laura Palese for her incredible design work. The end result is a dream come true: a coffee table–worthy book that showcases how delicious living a low-carb lifestyle can truly be.

NOTES

CHAPTER 1: THE HIDDEN SUGAR EFFECT

1. CDC: Adult obesity facts. (2016, September 1). https://www.cdc.gov/obesity/data/adult.html.

2. Olshansky, S. J., D. J. Passaro, R. C. Hershow, J. Layden, B. A. Carnes, J. Brody, et al. (2005). A potential decline in life expectancy in the United States in the 21st century. *New England Journal of Medicine* 352(11): 1138–1145. (2014, August). Overweight in children. www.heart.org/HEARTORG/HealthyLiving/HealthyKids/ChildhoodObesity/Overweight-in-Children_UCM_304054_Article.jsp#.Wleko1MrKCg.

3. *USDA Dietary Guidelines 2015–2020.* Appendix 7, Nutritional goals for age-sex groups based on dietary reference intakes and dietary guidelines recommendations. (2016, January).

4. Menke, A., S. Casagrande, and L. Geiss (2015). Prevalence of and trends in diabetes among adults in the United States, 1988–2012. *Journal of the American Medical Association* 314(10): 1021–1029.

5. Martin, C. K., D. Rosenbaum, H. Han, P. J. Geiselman, H. R. Wyatt, J. O. Hill, et al. (2011). Change in food cravings, food preferences, and appetite during a low-carbohydrate and low-fat diet. *Obesity* 19(10): 1963–1970.

CHAPTER 2: HOW ATKINS WORKS

1. Schwingshackl, L., G. Hoffmann, T. Kalle-Uhlmann, M. Arregui, B. Buijsse, and H. Boeing (2015). Fruit and vegetable consumption and changes in anthropometric variables in adult populations: a systematic review and meta-analysis of prospective cohort studies. *PLOS ONE* 10(10): e0140846. doi:10.1371/journal.pone.0140846. L. Dauchat, P. Amouyel, S. Hercberg, and J. Dallongeville (2006). Fruit and vegetable consumption and risk of coronary heart disease: a meta-analysis of cohort studies. *Journal of Nutrition* 136(10): 2588–2593. jn.nutrition.org/content/136/10/2588.abstract. H. Boeing, A. Bechthold, A. Bub, S. Ellinger, D. Haller, A. Kroke, et al. (2012). Critical review: vegetables and fruits in the prevention of chronic diseases. *European Journal of Nutrition* 51(6): 637–663.

CHAPTER 3: LET'S GET STARTED

1. U.S. Food and Drug Administration. (2017, February 10). How to understand and use the nutrition facts label. www.fda.gov/Food/IngredientsPackagingLabeling/LabelingNutrition/ucm274593.htm#overview.

2. American Heart Association. (2016). The American Heart Association recommendations for physical activity in adults. http://www.heart.org/HEARTORG/HealthyLiving/PhysicalActivity/FitnessBasics/American-Heart-Association-Recommendations-for-Physical-Activity-Infographic_UCM_450754_SubHomePage.jsp.

3. Harvard Health Publications, Harvard Medical School. (2011, February). Mindful eating. www.health.harvard.edu/staying-healthy/mindful-eating.

4. Turner-McGrievy, G. M., and D. F. Tate, (2013). Weight-loss social support in 140 characters or less: use of an online social network in a remotely delivered weight-loss intervention. *Translational Behavioral Medicine* 3(3), 287–294. R. R. Wing and R. W. Jeffery (1999). Benefits of recruiting participants with friends and increasing social support for weight loss and maintenance. *Journal of Consulting and Clinical Psychology* 67(1): 132–138.

CHAPTER 4: ATKINS YOUR WAY

1. Martin, C. K., D. Rosenbaum, H. Han, P. J. Geiselman, H. R. Wyatt, J. O. Hill, et al. (2011). Change in food cravings, food preferences, and appetite during a low-carbohydrate and low-fat diet. *Obesity (Silver Spring)* 19(10): 1963–70. C. Heimowitz, M. Abdul, Q. Hu, N. Le, K. Bingham, V. Cox, et al. (2017). Changes in food cravings during dietary carbohydrate-restriction. *FASEB Journal* 31(5). www.fasebj.org/content/31/1_Supplement/643.23.

**CHAPTER 5: LIVING A LOW-CARB
AND LOW-SUGAR LIFESTYLE**

1. Jones, P. J., V. K. Senanayake, S. Pu, D. J. Jenkins, P. W. Connelly, B. Lamarche, et al. (2014). DHA-enriched high-oleic acid canola oil improves lipid profile and lowers predicted cardiovascular disease risk in the canola oil multicenter randomized controlled trial. *American Journal of Clinical Nutrition* 100(1): 88–97.

2. Cardoso, D. A., A. S. Moriera, G. M. De Oliveria, L. R. Raggio, and G. Rosa (2015). A coconut extra virgin oil–rich diet increases HDL cholesterol and decreases waist circumference and body mass in coronary artery disease patients. *Nutrición Hospitalaria* 32(5): 2144–2152.

3. Marco, M. L., D. Heeney, S. Binda, C. J. Cifelli, P. D. Cotter, B. Foligné, et al. (2016). Health benefits of fermented foods: microbiota and beyond. *Current Opinion in Biotechnology* 44, 94–102.

4. Kong, A., et al. (2012). Self-monitoring and eating-related behaviors are associated with 12-month weight loss in postmenopausal overweight-to-obese women. *Journal of the Academy of Nutrition and Dietetics* 112(9): 1428–1435.

CHAPTER 6: BREAKFAST

1. Giusti, M. M. (2015). Anthocyanins. *Advances in Nutrition* 6: 620–622.

CHAPTER 7: SNACKS AND SIDES

1. Round, J. L. and S. K. Mazmanian (2009). The gut microbiota shapes intestinal immune responses during health and disease. *Nature Reviews Immunology* 9(5): 313–323.

CHAPTER 10: APPETIZERS

1. Salem, M. B., H. Affes, K. Ksouda, R. Dhouibi, Z. Sahnoun, S. Hammami, and K. M. Zeghal (2015). Pharmacological studies of artichoke leaf extract and their health benefits. *Plant Foods for Human Nutrition* 70(4): 441–453.

2. Weil, A. (2016, November 1). Curcumin or turmeric? https://www.drweil.com/vitamins-supplements-herbs/herbs/curcumin-or-turmeric/.

CHAPTER 11: 15-MINUTE MEALS

1. Hamidpour, M., R. Hamidpour, S. Hamidpour, and M. Shahlari (2014). Chemistry, pharmacology, and medicinal property of sage (salvia) to prevent and cure illnesses such as obesity, diabetes, depression, dementia, lupus, autism, heart disease, and cancer. *Journal of Traditional and Complementary Medicine* 4(2): 82–88.

CHAPTER 13: JUST DESSERTS

1. Brookshire, B. (2014). Cocoa antioxidant sweetens cognition in elderly. *Science News*. https://www.sciencenews.org/article/cocoa-antioxidant-sweetens-cognition-elderly.

INDEX

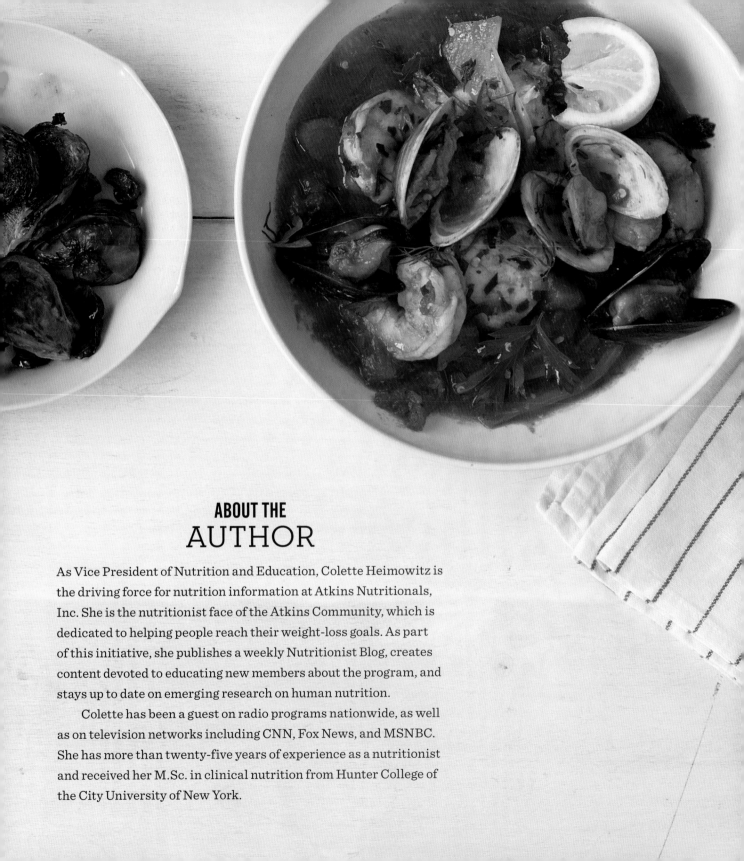

ABOUT THE
AUTHOR

As Vice President of Nutrition and Education, Colette Heimowitz is the driving force for nutrition information at Atkins Nutritionals, Inc. She is the nutritionist face of the Atkins Community, which is dedicated to helping people reach their weight-loss goals. As part of this initiative, she publishes a weekly Nutritionist Blog, creates content devoted to educating new members about the program, and stays up to date on emerging research on human nutrition.

Colette has been a guest on radio programs nationwide, as well as on television networks including CNN, Fox News, and MSNBC. She has more than twenty-five years of experience as a nutritionist and received her M.Sc. in clinical nutrition from Hunter College of the City University of New York.